P9-BYG-970

The Healing Foods

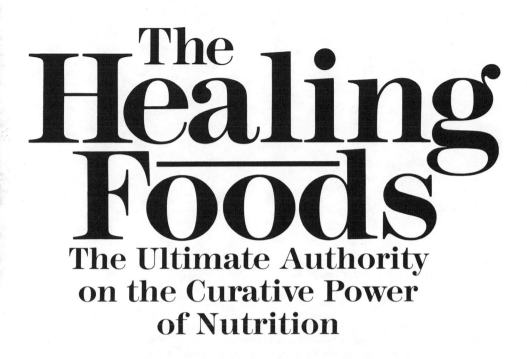

The Healing Foods

The Ultimate Authority on the Curative Power of Nutrition

By Patricia Hausman &
Judith Benn Hurley

A DELL TRADE PAPERBACK

A DELL TRADE PAPERBACK

Published by
Dell Publishing
a division of
Bantam Doubleday Dell Publishing Group, Inc.
666 Fifth Avenue
New York, New York 10103

If you purchased this book without a cover you should be aware that this book is stolen property. It was reported as "unsold and destroyed" to the publisher and neither the author nor the publisher has received any payment for this "stripped book."

Copyright © 1989 by Patricia Hausman

All rights reserved. No part of this book may be reproduced or transmitted in any form or by any means, electronic or mechanical, including photocopying, recording, or by any information storage and retrieval system, without the written permission of the Publisher, except where permitted by law. For information address: Rodale Press, Inc., Emmaus, Pennsylvania.

The trademark Dell® is registered in the U.S. Patent and Trademark Office.

ISBN: 0-440-50338-8

Reprinted by arrangement with Rodale Press, Inc.

Printed in the United States of America

Published simultaneously in Canada

February 1991

10 9 8 7 6 5 4 3 2

RRH

NOTICE

This book is intended as a reference volume only, not as a medical manual or guide to self-treatment. If you suspect that you have a medical problem, we urge you to seek competent medical help. Keep in mind that nutritional needs vary from person to person, depending on age, sex, health status, and total diet. The information here is intended to help you make informed decisions about your diet, not as a substitute for any treatment that may have been prescribed by your physician.

For Betsy and for Patrick

CONTENTS

ACKNOWLEDGMENTS

Many thanks to Anita Liss for her research assistance and work on the menu plans; to Debora Tkac and William Gottlieb for their editorial stewardship; to Jane Sherman and Roberta Mulliner for their help in converting the manuscript into book form; to JoAnn Brader for giving each recipe a careful test; and to Betsy Filsinger, who took care of anything and everything else.

Patricia Hausman
Judith Benn Hurley

INTRODUCTION

Accentuate the Positive

We could not be happier with where nutrition is taking us these days. A new era has dawned. We call it a renaissance—a renewed interest in the healing potential of food. And as you will see, it's a return to *positive* messages about the important role that these healing foods can play in helping to keep us healthy and well.

In the coming years, we know you will be hearing more and more about these friendly foods and nutrients. Among the current favorites are:

- Fish that provide "the good fat" friendly to our hearts.
- High-fiber foods that help maintain better levels of both blood sugar and blood cholesterol.
- Great sources of calcium and vitamin D that provide the right stuff to our bones.
- Foods rich in carotene, vitamin C, fiber, and selenium—all important cancer-fighting nutrients.

And these are just the best-known examples. As you will discover in *The Healing Foods,* lots of other foods also show health-boosting potential. If this carries a ring of "boring diet," allay your fears—immediately! We, too, have had our fill of rigid diets. This book is designed to give you choices. The key is *flexibility.*

A Prime Example

How can healing foods benefit you? Well, perhaps your blood cholesterol level is too high. Lowering it would do much for your health. But the standard cholesterol-lowering diet, with strict limits on meat and milk fats, may not appeal to your palate at all. If so, rest assured that you are not alone. For as much as we realize that cutting back on meat and milk fats does lower cholesterol, we also know that this method is often an unpopular one.

The Healing Foods offers you a more positive strategy for reducing a high cholesterol level–one that emphasizes foods with cholesterol-lowering power. This gives most cholesterol watchers greater freedom in making food choices. It can also greatly simplify life because a single healing food–oat bran–can make a big difference. Taken in the right amounts, it can lower cholesterol dramatically.

Of course, oat bran alone won't accomplish everything. Probably no food or supplement can completely counteract the hazards posed by risky habits. As long as we realize that an alternative such as oat bran *reduces but does not eliminate* the risk posed by diets high in saturated fat and cholesterol, we think that the news here is good. And needless to say, if you avoid troublesome foods in addition to eating the healthful ones that are featured here, you'll be living for maximum good health.

By the way, the news doesn't stop with oat bran. There are other options. Other foods also contain the cholesterol-lowering substance found in oat bran. So the chances are good that you can find some appealing foods from the choices we'll give you.

The Supplement Option

Supplements are as much a part of the flexible approach to nutrition as is food. Sometimes none of the food choices are appealing or practical. The meat-and-potatoes lover, for instance, often eats few vegetables rich in carotene –the plant form of vitamin A that shows much promise for preventing cancer.

The solution, obviously, is to consider a supplement. If your diet doesn't contain much of an important nutrient, it's better to take a supplement than to miss out on its special benefits. It is simply a better option than attempting to eat foods you don't like, because in our experience, this approach usually fails before long.

A Personalized Approach

There are too many recommendations. Too many diets. Too many foods to avoid; too many others to remember to include every day. Too many noes; too many nevers. If you've ever had the feeling that "there's nothing left to eat," or that following all the advice you hear requires a graduate degree in nutrition, we can understand. Trying to do what's good for you can be downright confusing!

One day, for instance, nutritionists advocate Swiss cheese as a good source of bone-building calcium. The next day they warn against its cholesterol-raising effects. There has to be a better way. In our book, there is.

Our solution is a more personalized approach, carefully tailored to your needs. Do you have a problem with gallstones? Angina? We'll show you how to eat to alleviate your problem. Or maybe your interest is just in giving your digestive tract or heart more healthful security. We'll show you how to do that, too.

Keeping nutrition simple is as important to us as keeping track of the latest research findings. We've made this book as simple as possible without sacrificing results.

Use this book in whatever way best serves you. Within these pages you'll find:

- All the foods that have been scientifically shown to enhance healthful living.
- The special conditions that can be helped by eating certain foods.
- The specific roles that vitamins and minerals play in keeping you healthy.

The entries are organized in alphabetical order for easy access, beginning with acerola and ending with yogurt. In the food entries, you will find nutritional profiles of the best foods, along with recipes and information about selection, storage, and cooking. Each special condition section explains the causes and symptoms of some of our most common health problems and offers nutritional strategies for preventing and treating them. Some also contain seven-day meal plans–all low to moderate in calories and high in vitamins and minerals–to guide you along. Finally, in the Appendix, you'll find a complete listing of all the foods high in the essential vitamins and minerals.

We hope that within these pages you will find a positive, personalized, flexible approach that makes better nutrition a pleasure instead of a burden. It's the best way we've found to accentuate the positive–and make good nutrition something that can be practiced for a lifetime.

ACEROLA

Good Things in a Small Package

2 calories per fruit

Is it a berry or is it a cherry? Actually, it's both. The tart and exotic acerola berry is also known as the West Indian cherry. Nutritionists know it for its vitamin C, with a single berry packing a generous 81 milligrams. That's 25 percent more than the official recommended allowance in each tiny fruit. You can't get this much of your daily vitamin C allowance from just a bite or two of an orange!

The acerola's distinction as a powerhouse of vitamin C has obscured an equally important fact: Acerola berries are low in calories, weighing in at only about 2 apiece. But unless you love lemons, you will find the acerola so tart that you must add sweetening. Instead of sugar, try thawed apple juice concentrate, remembering that this, too, will add calories. Even with the added sweetener, however, you'll still have a winner as far as fat, cholesterol, and sodium are concerned.

At the Market: In the United States, most acerola is marketed dried. To test for freshness, shake the package. Do you hear a rattle? If you do, the acerola should be good.

Kitchen Tips: Once you have it home, store acerola in a tightly covered glass jar. Keep it in a cool place and out of the light. Every now and then, inspect the jar for moldy berries and discard any that you find.

Accent on Enjoyment: To prepare acerola, you can use your imagination or try some of our favorites.

- Crush the acerola into tiny pieces with a rolling pin and use like raisins. Allow for its extra tartness by adding more sweetener to the recipe.
- Steep the crushed, dried fruit in boiling water and enjoy as tea. Of course, the heat will affect vitamin C, but the flavor will still be there.
- Add acerola to conserves, preserves, and fruit butters or use the acerola tea in making jelly.
- Give a new tart flavor to fruit pies, punches, hot-mulled beverages, relishes, and marinades for pork or game by seasoning with acerola.

We have to hand it to the Alaskans, by the way, for coming up with the most unique use of acerola that we know of. They collect fresh berries, simmer them, and dry the puree in the sun or oven. The dried puree is then crushed into a powder with a rolling pin and used to fortify bread doughs and pancake and waffle batters with extra nutritional value.

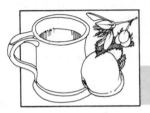

Mulled Apple Juice

1 tablespoon dried,
  minced acerola
2 teaspoons dried, minced
  lemongrass
1 cinnamon stick
2 teaspoons dried, minced
  orange peel
2 cups water
2 cups apple juice

Combine all ingredients in a medium saucepan. Simmer over medium heat for about 5 minutes, then strain and serve hot.

Makes 4 servings

ALFALFA SPROUTS

Three-Star Superfood

10 calories per cup

Sometimes it's not what you have that counts but what you don't have. Sprouts are a perfect example. Although low in protein, vitamins, and minerals, they rate the superfood label because they balance the scales with three other attributes: amazingly few calories, no fat, and virtually no sodium.

At the Market: The best-tasting sprouts measure 2 to 2½ inches in length. A truly fresh bunch will have no liquid at the bottom of their container and will smell fresh, too. As a general rule, sprouts stay fresh for about a week, but they must be refrigerated. We prefer to transfer them from the store packaging into a container that protects against crushing.

Kitchen Tips: Sprouts taste best when eaten raw–be it on sandwiches, in garnishes, or atop a salad. But as any sprout lover has discovered, their threadlike consistency makes them prone to mat up if tossed with other salad ingredients. Instead, arrange the sprouts in a ring around the salad or set them on top. Then drizzle the sprouts with some salad dressing; lemon-tahini dressing is great!

Accent on Enjoyment: Though raw is right for us, we understand if you tire of raw sprouts. Here are some novel uses to try:

- Grind or chop them and add to bread doughs.
- Add to soups and stews–but not until cooking is finished.
- Eat them with chopsticks for a change of pace.

We fully expect that once you try alfalfa sprouts, you'll get hooked. Then you'll want to grow your own, for no store-bought sprouts can compare to a superfresh, homegrown batch. All you will need to get started is a bean and seed sprouter, and before long, you'll be gardening away in your own kitchen.

Spring Rice Salad with Alfalfa Sprouts

2 cups cooked rice
½ cup snow peas
2 scallions, minced
½ cup shredded fresh
    spinach
1 tablespoon olive oil
    juice and pulp of 1
    lemon
½ teaspoon dried basil
½ teaspoon dried
    oregano
1 teaspoon Dijon
    mustard
2 cups alfalfa sprouts

In a large salad bowl, combine rice, peas, scallions, and spinach.

In a small bowl, whisk together oil, lemon juice and pulp, basil, oregano, and mustard.

Toss half of the dressing with the rice mixture, then arrange sprouts atop rice and drizzle the remaining dressing over them. (Sprouts are not tossed with rice because they tend to mat and tangle when mixed.) Serve at room temperature in individual salad bowls.

Makes 4 servings

ALLERGY

Its Agony and Its Ecstasy

It's an experience that a hostess never forgets.

The dinner party couldn't be going better. The guests are perfectly matched and are chatting away merrily without noticing the time. Everyone loves the food. All that's left is dessert.

You dash into the kitchen to get some coffee and tea for your guests, as well as the fresh-baked banana bread you bought a few hours ago at your favorite neighborhood bakery. The guests ooh and aah at the sight and smell of it.

Then one pipes up with a question. "Does this have any nuts in it?" he asks, pointing to the bakery's handiwork.

You know it doesn't, but to reassure him you cut off a piece, inspect it carefully for nuts, and seeing none, shake your head. "Not a nut in sight," you reply.

"That's what you think," he retorts 30 seconds later. You turn to him, stunned to see his face covered with big red hives. Before you can panic, he blurts out, "Someone get me some water—fast."

You run for a glass of water while he searches through his pocket for an antihistamine pill. He pops it in his mouth, takes a deep breath, and sighs, "Don't feel bad. I shouldn't have taken the chance."

You're sure you didn't see any nuts. But your thoughts are on your acutely sick guest, who excuses himself to lie down while he waits for the antihistamine to work. Two hours later he emerges from the guest room, and you're relieved to see that the red blotches and hives on his skin have started to fade. He looks tired but says he's much less sick to his stomach than he was. "Don't worry. I'll be fine," he says. But for the rest of the evening, worrying is the only thing you seem able to do.

Tracking Down the Troublemaker

First thing the next morning, you call the bakery to check on the ingredients. "We don't put nuts in our banana breads," says one of the bakers. She pauses. "Of course, we do use a little almond butter—to give it a distinctive flavor."

You can't believe that a little bit of almond butter could have touched off such a big reaction in your nut-allergic guest. But the memory of last night won't leave you, so you phone him at work to ask about the possibility.

5

"It not only is possible, with me it's a sure bet," he replies. "Almond butter has done me in before, and I'm sure it will again." Laughing, he continues, "It reminds me of my yearly Christmas crisis."

"What's that?" you ask.

"I used to have a reaction virtually every year at Christmastime. Someone would always put almond extract into the cookies and not realize that when I asked if nuts had been used, extracts counted, too. A minute later, I'd be sick, but it would be too late. Now I have a better approach. I never eat the cookies at the office parties. Better to offend someone than ruin everyone's good time with one of my reactions."

Allergy or Otherwise?

Some people think that any adverse reaction to food is an allergy. Not so. An allergic response is but one of many possible explanations for an adverse reaction to food. Whether or not the problem is an allergy depends on *why* your body isn't able to handle the problem food.

When an allergic reaction to food occurs, the immune system secretes unusually high levels of an antibody called IgE. By doing so, the immune system is reacting as if the offending food were as foreign and unwelcome as an infection. If elevated levels of IgE are found in the blood after an attack, that's excellent proof that an allergic reaction has occurred.

Of course, this type of test can't always be done after a reaction. An experienced allergist, however, can consider other clues to judge whether or not to suspect food allergy. There are several factors to consider.

Family history of allergy. Allergies occur in people who have a genetic trait called atopy. It affects about one in five people. If you or other family members already are known to have this trait because of allergies to pollen, dust, or ragweed, for instance, you are clearly a potential victim of food allergy.

Speed of reaction. Often, a reaction occurs soon after an offending food is eaten. Therefore, a reaction that is unusually rapid suggests allergy.

Amount eaten. You may find that certain foods disagree with you only if you eat considerable amounts. But if you react to even a tiny amount or react after touching (but not eating) the problem food, this, too, makes allergy a likely explanation.

Symptoms and response to antihistamine drugs. The classic allergic symptoms of hives and itching, rashes, and digestive upset result when the IgE antibodies involved in an allergic reaction secrete a substance called histamine. Should a reaction to food include these symptoms, and if the symptoms respond to an antihistamine medication, chances are excellent that the problem is an allergy.

Age at onset. Food allergies can begin at any age, but they most commonly start in infancy or childhood. A reaction that first occurs late in life is less likely to be a true allergy.

Testing for Trouble

Naturally, direct testing to confirm a suspected food allergy is preferred when possible. But it's not always as simple as it may sound. Allergy testing has proved to be a controversial subject, with some allergists insisting that the concept has been widened too far to include tests that offer little or no valuable information.

According to Dean D. Metcalfe, M.D., of the National Institute of Allergy and Infectious Diseases, three types of allergy test have proved their worth.

The familiar skin test. This tests for the appearance of inflammation after the skin is pricked and exposed to an extract of the suspected food. This test is simple, quick, low in cost, and generally accurate. Occasionally, however, it causes a severe reaction. It also cannot be used when certain skin diseases, such as eczema, exist.

The elimination diet. This test is designed to see if allergic symptoms disappear when a food is removed from the diet and reappear if the food is eaten again. When skin testing cannot be done, an elimination diet is an alternative. (A sample diet can be found in "Be Your Own Allergy Detective.") Elimination diets provide useful information at a low cost, but they require effort and patience. Also, if the symptoms occur only rarely or are severe, other tests are favored over this type.

The RAST or ELISA blood tests. Performed by medical laboratories, these test for high levels of allergy antibodies after a patient's blood is incubated with a suspected food. These tests are safe and offer a good alternative when skin testing cannot be done or when results of a skin test are in question. As for accuracy, these tests rate well although, as with other tests, false-positive reactions can occur. Results are not available as quickly as with skin tests, of course, but the more significant disadvantage of RAST and ELISA is their hefty price tag.

Tainted Tests

Of course, an allergy test is good only when it is performed properly, and even then, a false-positive reaction will sometimes occur. Nonetheless, accepted allergy tests have a good (not perfect) record. Unfortunately, some tests that do

(continued on page 10)

Be Your Own Allergy Detective

Tracking down food allergies is detective work, pure and simple. That means, of course, that it takes effort and that there are no easy answers.

One of the time-honored approaches for finding food allergies is known as the elimination diet. You start by removing certain suspects from your diet, then add them back one at a time. If your immune system offers no protest, chances are good that you are not allergic to the food in question.

Try to avoid restaurants when using this diet, for you can't be sure what you are getting when eating out. Also be careful with any multi-ingredient product; for instance, a bread labeled corn or rye is likely to contain wheat flour, too.

Round One

Round One of the diet tests your tolerance to beef, pork, fowl, milk, rye, and corn. While on the diet, eat nothing that contains any of these in any form. Instead, use the list below to find foods allowed while this test is in progress.

Try the diet for two weeks. If you don't improve at all, move on to Round Two for two weeks. If that, too, doesn't help, it's time for Round Three.

Food Group	Permitted Foods
Beverage	Coffee (black), lemonade, tea
Cereal	Rice products
Fat	Cottonseed oil, olive oil
Flour (bread or biscuits)	Rice
Fruit	Grapefruit, lemon, pear
Meat	Lamb
Miscellaneous	Cane sugar, gelatin, maple sugar, olives, salt, tapioca pudding
Vegetable	Artichokes, beets, carrots, lettuce, spinach

If you do improve on the Round One diet, it's a good bet that you are sensitive to one of the foods that you have eliminated. But which one? To find out, start adding back the foods you have eliminated, but only one at a time. If your symptoms return when you add a food, eliminate it again. Do the problems vanish when you do? If so, congratulations. You have zeroed in on an offending food. Avoid it.

If you add a food back without problem for three days, cross it off your worry list and try another of the six suspects.

Round Two

In this round, you will be testing yourself for allergies to beef, lamb, milk, and rice. Avoid them in any form while this phase of the test is in progress. Although the eliminated foods have been changed, the method for following this diet is the same as for Round One. Use the list below to find your permitted foods.

Food Group	Permitted Foods
Cereal	Corn products
Fat	Corn oil, cottonseed oil
Flour (bread or biscuits)	Corn, 100% rye (ordinary "rye" bread contains wheat)
Fruit	Apricots, peaches, pineapple, prunes
Meat	Bacon, chicken
Miscellaneous	Cane sugar, corn syrup, gelatin, salt
Vegetable	Asparagus, corn, peas, squash, string beans, tomatoes

Round Three

This third and final diet will test for allergy to lamb, fowl, rye, rice, corn, and milk. As with Rounds One and Two, you must avoid these six foods in any form during the test. Again, follow this diet in the same way as you did the previous two, using allowed foods from the list below.

Food Group	Permitted Foods
Beverage	Coffee (black), lemonade, tea
Cereal	None
Fat	Cottonseed oil, olive oil
Flour (bread or biscuits)	Lima beans, potatoes, soybeans
Fruit	Apricots, grapefruit, lemons, peaches
Meat	Bacon, beef
Miscellaneous	Cane sugar, gelatin, maple sugar, olives, salt, tapioca pudding
Vegetable	Beets, lima beans, potatoes (white and sweet), string beans, tomatoes

not have a record for accuracy remain in use.

In 1980, the National Center for Health Care Technology asked that interested individuals and organizations submit comments about a variety of techniques that were being used to diagnose food allergy. Let's look at several of these controversial tests and what the American Academy of Allergy and Immunology (AAAI) had to say about them.

Putting Cytotoxic Testing to the Test

Cytotoxic (or leukocytotoxic) testing is a time-consuming, expensive test of how exposure to a food affects the white cells in your blood. A reduction in white cells or death of cells is considered a positive reaction.

According to the AAAI, cytotoxic testing "has never been proved effective by controlled studies, nor has a scientific basis for its use been demonstrated. . . . [Moreover,] numerous published controlled trials indicate that the

Man versus Mold

You may not have allergies to specific foods, but that doesn't mean that you are home free. Some of us are allergic instead to the molds that grow invisibly on food rather than the food itself. Unlike the severe reaction often caused by food allergies, mold allergy often appears as less-alarming (but more-chronic) complaints such as headaches and nasal congestion. Itching and pain in the ears is another common symptom that suggests allergy to mold.

If your doctor confirms that you are allergic to mold, managing it will be a challenge at first. Molds are persistent and pervasive troublemakers that grow wherever they can. In theory, many foods are potential sources. Your goal, however, is to avoid the worst offenders. Fortunately, certain foods are known to be favorites of food-borne mold. Here they are, followed by some tips on minimizing mold growth on fresh foods.

- Cheese of all kinds, including cottage cheese.
- Beer and wine.
- Sour cream, sour milk, buttermilk, and yogurt.
- Canned tomatoes and canned tomato products, including ketchup, chili sauce, and tomato paste, unless homemade.
- Mushrooms and sauerkraut.
- Vinegar and vinegar-containing foods, such as mayonnaise and other salad dressings, pickles, pickled beets, relishes, and green olives.

procedure is not effective for diagnosis of food allergy." Often, the AAAI points out, patients not only test positive for foods that don't produce symptoms but also test negative for those that clearly do trigger their allergies.

Philip Lieberman, M.D., and co-workers at the University of Tennessee submitted samples from the same patients twice for cytotoxic testing. The results were different each time! Dr. Lieberman also used the cytotoxic test on the blood of 15 patients who had already been proved allergic to certain foods. The cytotoxic test turned out positive for the offending foods only 4 times in 15. A success rate this low simply is not good enough.

A Provocative Debate

Like the well-regarded skin test, two other tests are designed to provoke symptoms when an allergic patient is exposed to problem foods. But unlike

- Canned juices, including frozen juice concentrates.
- Cider and homemade root beer.
- Dried fruits.
- Soured breads such as pumpernickel and rye, and coffee cakes and baked goods made with a large amount of yeast.
- Pickled, smoked, or cured meats and fish, such as bacon and delicatessen foods including sausage, frankfurters, corned beef, and pickled tongue.

To keep mold from developing after food is prepared, follow these suggestions.

- Eat only freshly opened canned foods.
- Choose meat or fish cooked within the past day.
- Avoid foods made from leftovers, such as meat loaf, hash, or croquettes.
- Prepare hamburgers from freshly ground meat.
- If using only freshly prepared meat is difficult, buy fresh meat, cook it promptly, and freeze until ready to use.

Above all, don't be discouraged about your mold allergy. If you take shots for your allergy, in time you may be able to eat some of the foods that used to cause you problems.

the skin test, these two "provocative methods" have few fans.

In "provocative and neutralization testing," the suspected allergen is to be injected under the skin in amounts great enough to provoke symptoms, and when these occur, a "neutralizing" dose of the same substance is then given as a sort of antidote. The AAAI could not find any well-designed experiments to support the value of this test but did find four such studies that found it to be ineffective.

Also designed to provoke allergic symptoms is the "sublingual provocative test." In this test, a few drops of a food extract are placed under the tongue rather than under the skin. Again, the AAAI found no evidence that this technique is valuable in diagnosing food allergies.

The Most Common Causes

Experts now believe that one or more of the proteins in an offending food triggers the allergic response in overly sensitive individuals. Although this means that countless protein-containing foods pose a potential threat, a handful of troublemakers tops the list of common food allergens.

- Fish and shellfish.
- Legumes, especially peanuts.
- Nuts (note that peanuts are legumes, not nuts).
- Eggs.
- Chocolate.
- Cow's milk.
- Citrus fruits.
- Tomatoes.
- Wheat.

Also a potential problem for the allergic individual is the mold that is found in food. (See "Man versus Mold" for more about when to suspect mold allergy and what to do about it.)

Color Me Allergic

Allergy-producing proteins and molds can explain many food allergies, but not all. In other cases, natural foodstuffs or molds are innocent but colorings or other ingredients added to food are guilty.

Here's a classic case of color allergy reported in the *Annals of Allergy* by Robert Desmond, M.D., and Joseph Trautlein, M.D., of the Hershey Medical Center in Pennsylvania. The victim, one of their medical students, was lucky in that he was never far from help when trouble struck.

The patient was a 25-year-old student with a long history of [allergy]
and asthma . . . on March 3, 1979, while eating dinner, [he] experi-
enced a severe tightening sensation in his throat accompanied by
shortness of breath. This rapidly progressed to complete inability to
swallow . . . [and many hives appeared. He] was taken to the
emergency room and treated [successfully]. While under observation,
symptoms reoccurred. . . . The only new item ingested by the patient
was cauliflower and cheese sauce in a commercial preparation.
      On April 12, 1979, while on rounds . . . in the Hershey Medical
Center, he experienced light-headedness, intense [itching] of the scalp
and a constricting sensation in his throat [and] was admitted [to the
hospital] and closely monitored. A careful food history taken by the
patient revealed the only food ingested that morning to be a glass of
orange juice and three yellow jelly beans. . . . He was treated [with
several drugs] including theophylline.
      On day two of the hospitalization he began experiencing periods
of light-headedness, shortness of breath, [and a] patchy rash. The
symptoms persisted and worsened and eventually were noted to
follow administration of the theophylline. This was discontinued
with subsequent resolution of symptoms.

At this point, the doctors were looking for similarities between the
theophylline medication, jelly beans, and cauliflower. They found that the first
two items contained the food dye tartrazine, better known as Yellow Dye No. 5.
They suspected that the cheese sauce did, too, given its bright yellow-orange
color.

Most people who are allergic to this common dye also cannot take aspirin.
Although in this case, the doctor-to-be could take aspirin without problem,
his allergy to the yellow dye was obvious. It was confirmed on two later occa-
sions, when he again suffered symptoms after eating products that contained
this dye.

Fortunately, more and more manufacturers of tartrazine-containing products are disclosing its presence on product labels. You can monitor food and
over-the-counter drugs yourself, but when given a prescription drug, be sure
to ask the doctor or pharmacist to check the product information for the use of
food colorings. Often there will be a brand of the medication available that
does not contain the problem dye.

A Is for Adrenalin

A is for allergy, antihistamines, and Adrenalin. Antihistamines are usually the first line of defense against allergy symptoms, including food allergies. Many are available over-the-counter, although your doctor may instead give you a prescription-strength product. The important thing is to use the medicine that gives you the most relief with the fewest side effects.

For those rare, life-threatening allergic reactions, Adrenalin is standard fare. It's what the emergency room typically gives to someone who is rushed in with a severe allergic attack.

If you ever have one of these extreme attacks, your doctor may want you to carry Adrenalin with you as a precaution. Sold only by prescription, it is usually packaged as a "bee-sting kit" for use by those who react severely to insect bites. The kit allows you to administer the Adrenalin yourself, saving the time it takes to get to the doctor or hospital. (Don't cringe at the thought. When a reaction occurs, you will probably have no trouble giving yourself a shot.)

Still squeamish about self-administering Adrenalin? There's a new product called the EpiPen. The EpiPen contains a shot of Adrenalin packaged in such a way that the drug will be administered almost automatically on receiving your cue. Whether you have a bee-sting kit or an EpiPen, be sure to replace it every so often. You'll find an expiration date stamped on the package.

By the way, Adrenalin is not always advised to fight a severe reaction. It can be dangerous to those who have heart conditions or use certain medicines. Your doctor, not you, should decide whether or not it's for you.

If It's Not Allergy

Just because a reaction to food isn't allergy hardly means that you're imagining things. There are lots of other problems that might explain why you suffer unpleasant symptoms after eating one or more foods. Let's look at one of the most common food reactions that is often described as an allergy but is actually something quite different.

You may be one of the many who always tolerated milk well, only to find in your fifties or later years that drinking it brings on gas pains and diarrhea that you never had before. These symptoms are classic signs of lactose intolerance—the inability to digest the sugar (lactose) that milk contains. The cause is not an allergy or any kind of reaction of the immune system. Rather, the problem results from a deficiency of an enzyme called lactase that is needed to digest

Getting to Know Food Families

If you suffer from a specific food allergy, chances are good that you are allergic to other foods, too. Once allergists have determined that you are allergic to a food, they know that other offenders are likely to be foods belonging to the same botanical family as the proven troublemaker.

The next surprise may be finding out that the food that gives you trouble has some close cousin that you would never think of as a relative. Can you believe that avocado and cinnamon belong to the same family? Ditto for cucumber and watermelon. Obviously, you will need to know which foods are related and watch for allergy to all family members.

Rest assured, however, that allergy to one member of a food family does not guarantee that its relatives will cause the same problem. Peanuts may do you in, but it doesn't always mean that their relatives do, too.

Allergy to more than one food within a family is more likely with plant foods. Nonetheless, there are people who are allergic to more than one member of an animal food family. This table matches each food family with its members. Foods belonging to the plant kingdom appear in the first group; those in the animal kingdom are listed in the second.

Plant Kingdom

Family Name	*Members*
Apple	Apple, pear, quince
Aster	Artichoke, chicory, dandelion, endive, escarole, lettuce, sunflower seeds, tarragon
Beet	Beet, chard, lamb's-quarter, spinach
Blueberry	Blueberry, cranberry, huckleberry, wintergreen
Buckwheat	Buckwheat, garden sorrel, rhubarb
Cashew	Cashew, mango, pistachio
Chocolate	Chocolate (cocoa), cola
Citrus	Citron, grapefruit, kumquat, lemon, lime, orange, tangerine
Fungus	Mushroom, yeast
Ginger	Cardamom, ginger, turmeric
Gooseberry	Currant, gooseberry

(continued)

Plant Kingdom–*continued*

Family Name	*Members*
Grains (cereal or grass)	Bamboo shoots, barley, corn, millet, oats, rice, rye, sorghum, sugarcane, wheat, wild rice
Laurel	Avocado, bay leaves, cinnamon, sassafras
Mallow	Cottonseed, okra
Melon (gourd)	Cantaloupe, cucumber, other melons, pumpkin, squash, watermelon
Mint	Balm (Melissa), basil, catnip, horehound, marjoram, mint, peppermint, rosemary, sage, savory, spearmint, thyme
Mustard	Horseradish, mustard, radish, turnip, varieties of cabbage (broccoli, brussels sprouts, cabbage, Chinese cabbage, cauliflower, collard greens, kale, kohlrabi, kraut, rutabaga), watercress
Myrtle	Allspice (pimento), clove, guava
Onion	Asparagus, chives, garlic, leeks, onion, sarsaparilla
Palm	Coconut, date
Parsley	Angelica, anise, caraway, carrot, celeriac, celery, celery seed, coriander, cumin, dill, fennel, parsley, parsnip
Pea	Acacia, beans (lima, navy, pinto, soy, string, etc.), licorice, peanut, peas (cowpeas, green), tragacanth
Plum	Almond, apricot, cherry, nectarine, peach, plum, wild cherry
Potato	All foods called pepper (except black and white) including cayenne, chili pepper, capsicum, green pepper, red pepper, eggplant, potato, tomato
Rose	Blackberry, developed berries (such as boysenberry, loganberry, youngberry), dewberry, strawberry, raspberry

Plant Kingdom

Family Name	*Members*
Walnut	Black walnut, butternut, English walnut, hickory nut, pecan

Animal Kingdom

Family Name	*Members*
Bird	All fowl and game birds – chicken, duck, goose, guinea, pigeon, pheasant, quail, turkey, etc.
Crustacean	Crab, lobster, shrimp
Fish	All true fish, either fresh-water or salt-water fish such as catfish, salmon, sardine, tuna, trout
Mammal	Beef, lamb, pork, rabbit, squirrel, venison, etc. There is a tendency for milk-sensitive people to be allergic to beef. If you are allergic to cow's milk, you may be allergic to the milk of other animals, such as goat, as well.
Mollusk	Abalone, clam, oyster, mussel

milk sugar comfortably. (For more on lactose intolerance, see page 276.)

To help clarify differences between the most common types of food reaction, Dr. Metcalfe offers some guidance:

- Food allergy is synonymous with food hypersenstivity. In these reactions, the body releases certain immune factors in response to ingestion of a food or food additive that does not bother a nonallergic person.
- Food intolerance is an inability to consume normal amounts of a food for reasons unrelated to the immune system. Lactose intolerance, for instance, falls under this category.
- Food poisoning is a reaction to a toxic ingredient in food that occurs naturally or as a result of contamination. Anyone can succumb to food poisoning, whereas true allergies can occur only in the 20 percent or so of the population who have the immune response that causes allergy.

ANEMIA

Nutritional Enemy Number One

No matter how well your life is going, anemia makes it hard to appreciate your good fortune. You feel tired and low on energy most of the time. You're irritable and have trouble concentrating. If you exert yourself, you gasp for breath. You feel numbness, tingling, or a sensation of coldness in your hands or feet. You don't have much interest in eating, and you seem unusually susceptible to infection.

After a few weeks of these symptoms, you visit the doctor's office. The nurse takes one look at your pale skin and suspects anemia. The doctor agrees and orders a blood test to assess your hemoglobin and hematocrit levels. These tests measure the amount of iron-carrying protein in your blood and the volume of red blood cells. Although invisible to you, these two factors greatly affect how you feel.

Sure enough, the lab tests confirm the suspicion. You are anemic. The next question to ask is why.

Anemia has many causes—some nutritional, others not. Many vitamins and minerals are involved in the process of building and maintaining healthy blood. In theory, a deficiency of any one might be causing your anemia. In reality, though, anemias that are nutrition related are overwhelmingly due to too little iron, vitamin B_{12}, or folate.

Sometimes deficiencies occur simply from a diet that contains too little of one or more of those nutrients. But in other cases, an underlying health problem that is preventing the body from getting or keeping a healthy store of the nutrient is ultimately at fault. In the sections that follow, we'll look at both dietary and nondietary factors that influence your iron, B_{12}, and folate nutrition. Let's start with iron.

Iron Deficiency—The Anemia That's Everywhere

Unlike many common health problems, iron-deficiency anemia is more a disease of youth than of old age. Its favorite victims are babies, children, teenage girls, and of course, pregnant women. And it is no stranger to any part of the world. Anemia is common in both rich and poor countries, although, not surprisingly, the problem is greatest in developing areas. In some underdeveloped areas, as many as 50 percent of the children and women of childbearing age may be affected.

Fortunately, however, the chances of anemia decrease once a woman passes menopause, as she no longer loses iron during menstruation. Anemia after menopause may be a warning sign of a more serious condition that is causing abnormal loss of blood. In these cases, as with anemic men, the doctor's first job is to rule out the presence of an underlying disease.

Tired Blood and Its Toll

The word anemia conjures up thoughts of fatigue and loss of energy. But although tiredness is one of the classic signs, it is hardly the only one. Chances are that you will feel depressed and irritable, too. And no wonder—who wouldn't be after a few weeks of feeling run-down all the time?

But the plot thickens. Your crankiness probably comes from more than feeling tired. New research tells us that iron may affect mood, too. In a thought-provoking editorial published in the *British Medical Journal,* D. P. Addy, M.D., cites a half-dozen studies that found that after iron supplementation, mood or learning ability improved among iron-deficient children. Dr. Addy, a British pediatrician in Birmingham, England, believes that iron affects the brain directly. "In some children," he concludes, "happiness may indeed be iron."

Running Scared?

We've known for years that anemia most commonly strikes young children and premenopausal women. What we have learned more recently, though, is that athletes, of all people, are also likely victims. In 1982, for instance, D. B. Clement and R. C. Asmundson reported that about three-quarters of female long-distance runners and one-quarter of their male counterparts were running a risk of anemia.

Hard as it was to imagine high-energy runners becoming anemic, further research has confirmed these findings. Perhaps nothing drove the message home as much as the report that standout marathoner Alberto Salazar had been suffering from iron deficiency! Needless to say, his running skills suffered, too.

Are you wondering how this can be? No one knows for sure why an athletic lifestyle increases the chances of anemia. We believe, however, that iron losses are a key cause of iron deficiency among otherwise energetic people. It's no mystery where athletes lose iron aplenty. Obviously, it's in the large amount of sweat that they generate during heavy exercise.

The Conditions That Contribute

Most of us, of course, are more likely to eat ourselves into an iron-deficient state than to sweat our way there. It's also more likely that a medical condition that compromises iron nutrition will be the culprit. Among the most common causes of iron deficiency are the following conditions.

- Poor iron absorption due to diseases of malabsorption, stomach surgery, or chronic diarrhea.
- Excessive blood loss from ulcers, heavy menstruation, cancer, or other internal bleeding.
- Pregnancy, particularly during the later months, when the baby's demands for iron from the mother are greatest.

And every now and then, an uncommon metabolic disease or medical procedure will do its part in causing iron deficiency.

Forecasting with Ferritin

Thanks to an important advance in laboratory testing, iron deficiency now can be detected before anemia actually develops. This kind of early detection constitutes a major breakthrough, for it allows nutritional problems to be found before they become severe. Although many have long considered "iron deficiency" to be synonomous with anemia, this new test enables us to make a valuable distinction between these two terms.

Iron deficiency refers to the stage before the development of the low hemoglobin or hematocrit readings that indicate anemia. In this preanemic stage, the body has too little iron stored away but has not yet become deficient enough to show signs of anemia. A blood ferritin test will tell whether or not your body has enough iron stored in its "bank account."

Iron-deficiency anemia develops after the body's bank account of iron is depleted. The hallmarks of anemia are low readings on the hemoglobin or hematocrit blood tests.

Obviously, a low score on the blood ferritin test sounds an early alert of impending trouble. It gives you a head start on correcting the problem before it progresses to a full-blown case of anemia.

This is the bright side of iron deficiency–that it doesn't have to lead to anemia. But, on the other hand, this less-severe condition is much more common than outright anemia. At their Paris research institute, Dr. P. Galan and colleagues tested almost 500 women of childbearing age. Only 6 were actually anemic, but 77 were iron deficient, based on results of the blood ferritin test.

The Absorption Advantage

Dr. Galan's group uncovered another surprising fact when they looked at how dietary iron intakes affected the women's blood test scores. The bottom line? They were unable to show a link between intake and nutritional status– that is, the total amount of iron in a woman's diet did not correspond to her chances of becoming iron deficient.

But these findings hardly let diet off the hook. What the researchers did show is that factors that influence the absorption of iron (rather than the total amount consumed) were important. In fact, the study showed that factors that increase iron absorption (iron's friends) along with factors that decrease absorption (iron's enemies) were more significant than the amount of iron itself. So let's take a look at just who these friends and enemies are.

Focus on Friendly Factors

One of iron's best friends is found in plant foods, while another is found in animal foods. That means that vegetarians and nonvegetarians alike can take effective steps to improve iron absorption.

In the plant world, iron's best friend is vitamin C. In their classic paper on iron absorption, Elaine Monsen, Ph.D., and co-workers reported that the iron in a meal is well absorbed as long as 75 milligrams of vitamin C are also present. (See "The C Solution" for foods that provide at least this much of the vitamin.)

As an alternative, said Dr. Monsen and her colleagues, even a modest-size serving (more than 3 ounces) of meat, poultry, or fish will also make the iron in a meal highly absorbable. Meats contain heme iron–a special form of iron that not only is unusually well absorbed but also helps you absorb iron from other

The C Solution

Looking for a natural way to enhance your absorption of iron from food? Including at least 75 milligrams of vitamin C with a meal helps you get the most from its iron. So take your pick from any of the following choices—all provide at least the minimum amount of vitamin C needed to maximize iron absorption.

1 cup broccoli
1 cup brussels sprouts
½ cantaloupe
1 cup cauliflower
1 cup collard greens
1 cup cranberry juice cocktail
1 cup grapefruit juice (fresh or from concentrate)
1 cup kale
1 cup orange juice (fresh or from concentrate)
1 cup papaya chunks
1 cup pineapple juice
1 cup fresh strawberries
½ package frozen strawberries (10-ounce package)

foods. Only meats contain heme iron. Still another alternative is to include both a modest amount of vitamin C (25 to 75 milligrams) and a very small amount of meat (1 to 3 ounces).

A third factor also possibly gives iron absorption a boost, but nutritionists are reserving judgment until more studies are done. This is the acid factor. Certain acidic substances found in citrus fruits, sauerkraut, beer, and other foods may lend a hand with iron absorption by converting it to a form that the body can absorb more easily.

And, as you'll see in the next section, iron needs all the help it can get to fend off the effects of its enemies.

Identifying Iron's Enemies

If you're concerned about factors that interfere with your iron nutrition, you'll be happy to learn about the work of the International Center for Control of Nutritional Anemia, affiliated with the University of Kansas Medical Center. A research group of doctors and scientists at the center has made a concerted effort to track down the factors that inhibit our absorption of iron. Here are some of their key findings.

- Tea strongly inhibited absorption of iron from a hamburger meal. Taking a cup of tea with the test meal reduced iron absorption by almost two-thirds.
- Tea's strongest rival–coffee–also inhibited iron absorption if taken at meal-time, but not as much. A cup of coffee given with the hamburger meal reduced the amount of iron absorbed by about 40 percent. Coffee consumed at least an hour before the meal did not inhibit iron absorption, but if taken within an hour after the meal, absorption was reduced as much as when the coffee was consumed at mealtime.
- Soy flour contains both enhancing and inhibiting factors. Its positive influences on iron absorption compensate partially, but not completely, for the inhibiting factors it contains.
- Substances present in five different legumes (soybeans, black beans, lentils, split peas, and mung beans) interfered with absorption of most of their iron. Nutritionists believe that absorption of iron from food in general averages about 10 percent, but only 1 to 2 percent of the iron in these legumes were absorbed.
- Dairy products and egg yolk appear to reduce absorption of nonheme iron, but not of heme iron. The nonheme form, of course, is found in all iron-containing foods, while the heme form occurs only in flesh foods.

In addition, nutritionists have long believed that the oxalates found in certain foods (most notably spinach) reduce iron absorption. Although the iron in these foods may be poorly absorbed, the iron in other foods you eat at the same time is believed safe from their effects.

Last but not least is the issue of whole grain foods. Nutritionists have pointed out that the fiber and phytate that they contain can reduce iron absorption. We don't doubt that it can, but at the same time, we're impressed with a number of studies that did not find deficient iron nutrition when the subjects ate diets rich in bran or other fiber. "Adequate iron nutrition is attainable with mixed diets high in wheat bran," says Eugene R. Morris, an authority on iron nutrition at the U.S. Department of Agriculture. But if you use bran frequently, we'd suggest taking a multimineral supplement just in case.

Avoiding the other foods that inhibit iron absorption may also be impractical or unappealing to you. Moreover, many of us can eat these foods without depleting iron stores. So what should you do? If you know that your iron nutrition is fine with your current diet, you don't have much to gain by worrying about these interactions.

If, on the other hand, you are iron deficient, do what you can to apply these findings to your dietary lifestyle. If you are a coffee or tea drinker, for instance, try not to schedule your favorite beverage within an hour or so of a meal or iron supplement. If you are a vegetarian, don't depend on legumes for your iron. Above all, try to temper the ill effects of these influences by including one or more iron friends in your diet or supplement program.

Vitamin B_{12} and Vegetarians

Vegetarianism has both its supporters and critics. Fortunately, the supporters are gaining in their efforts to call attention to the many advantages of a well-balanced vegetarian diet. We're very impressed with those benefits. But at the same time, we don't want to imply that all vegetarian lifestyles are risk free.

Many nutrients in animal foods also occur in plant foods, and vegetarians usually can get enough from nonflesh sources. But vitamin B_{12} is an exception: Only animal products are known to contain it. That poses no problem for the vegetarian who eats dairy products or eggs. But those who eat only plant foods may eventually develop B_{12} deficiency. It usually takes at least several years of a strict vegetarian diet before the deficiency develops in adults. However small the risk, we don't think it worth taking, and do recommend B_{12} supplementation in this case.

We're particularly concerned that vegetarian children have a reliable source of B_{12}. Here is a story about one-year-old Edward, who didn't. It's excerpted from a report by R. C. Gambon and co-workers of Children's Hospital in Bern, Switzerland.

> *The 35-year-old mother had been living on a diet based on plant food only, with strict exclusion of all animal products (meat, milk, eggs) for seven years before the birth of the twins. . . . Both twins were exclusively breast-fed from birth.*

The Supplement Alternative

For preventing iron deficiency, supplementation offers an alternative when you can't always manage an iron-friendly diet. Once iron-deficiency anemia develops, however, supplements are usually the only simple alternative for treating it. No matter how many iron-rich foods you choose, then, you are unlikely to take in enough iron to replenish your "iron bank" and meet your ongoing need for iron. What's more, you will probably want to get back on your feet as quickly as possible, and the extra iron in a supplement can help you do that.

Development was reported to be normal for both during the first months of life. They smiled at 6 weeks of age and reached for toys at 3 months. Growth and psychomotor development were equal in both twins until the age of 8 months, when the patient . . . started to vomit frequently after feedings. Then the mother noted a gradual change in his behavior. He stopped smiling and socializing, his activity decreased rapidly, spontaneous movements were slow. He was no longer able to sit or to turn over, and despite frequent feedings seven times a day he began to lose weight. Sleeping periods became longer. He stopped vocalizing and became lethargic. At 11 months of age the infant was referred for investigation. Neither twin had received any vitamin supplementation.

It didn't take long for the doctors to diagnose B_{12} deficiency. They started Edward on B_{12} supplementation, and within a week he was much better. Two weeks later he was released from the hospital, although he continued to take a supplement, of course. Fortunately, he did not show any signs of permanent damage to his brain or nervous system. And the doctors later learned that the children's grandmother had been feeding small amounts of meat to Edward's twin brother, which explained why only one of the twins became deficient.

Why let a baby take a chance like this?

Supplementation sounds great, and it's simple and inexpensive, too. But sometimes there are side effects. At the higher doses used to treat anemia, you may find that an iron supplement causes nausea or digestive discomfort. If so, try taking it with meals or check with your doctor about reducing the dose.

You may also find that iron supplements tend to be constipating. Again, the higher the dose, the more likely the problem. Our recommendation is to try some bran or other fiber-rich foods. Of course, you may be concerned that the extra fiber will interfere with iron absorption. Just ask your doctor to take a simple blood test to determine if your iron status is getting better or worse or staying the same when you add fiber to the regimen. More likely than not, the therapeutic dose of an iron supplement will more than make up for any iron lost to the extra fiber.

The Other Anemias

Too little iron is the most common dietary problem leading to anemia, but it's hardly the only one. Vitamins, too, are needed to prevent anemia, especially two that belong to the B complex—vitamin B_{12} and folate.

With a microscope, you can see that blood deficient in vitamin B_{12} or folate looks very different from blood that is lacking in iron. When iron deficiency is to blame, the red blood cells are unusually small, but when too little of these B vitamins is the problem, the cells are abnormally large and irregularly shaped. The technical name for this condition is nutritional megaloblastic anemia. Among its many symptoms are fatigue, sore tongue, pallor, weight loss, tingling sensations, back pain, digestive upset, irritability, and depression.

The most common causes of megaloblastic anemia are alcohol, alcohol, and alcohol! As you might guess, alcohol abusers tend to have vitamin-poor diets, and anemia might be expected as a result. But there's another reason, too. Alcohol apparently encourages excretion of B vitamins, resulting in an increase in need that often goes unmet. In fact, when David Savage, M.D., and John Lindenbaum, M.D., tested alcoholics admitted to Harlem Hospital in New York City, they found that one out of three showed laboratory signs of this condition.

Of course, not all victims of vitamin B_{12} or folate deficiency have an alcohol problem. In fact, some are teetotalers! But if they take in too little of these B vitamins, they, too, may develop megaloblastic anemia.

As a practical matter, however, those at highest risk for diet-induced B_{12} deficiency are vegetarians who eat no animal products, the only documented source of B_{12}. Years of eating such a diet can slowly deplete the B_{12} bank and lead to serious health problems. But people who eat animal foods and strict vegetarians who take a B_{12} supplement generally do fine, as the body conserves B_{12} well. Unfortunately, the picture is not so rosy for folate.

Focus on Folate

Folate, also known as folic acid, is one of the nutrients that has become most endangered in our modern food environment. Although fresh fruits and vegetables are good sources, our decreasing use of fresh produce may jeopardize our chances of getting enough to meet our needs. Also, as food is cooked, folate is lost. While severe deficiency remains rare in the United States, nutritionists now believe that mild or "borderline" folate deficiencies affect more than a few individuals, and that the elderly are at special risk. Here's why.

- Older individuals may have dental problems that favor consumption of soft, overcooked food—the kind that is likely to be low in folate from excessive cooking.
- Certain drugs may interfere with folate nutrition, and the elderly use more medications than other segments of the population.
- The ability to absorb folate from food may decrease with age. Research has found low folate levels even among elderly people eating diets considered adequate in this nutrient.
- Our bodies store only a two- to four-month supply of folate, making deficiency more likely than in the case of nutrients that are stored in larger amounts.

If diagnosed early enough, the effects of deficiency on the brain and nervous system can be reversed by boosting folate intake. If eating more fresh fruits and vegetables isn't practical, multiple-vitamin products containing folate are widely available, as are fortified foods that contain 100 percent of the recommended allowance. Although folate has little toxicity at high doses, nutritionists do not recommend taking large amounts except in severe cases. There is a small risk (but not one worth taking) that a high dose will disguise the presence of vitamin B_{12} deficiency.

There's no need to be in the dark about your folate nutrition. Tell your doctor if you would like a test of your blood folate level. If you regularly take anticonvulsant drugs (such as Dilantin), anticancer drugs, birth control pills, cortisone, sleeping pills, or sulfa drugs, your doctor may have already ordered the test as a way of monitoring the effect of your medication on this important B vitamin.

Iron-Friendly Meal Plans

Eating more iron-rich foods was once considered the only logical way to prevent or treat iron deficiency. But today, there are additional considerations. We now know that including a source of vitamin C or a small amount of flesh food while limiting coffee and tea with meals can help ensure that your iron stores are adequate.

That's because your body can make you do with less iron when it has friends to help it use the iron that is available. Accordingly, we prefer to think of the optimal diet as "iron friendly" rather than "iron rich."

Here we have combined all four recommendations into a simple weekly menu plan that is very iron friendly. If your diet doesn't look anything like our iron-friendly meal plans, you can take a multivitamin tablet with iron as a sensible preventive measure.

Day 1

Breakfast
⅔ cup Total cereal
1 orange
2 pieces raisin bread
½ cup skim milk

Lunch
3 ounces chicken breast (without skin)
2 slices Italian bread
1 cup honeydew melon
1 cup skim milk

Snack
1 apple
1 ounce cheddar cheese

Dinner
1 cup oysters
¾ cup cooked eggplant
1½ cups raw celery
1 cup raw green pepper
1 fresh tomato
1 cup fresh pineapple chunks with ½ cup vanilla low-fat yogurt

Day 2

Breakfast
1 cup Team cereal
1 orange
1 slice Italian bread
1 teaspoon margarine
1 cup skim milk

Lunch
¾ cup fresh spinach
6 cucumber slices (with peel)
1 fresh tomato
3 ounces steamed scallops
¼ cup seedless raisins
¼ cup pumpkin seeds
1 cup skim milk

Snack
1 apple
1 ounce cheddar cheese

Dinner
4 ounces chicken breast (without skin)
1 simmered chicken liver
½ cup peas
½ cup brown rice
1 cup pineapple juice

Day 3

Breakfast
⅔ cup Most cereal
½ white grapefruit
1 slice Italian bread
1 teaspoon jelly
1 cup skim milk

(continued)

Lunch
  2 ounces water-packed tuna
  ½ tablespoon reduced-calorie mayonnaise
  ½ cup canned peas
  ½ cup butterhead lettuce
  1 fresh tomato
  1 tablespoon low-calorie salad dressing
  1 cup skim milk

Snack
  ½ cup fresh orange sections

Dinner
  2½ ounces lean sirloin steak (trimmed of fat)
  ⅓ cup unsweetened applesauce
  1 cup lima beans
  ½ tablespoon margarine
  1 cup skim milk
  1 ounce black walnuts

Day 4

Breakfast
  ⅔ cup Product 19 cereal
  1 apple
  2 pieces Italian bread
  1 tablespoon jelly
  1 cup skim milk

Lunch
  3 ounces ground round patty with 1 slice low-fat cheese
1½ cups tossed salad
  2 tablespoons low-calorie salad dressing
  2 pieces Italian bread
  1 cup tomato juice

Snack
  1 cup fresh strawberries with ½ cup vanilla low-fat yogurt

Dinner
  4 ounces Cornish hen (without skin)
  1 whole wheat roll
  ¾ cup brussels sprouts

1 tablespoon margarine
1 cup skim milk
1 cup cantaloupe

Day 5

Breakfast
⅔ cup Most cereal
1 fresh tangerine
1 piece raisin bread
1 cup skim milk

Lunch
1 cup fresh spinach
¼ cup dry bread crumbs
9 cucumber slices (with peel)
1 apple
1 cup raw broccoli
½ cup raw cauliflower
2 tablespoons low-calorie salad dressing
1 cup low-fat yogurt

Snack
½ cup dates

Dinner
2 simmered chicken livers
¼ cup onions
½ cup brown rice
½ cup Great Northern beans
1 cup skim milk
½ tablespoon margarine
1 piece watermelon

Day 6

Breakfast
1 cup strawberry shake (¾ cup skim milk, 5 frozen strawberries)
1 ounce Total cereal
½ cup milk

Lunch
1 cup fresh spinach
½ cup green beans
½ cup navy beans

(continued)

2 pieces tofu (soybean curd)
6 cucumber slices (with peel)
⅓ cup raw celery
¼ cup shredded carrot
¼ cup shredded cheese
2 tablespoons low-calorie salad dressing

Snack
¼ cup raisin-nut mix

Dinner
3 ounces veal cutlet
½ cup mashed potatoes
½ cup peas
1 tablespoon margarine
¾ cup orange juice
1 cup fresh raspberries with ½ cup frozen low-fat yogurt

Day 7

Breakfast
1 cup farina
1 tangerine
1 slice Italian bread
½ tablespoon jelly

Lunch
2 tomatoes stuffed with 1 cup canned clams, ½ cup low-fat cottage cheese, 1 tablespoon reduced-calorie mayonnaise
¾ cup orange juice

Snack
½ cup dried apricots

Dinner
3 ounces calves' liver
½ cup lima beans
1 small boiled potato
1 tablespoon margarine
1 cup skim milk
1 cup fresh strawberries

ANGINA

How to Mend a Broken Heart

(See also *Cholesterol; Triglycerides*)

The pain of angina is almost as old as man himself. William Harvey, a pioneer in the history of modern medicine, referred to it as "an oppression in the breast." Two thousand years ago, Roman philosopher Lucius Annaeus Seneca wrote that the sudden attacks of pain were "very short, and like a storm." But the pain was so intense, said Seneca, that "to have any other malady is only to be sick. To have this is to be dying."

Well, not quite. Modern medicine has made enormous progress against angina pectoris, also known simply as chest pain. A wealth of knowledge about its causes and treatment has brought a degree of relief that Seneca could only have dreamed about. In fact, much of this new information has become available only in the last few decades. And the best time to put the new findings to use is right now!

As any angina sufferer can tell you, the pain usually begins near the heart and stomach, but it may spread–to the neck, jaw, back, abdomen, and arms, for instance. Most commonly, an attack is triggered by smoking, eating, exertion, anxiety, or exposure to cold; often it subsides with rest. Because the triggering factors are known to increase the heart's need for oxygen, doctors have long suspected that angina was a cry for help from an overtaxed heart.

A Mystery No More

Another curiosity about angina was that it develops with age. Activities performed with "no sweat" during our youth can bring on protests from the heart in later life. It was a mystery that put medical detectives to work. And today, the case has been pretty much closed. Research has repeatedly shown that angina is related to hardening of the arteries, the underlying cause of most heart attacks. Thousands of studies make this link clear, but we will cite just a few of the more recent ones.

• Dr. Marianne Hagman and her colleagues at the University of Gothenburg in Sweden compared angina sufferers to almost 6,000 men free of chest pain. The results linked angina to high blood cholesterol, high blood pressure, smoking, overweight, diabetes, and lack of exercise–in other words, the same factors known to increase the chances of having a heart attack.

- Dr. O. Kusa's research team at the Institute for Cardiovascular Diseases in Bratislava, Czechoslovakia, showed that the severity of angina was linked to the ratio between two blood fat measurements, HDL (high-density lipoprotein) cholesterol and total cholesterol. In their patients, angina worsened as the levels of these two fats became more and more imbalanced. At the same time, other researchers were finding that this same cholesterol imbalance best predicted the chance of having a heart attack. It was yet another clue that angina and heart attacks are the work of the same unfriendly process.
- The link between angina and hardening of the arteries was proved the high-tech way by Dr. Shlomo Eisenberg and his co-workers at Hadassah University in Jerusalem. Using a sophisticated test called angiography, this group showed that two-thirds of angina sufferers had arteries hardened enough to put their hearts at risk.
- Dr. Leif Lapidus and his co-workers, also of the University of Gothenburg, wanted to determine whether risk factors for angina differ between women and men. They found women suffering from angina tended to have high levels of triglycerides—another blood fat long suspected of promoting hardening of the arteries.

But troubled arteries aren't the only cause of angina. Sometimes it strikes even when these important blood vessels are in good shape. With a little further exploration, the problem sometimes proves to be too much thyroid hormone, severe anemia, syphilis, or a disease of the heart itself rather than its arteries. Still, all of these other causes account for only a minority of the two million or so Americans who experience angina.

Angina attacks can be both painful and frightening, but there is a bright side. After all, for some of us, angina is a signal that warns us of underlying trouble before a worse fate—heart attack—actually occurs.

Needless to say, angina sufferers should take care to get enough rest and to avoid stress as much as possible. In some cases, the doctor will prescribe drug treatment and perhaps surgery. If the angina seems to be the sign of hardened arteries, nutritional approaches will be a first order of business. (Turn to the sections on cholesterol, beginning on page 136, and triglycerides, beginning on page 395, for how-to advice.)

APPENDICITIS

Another Victory for Vegetables

Probably no one is as blasé about the value of nutrition as children are, and understanding why is easy. A child's experience with disease is often limited to colds and other benign infectious diseases. They give little thought to the chronic diseases that adults fear most, the diseases where nutrition is most likely to play a role. But now it appears that nutrition does affect at least one disease that strikes children and young adults far more than older people.

For decades now, health experts have been debating whether nutritional factors are to blame for appendicitis. The idea dates back to World War II, when observant British doctors such as John Black, M.D., noticed that their many appendicitis patients were almost exclusively Japanese soldiers who were receiving British rations instead of their usual diet. Dr. Black and the surgeon he worked with believed that the "epidemic" was due to the sudden dietary change.

In other populations, though, rates of appendicitis actually decreased during the war. According to Alexander R. P. Walker of the South African Institute for Medical Research, the appendicitis rate in the English Channel Islands and Switzerland fell during wartime. The war had forced residents there to make dietary changes, too.

The Fiber Faction

Of all possible dietary explanations for appendicitis, a low fiber intake has been suspected most. The case for a protective effect from fiber rests on facts such as these.

• Appendicitis tends to be more common in countries where the diet is low in fiber.
• During the war, when appendicitis rates fell, residents of Switzerland and the English Channel Islands were eating more fiber (and less fat) than usual.
• Surveys in African cities by Denis Burkitt, M.D., have shown that appendicitis is ten times more common in whites than in blacks. In Africa, of course, the former are more likely to follow a Western-type diet.

• Some research shows that children who develop appendicitis eat less fiber. Jean Brender, Ph.D., and associates at the University of Washington School of Public Health reported in 1985 that children who had eaten the diets richest in fiber were only half as likely to develop the disease.

Go for the Green

Despite the enthusiasm for the fiber theory, the most comprehensive study that we found failed to link fiber or whole grain foods to appendicitis. D. J. P. Barker and his co-workers at the University of Southampton studied the typical diet available to about 50,000 appendicitis victims living in England and Wales. A generous intake of green vegetables and tomatoes–not whole grain foods or total fiber intake–showed up as a protective factor against the disease.

Dr. Barker and his associates are sold on the idea that the effect of these foods is real. They speculate that these vegetables affect the bacteria in the appendix in a way that helps protect against infection. We like these findings for a more practical reason. Taking advantage of them requires no explanation; you don't need a nutritionist to help you identify green vegetables or tomatoes.

Informed Dissent

Although impressed with these findings regarding vegetable consumption, Dr. Barker considers diet to be a secondary factor in appendicitis. His research team has pursued lots of other leads, too; the results show that hygienic factors such as overcrowding and lack of hot water best account for appendicitis in the United Kingdom. Dr. Barker believes that sanitation and exposure to infection are what matter most.

Anyone who has been following the issue in the British medical press knows that right now, the nutrition-versus-infection debate is at a fever pitch. Moreover, settling the debate will be tough. Appendicitis victims usually undergo appendectomy, making it impossible to test whether changing diet after the first attack helps prevent a second. So we suspect that the debate will be with us for quite a while.

Meanwhile, if we had to predict what the answer will be, we'd venture a guess that both will turn out to play a part. But no matter how the debate turns out, Mom and Dad, the "advice" you're already giving your kids is just right: Eat your vegetables.

APPLES

Working Each Day
to Keep Cholesterol at Bay

81 calories per medium apple

For years, nutritionists wondered how apples ever became known for keeping the doctor away. Not that they had anything against the apple, it just seemed so much less nutritious than a heavy hitter such as the orange. After all, oranges are loaded with vitamin C; apples, by contrast, aren't rich in any vitamins or minerals.

But times change. Today, nutritionists appreciate fiber like never before. And the apple is rich in the soluble form of fiber. In fact, it's one of the best sources of soluble fiber in the supermarket.

Unlike insoluble fibers, soluble fibers aren't thought to play a part in treating digestive disorders or preventing cancer. Instead, they have other talents. These forms of fiber help to prevent sharp swings in your blood sugar level. Naturally, the diabetes experts have taken notice. In the process, they've documented that soluble fiber also has an impressive ability to lower blood cholesterol levels.

At the University of Kentucky School of Medicine, where diabetes expert James W. Anderson, M.D., has been remarkably successful in treating diabetics with high-fiber diets, the news about cholesterol has been just as, well, heartening. Researchers there found that blood cholesterol levels fell an average of 30 percent when patients switched to the high-fiber diet. Dr. Anderson has estimated that about half the drop was caused by the generous amounts of soluble fiber in the new diet. According to Dr. Anderson, "gummy, water-soluble fibers" are best for lowering cholesterol. Pectin, the best-known form of fiber in apples, falls into this category.

Of course, it takes more than an apple a day to reap the benefits of a diet rich in soluble fiber. But if you usually eat lots of fruits and vegetables, you're probably taking in enough soluble fiber to make a difference. If you don't usually eat this way, use the list in "The Soluble Fiber Solution," on page 140, to find the very richest sources of soluble fiber, and incorporate four or more servings of these into your daily diet.

And don't forget some other attributes of the apple that are good for your heart: It has virtually no saturated fat, cholesterol, or sodium.

Baked Apple in a Flash

Here's a quick idea for a tasty and nutritious snack.

Peel the top third of a good cooking apple, and core it. Wrap it in plastic wrap, then microwave on full power for about 2½ minutes. (The apple will be very hot!) Let it stand for 2 minutes, then season to taste.

For a real treat, top with some frozen vanilla yogurt, cinnamon, and raisins.

In addition to fiber and its heart-healthy properties, the apple boasts one other distinction. Dentists have long advocated apples for their possible tooth-cleaning properties. At the University of Oslo, dentists J. M. Birkeland and L. Jorkjend put the idea to the test. They had one group of children eat a bun and another group eat a bun and an apple. Less food stuck to the teeth of those who ate both the apple and the bun, suggesting that apples do help clear away food debris. Presumably this helps to prevent tooth decay.

At the Market: There are many varieties of apples, but regardless of variety, the fruit should be firm, fragrant, and free of bruises. Look for apples that are bright in color for their particular variety. Freshly picked apples tend to be the most flavorful and crisp.

Although fresh-picked tastes best, apples store fairly well in the refrigerator, though not nearly as long as at room temperature. If you want to keep apples for a long time, gently place them in a plastic bag and spray with water from a plant mister once a week. They may last four to six weeks this way, depending on variety.

Kitchen Tips: Most cooks have their own opinions on which apple varieties make the best pie. But despite the disagreement, everyone considers Red Delicious to be good only for eating raw or for using in salad. (Once you cut raw apples, by the way, toss the pieces in a little lemon juice to discourage browning.)

Accent on Enjoyment: Finding uses for apples in cooking is easy. You can:

• Peel and slice them for fillings.
• Core them, then chop or grate for stuffing or mincemeats.
• Core them, then cut into rings for fritters.

- Cook and strain them to make applesauce.
- Slice them and sauté with cabbage for a quick, high-fiber side dish.
- Add small amounts to stir-fries and meat dishes.
- Cut them into wedges and sauté them, then season with spices of your choice and serve as an accompaniment to meat and game.

Sautéed Apples with Toasted Walnuts

1 tablespoon sweet butter
4 cooking apples, such as Granny Smith, cored and thinly sliced
2 tablespoons lime juice and pulp
¼ cup white grape juice
1 teaspoon lime peel
1 tablespoon maple syrup
½ teaspoon vanilla extract
1 allspice berry, ground pinch of freshly grated nutmeg
2 tablespoons chopped walnuts

In a large nonstick skillet, melt butter over medium heat.

Toss apples with lime juice and pulp. Add apples to the skillet and sauté for about 2 minutes. Then cover with crumpled aluminum foil and simmer until the slices are just tender, about 4 minutes. Use a slotted spoon to transfer apples to individual serving dishes.

Add grape juice, lime peel, maple syrup, vanilla, allspice, and nutmeg to the skillet and boil, stirring constantly, until the mixture becomes a syrup, about 2 to 3 minutes.

Toast walnuts by heating them in an ungreased nonstick skillet, shaking constantly, until they begin to brown and are fragrant.

Pour syrup over apples, sprinkle with walnuts and serve warm.

Makes 4 servings

Fresh Apples with Barley and Pine Nuts

¼ cup pearled barley
1 cup water
3 bay leaves
3 apples, cored and
    sliced
2 teaspoons lemon juice
1 teaspoon peanut oil
½ teaspoon dried
    rosemary, crushed
3 tablespoons pine nuts
¼ cup plain low-fat
    yogurt

In a small saucepan, combine barley, water, and bay leaves. Bring to a boil and continue to boil, uncovered, for 5 minutes. Remove from heat, cover, and let stand for about 1 hour, or until all the liquid has been absorbed. (This yields about a cup of barley.)

Meanwhile, in a large serving bowl, toss apples with lemon juice.

In a medium nonstick skillet, heat oil and rosemary over medium-high heat. Scoop in barley and pine nuts and sauté until barley grains are separate and almost dry, about 4 to 5 minutes.

Add barley, pine nuts, and yogurt to apples and toss well. Serve warm or at room temperature with grilled meats or poultry.

Variation: Substitute cooked rice for barley.

Makes 4 servings

APRICOTS

Carotene without the Carrot

40 calories per 3 halves (canned, juice-packed)
23 calories per 3 halves (canned, water-packed)
83 calories per 10 halves (dried)
51 calories per 3 medium apricots (fresh)

If you're having trouble getting those you love to eat more vegetables, perhaps you need to try a new tactic. Why not offer foods that have the nutrition of vegetables but the sweet taste of fruit? Our favorite of these is the apricot.

Like vegetables that are yellow to orange in color, apricots are a store-house of carotene—the plant form of vitamin A. Carotene has taken the nutrition world by storm since being linked to cancer prevention several years ago. In their landmark study, Richard Shekelle, M.D., and his co-workers at Rush-Presbyterian-St. Luke's Medical Center in Chicago compared lung cancer rates among those on both high- and low-carotene diets. Of 500 men in the high-carotene group, only 2 developed lung cancer, but among 500 men with low intakes, 14 did.

According to Peter Greenwald, M.D., director of the National Cancer Institute's (NCI) Division of Cancer Prevention and Control, other studies also show a protective effect from carotene, not only against cancer of the lung but also cancer of the stomach, bladder, esophagus, and throat. As a result, the NCI is now sponsoring more than a dozen studies to confirm carotene's role as a protective nutrient.

You can meet your carotene quota with apricots alone. Three raw fruits or ten dried apricot halves will give you half the recommended allowance. And whether canned, fresh, or dried, apricots have little or no fat, sodium, or cholesterol, which is a plus for your heart. Dried apricots offer another bonus for a healthy heart—plenty of potassium. In fact, an easy-to-eat handful of ten dried apricots provides as much potassium as a medium-size orange or a banana.

Potassium isn't dried apricot's only mineral. The same serving of ten halves has 20 percent of the recommended iron allowance for men and postmenopausal women and is a moderate source of copper, with about 10 percent of the recommended allowance. Of course, the higher concentration of minerals in dried apricots has its price—more calories than apricots that are raw or canned in juice.

41

At the Market: The ideal fresh apricot has a golden orange color. A pink blush indicates sweetness. If harvested while too immature, an apricot may never fully ripen or reach peak flavor. When ripe, apricots feel soft. Avoid shriveled apricots. When shopping for canned apricots, always check labels to be sure that the contents are packed in juice, not in heavy syrup. In choosing dried apricots, look for ones that aren't too shriveled.

Kitchen Tips: At home, treat apricots as you would fresh peaches. Leave them at room temperature until fully ripe, then refrigerate them in perforated plastic bags. Transfer canned apricots to a well-sealed container after opening and store them in the refrigerator. Dried apricots should also be stored there, in covered glass jars.

To cook dried apricots, simmer them in orange juice or water until tender. Then season to taste with cinnamon or the spices of your choice. (Spices that go well with pumpkin and apples tend to complement apricots, too.)

Accent on Enjoyment: Raw apricots lend themselves nicely to toppings and cooked foods. They can be:

- Pureed with raspberries and used atop tarts, fruit, or vanilla yogurt.
- Added to preserves, chutneys, or conserves.
- Halved, pitted, and simmered in juice until tender, then sprinkled with crushed gingersnaps and served warm. (Better yet, top with a scoop of frozen yogurt).

Should you find yourself with apricots that are shriveled or bruised, you can make apricot nectar. Simply peel and pit the apricots, then run them through an electric juicer. Chill and drink or use in marinades, punches, or sorbets.

Canned apricots, too, can be used creatively in cooking.

- Put them in a saucepan with spiced cider and simmer them until fragrant.
- Slice them and stir-fry with chicken, or chop them and add to poultry stuffings.
- Slice decoratively and use to top cakes instead of icing.
- Add them to fruit salads and compotes.
- Arrange on a cheese tray.

Finally, we'd like to mention some ideas for cooking with dried apricots.

- Add dried figs and prunes to the apricots. Then simmer and serve as a terrific condiment with roast meat.

- Slice dried apricots and add along with green pepper and onion to stir-fried chicken. The dish is as delicious as it is colorful.
- Chop and add to muffin and quick bread batters to boost nutritional value and add a fresh, tart flavor.
- Look for apricot leather to serve at snack time. These thin sheets of pressed, dried apricots are the perfect easy-care snack.

Whether you are working with raw, canned or dried apricots, remember one more family secret: Apricots are delicious with almonds. To the botanist, that's no surprise; both are members of the same family.

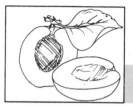

Apricot on the Half-Shell

10 fresh apricots
½ cup orange juice and
    pulp
    pinch of ground
      cinnamon
2 drops almond extract
2 teaspoons maple
    syrup
3 tablespoons low-fat
    cottage cheese,
    pressed through a
    sieve
    orange peel for
      garnish

Use a sharp paring knife to slice apricots in half, then remove the pits and stems.

In a large bowl, combine orange juice, cinnamon, almond extract, and maple syrup. Add apricots and toss until they're well coated. Then let them marinate at room temperature for 30 minutes.

Preheat broiler.

Remove apricots from the bowl, reserving marinade. Fill each apricot half with about ½ tablespoon of cheese and set on a baking sheet. Broil until lightly speckled brown, about 4 minutes.

Meanwhile, in a small saucepan, heat marinade over high heat until thick and reduced by half.

Arrange apricot halves in small dessert dishes and drizzle some sauce over each. Garnish with orange peel and serve warm for dessert, breakfast, or brunch.

Makes 4 servings

ARTICHOKES

The Assets Add Up

53 calories per medium artichoke

Artichokes have a little bit of a lot of good things. And all of these little things add up to one wholesome food. Among the nutrients that artichokes contain in small but significant amounts are calcium, iron, phosphorus, niacin, and vitamin C. In addition, they are good sources of two minerals, magnesium and potassium.

Although fat free, artichokes do have more naturally occurring sodium than most fruits and vegetables. If you are on a sodium-restricted diet, take note: One medium cooked artichoke contains 80 milligrams of sodium. Of course, this is still low when compared to many processed foods.

At the Market: Picking out a good artichoke isn't difficult. A good one is uniform in appearance, olive green in color, and marked by leaves that are tightly closed. For steaming, round artichokes are the best. The outside appearance of an artichoke, however, is not the sole test. The so-called winter-kissed artichoke may have a bronze, blistered exterior, but as long as the leaves are closed and the inside is green with a fresh appearance, it should be good to eat.

Leaves that have started to open up or have a soft consistency are signs that an artichoke is no longer fresh. If you have any doubts, hold the artichoke up to your ear and squeeze it. If it squeaks, it is still okay.

Kitchen Tips: Uncut fresh artichokes can be refrigerated for about a week. Keep them in tightly closed plastic bags to retain moisture. Artichoke bottoms freeze very well.

You can prevent discoloration of artichokes during preparation with two simple steps. First, use a stainless steel knife or scissors–not a carbon steel knife–to cut them. Second, add lemon juice to the cooking water.

Steaming is favored for cooking artichokes. Depending on size, cooking time may vary from 30 to 60 minutes. When fully cooked, a leaf can be easily pulled away. Dip the leaves in vinaigrette or your favorite sauce. To extract the meat from a leaf, pull the lower part of the leaf through your teeth.

Accent on Enjoyment: For a special occasion, fill whole steamed artichokes with crabmeat stuffing and bake until cooked through. Or consider these ideas:

- Look for tiny, whole artichokes, which can be halved and grilled.
- Marinate artichoke hearts in an herbed vinaigrette, then serve on lettuce leaves.
- Use a spoon to scrape the pulp from the leaves, then puree in a food processor or blender and use in soups or sauces.

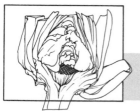

Artichoke Bottoms and Shrimp with Shallot Vinaigrette

1 pound large shrimp
 (about 24)
juice and pulp of 1 lime
1 teaspoon balsamic
 vinegar
2 teaspoons olive oil
2 shallots, minced
1 tablespoon fresh thyme
 or 1 teaspoon dried
 thyme
8 artichoke bottoms,
 quartered
6 large Swiss chard
 leaves, chopped
2 scallions, minced

Peel and devein shrimp and steam in 1 inch of boiling water until curled and cooked through, about 5 minutes.

In a small bowl, whisk together lime juice and pulp, vinegar, oil, shallots, and thyme.

In a large serving dish, toss together artichokes and dressing. Add shrimp, chard, and scallions and toss well. Serve at room temperature or chilled.

Makes 4 servings

ARTHRITIS

The Nutrition Connection Comes of Age

Mention the words *nutrition* and *arthritis* in the same sentence and you're sure to get at least a skeptical look (or worse) from your doctor. For centuries, it seems, most doctors have believed that anyone who considers the two related is at best misinformed–and at worst a huckster.

We confess that we were hardly immune to this attitude ourselves. For many years we were swayed by conventional biases against any proposed link between nutrition and arthritis. But recently, several reputable reports linking rheumatoid arthritis (RA) to diet have been published, challenging us to reconsider.

The facts that follow are based on reports with patients suffering from RA, not from osteoarthritis. The latter is the most common form of the disease that comes from wear and tear on the joints as a result of injury. It differs from RA in that little or no inflammation occurs around the joints.

RA: Symptoms and Signs

Rheumatoid arthritis is an autoimmune disease, and as such is related to such conditions as Graves' disease, a thyroid disorder, and systemic lupus erythematosus (SLE), a condition affecting the skin and other vital organs. The common feature of these disorders is an odd sensitivity of the immune system–one that causes it to attack the body's own tissues as unwelcome foreign substances.

Making the diagnosis of an autoimmune disease is no simple matter, and it's a job best left to a professional.

The symptoms of rheumatoid arthritis vary with the stage of the disorder. At first, those affected complain of fatigue and feeling sore, achy, and stiff. Because the disease involves a stiffening of joints, RA patients may eventually find themselves unable to move their limbs fully without trouble. Some lose weight or develop anemia; experience inflammation in the eye area or develop lumps beneath the skin. The latter most commonly occur around the elbow.

The course of the disease varies from one person to the next. For some time it may come and go, but at some point, the symptoms may become permanent.

46

The Allergy Angle

Living with RA understandably makes one attentive to triggers that make the symptoms worse. Richard Panush, M.D., of the University of Florida, notes that 30 percent of his RA patients claimed that certain foods contributed to their symptoms. Rather than dismiss their observations, Dr. Panush pursued their claims—this time under the kind of stringent conditions that scientists demand. He gave the patients their suspect foods, but disguised the foods in capsules so that neither the doctor nor the patient knew which foods they were being exposed to.

Dr. Panush found food was unrelated to symptoms in 10 of the 15 patients he studied; two others had borderline reactions. Notable, however, is that several of the patients clearly did react to various foods with a worsening of their RA symptoms.

Which foods are the troublemakers? Unfortunately, even the few doctors who are convinced that food can be an offender can't answer across the board. The list of alleged trigger foods varies from one person to the next.

Consider, for instance, another report of the food-RA link. In this one, Deepa Beri of the All-India Institute of Medical Sciences in New Delhi treated RA patients with a very limited starter diet of fruits, vegetables, oil, and sugar. One at a time, suspect foods such as rice, wheat, legumes, milk, and meat were added. Of the 14 participants, 10 experienced a worsening of symptoms when one or more of the test foods was given.

As you might guess, the culprits varied among these ten reacting patients. Four appeared sensitive to wheat and rice, two to rice only. Of the remaining four, each had a unique set of trigger foods. One was bothered only by legumes, another by legumes and meat, a third by dairy foods and meat, and the fourth by legumes, wheat, and milk. How's that for a perfect example of the old saying that one man's meat is another's poison!

The Fish Theory Holds Water

Fish has long earned praise from nutritionists. Its outstanding nutrient profile and low calorie count make it an ideal healing food. As if that weren't enough, preliminary research has also linked the fat in fish to improvement of RA symptoms.

The secret ingredient is the omega-3 fatty acids found in fish oils. Omega-3's have grabbed the limelight in recent years for the promise they show in preventing heart disease. And now British scientist J. M. Kremer has charted new territory by testing fish oil as a treatment for RA. Dr. Kremer asked RA patients to take capsules that contained either a fake pill or the omega-3 fatty acid known as EPA (eicosapentaenoic acid). Neither the researchers nor the patients knew who had the blank capsules and who had the fish-oil capsules, which provided 1.8 grams of EPA a day.

The results were promising. Those who were taking the fish oil had a significant lessening of the tenderness in their joints. Moreover, when they were removed from treatment, their symptoms rebounded—another sign that the effects of the fish oil were real.

Researchers, of course, want to confirm these findings. But they are already speculating that fish oil helps reduce inflammation by helping the body make substances called prostaglandins that have a favorable effect on inflamed tissue.

You'll find details on the omega-3 content of different fish, by the way, in "Fish Oil Facts," on page 138.

A Call for Open Minds

These findings are sure to be controversial among scientists. And those in the forefront of this research are prepared for the big debate. But they urge that it be based on an objective look at the facts, not on the long-held bias against the idea that food contributes to RA.

In our view, Gardner Moment, Ph.D., professor emeritus of biology at Goucher College in Towson, Maryland, said it best. Dr. Moment recently published an editorial on food-related arthritis in a medical journal in which he urges us to expect—rather than resist—new findings that challenge conventional wisdom. "It should be remembered," he wrote, "that science has been full of surprises in the past and there is no reason to imagine that the supply of surprises has been exhausted."

Surprises in nutrition and arthritis probably are on the way. As far as we're concerned, such surprises are welcome; it's helping even a minority of patients—not defending conventional wisdom—that matters most.

ASPARAGUS

All-in-One Protector Food

44 calories per cup (cooked)

If you love asparagus, you don't need an excuse to indulge your passion. It is not only a gourmet's delight but also one of our most healthful foods. It's a rare food that has so many protective nutrients with so few calories.

Few people know as much about preventing cancer as Bruce N. Ames, Ph.D., the University of California biochemist who invented a simple, inexpensive test that uses bacteria rather than animals to determine whether a chemical may cause cancer. Writing in *Science* magazine a few years ago, Dr. Ames cited three food-based nutrients that can help us defend ourselves against cancer agents. These three, of course, include two vitamins–carotene (actually provitamin A) and vitamin C–and the mineral selenium. Asparagus is chock-full of all three!

If you're still not sold on asparagus, consider its benefits to your heart. With no fat, cholesterol, or sodium to speak of, as well as modest amounts of cholesterol-lowering fiber, asparagus is ideal for heart-healthy menus. Combine it with other vegetables, beans, and legumes, says heart expert W. Virgil Brown, M.D., of the Mount Sinai School of Medicine in New York City, and you have just the kind of diet that is "consistently associated with a reduced incidence of cardiovascular disease." Not to mention how great this gourmet vegetable tastes!

At the Market: Here are a few tips for choosing asparagus at its best.

- The tips should be tightly pointed and purplish in color. If they are starting to open or are soft, the asparagus is past its prime.
- The spear of the asparagus should be smooth and firm.
- Asparagus that has a strong odor is too old.
- Sand in the tips is difficult to wash out, so look for spears that don't have sand clinging to them.
- The thickness of the asparagus does not affect its flavor.

Kitchen Tips: Refrigerate asparagus as soon as you bring it home; keep it loosely wrapped in plastic or a paper bag. To enjoy fresh asparagus year round, blanch it immediately after buying it, then wrap it tightly in aluminum foil or place it in an airtight container. It can then be frozen for up to 12 months.

To prepare asparagus, snap off, rather than cut away, the tough white section; it is usually hard to eat and lacking in flavor. Use a sharp paring knife to remove the points on the spears; sand usually lurks underneath. Next, steam the spears, starting with the thickest ones. Thinner spears will need less cooking time. Because the tips cook more rapidly than the spears, a vertical asparagus cooker that keeps the tips above the bubbling water is a good idea. The stalks should be flexible but not limp.

Accent on Enjoyment: Toss the cooked spears with:

- A bit of soy sauce, minced garlic, and ginger.
- Lemon, tarragon, and olive oil.
- Pasta of your choice.

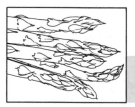

Vermicelli with Asparagus and Slivered Chicken

½ pound chicken
   cutlets, pounded to
   an even thickness
1½ teaspoons coarse
   mustard
3½ ounces vermicelli
1 pound fresh asparagus
   (about 26 spears),
   tough ends
   removed and
   spears chopped
   into 1-inch lengths
juice and pulp of
   1 lemon
2 teaspoons hazelnut
   or olive oil
pinch of freshly
   grated nutmeg
2 tablespoons freshly
   grated Parmesan
   cheese

Preheat the broiler or grill.

Rub chicken with 1 teaspoon mustard, then broil or grill until cooked through, about 4 to 5 minutes on each side.

Meanwhile, cook vermicelli in boiling water for 4 minutes, then add asparagus and boil for 4 minutes more. Drain.

When chicken is cool, tear it into slivers with your fingers.

In a small bowl, combine lemon juice and pulp, oil, ½ teaspoon mustard, and nutmeg.

In a large serving bowl, toss together chicken, vermicelli and asparagus with the dressing. Sprinkle with Parmesan and serve warm.

Makes 4 servings

BANANAS

A Powerhouse of Potassium

100 calories per medium banana

If potassium is on your mind, then the banana should be on your menu. Of all sources of this sought-after mineral, this much-loved fruit is among the most popular. In fact, a banana a day is often part of the doctor's orders.

Why? Originally, the reason was to guard against potassium depletion sometimes caused by blood pressure medications belonging to the thiazide family: Aldactazide, Apresoline, Diuril, HydroDiuril, Rauzide, and Ser-Ap-Es are among its best-known brand names.

Recently, though, a second benefit has emerged. It now appears that potassium itself plays a role in controlling blood pressure! In a classic study, researchers compared the average blood pressure of inhabitants of two Japanese villages. The average pressure differed dramatically even though sodium intakes were similar in both villages. Stumped at first, the researchers found that the villagers with the healthier pressure also had higher potassium levels.

And while we're on the subject of heart health, we should mention another benefit of the banana. Two small bananas provide about as much fiber as a slice of whole wheat bread. But unlike bread, bananas contain a significant amount of soluble fiber. As shown in pioneering studies by Ancel Keys, Ph.D., and his co-workers at the University of Minnesota, diets rich in fruits, vegetables, and legumes help lower blood cholesterol, and their soluble fiber has earned credit for doing the job.

Finally, here's another heart-healthy note: Bananas contain almost no sodium. And if vitamins, too, concern you, take heart that the banana is a modest source of vitamin C.

At the Market: When choosing bananas, look for yellow, unblemished skin—with or without brown specks. Single bananas may be bargain priced but will not last as long as those still in bunches.

Kitchen Tips: Store bananas at room temperature until ripe. Once ready to eat, refrigerate them to prevent further ripening. The skin will turn black but the flesh will remain fresh.

Accent on Enjoyment: Needless to say, a ripe banana is perfect to eat right after peeling; it can also be sliced and added to fruit and chicken salads. After putting bananas in a salad, we like to top it off with some peanuts. And here are some of our other favorites.

- For a nutritious treat, peel ripe bananas, wrap them in plastic wrap, and freeze. Eat them like Popsicles or puree them with a small amount of skim milk to make a low-fat frozen dessert.
- Slice bananas into spears or coin-shaped pieces and sauté in orange juice with a pinch of cinnamon or nutmeg.
- Bake banana pieces after tossing with lime juice and honey; let them cook just until tender.
- Mash bananas and add to batters for muffins and quick bread.

When you want your banana-containing dishes to look as great as they taste, toss in a little lemon juice first to help prevent browning.

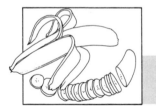

Banana Coins with Lime and Tangerines

juice and pulp of 1 lime
2 drops vanilla extract
  pinch of ground
  cinnamon
2 tangerines, seeded and
  sectioned
4 bananas, sliced into
  coins
1 tablespoon shredded,
  unsweetened
  coconut

In a small bowl, combine lime juice and pulp, vanilla, and cinnamon. (It's best to use a small whisk or fork so cinnamon doesn't clump up.)

In a large bowl, combine tangerines, bananas, and coconut. Pour lime mixture over them and toss well, until all the fruit is coated. Serve at room temperature or slightly chilled in small sundae dishes, for dessert or breakfast.

Makes 4 servings

BARLEY

One of the Great Grains

170 calories per cup (cooked)

If you're a novice with grains other than rice, you've probably wondered how "pearled" barley differs from other forms. To explain it simply, pearling is to barley as polishing is to rice. The pearling press removes the hull and the bran. Yet it leaves a tasty, low-fat food that fits into almost any healthy menu, including weight-loss diets!

Researcher Lauren Lissner and her colleagues helped usher in this happy news in 1987. Their goal was to see whether low-fat diets promoted weight loss better than diets containing moderate to high levels of fat. After two weeks on a low-fat diet, their female subjects each lost a pound; on higher-fat diets their weight either increased or stayed the same. That means foods such as barley rated best!

In addition to its low fat and sodium content, pearled barley also has respectable levels of fiber and protein. Of course, unblocked (unhulled) barley has more fiber than pearled. Its very heavy texture, however, doesn't appeal to most palates.

At the Market: Good barley is creamy ivory to taupe in color and unblemished. When choosing barley, look for grains that are stubby and fairly even in size. This allows for best results when cooking.

Kitchen Tips: Store barley in covered jars in a cool, dry place such as the refrigerator.

To make 1 cup of cooked barley, combine ¼ cup of the raw grain and 1 cup water in a small saucepan. Boil for 5 minutes, then cover the pan and let it stand for about an hour.

Accent on Enjoyment: You can use cooked barley in any of the following ways.

• Use it as a substitute for rice in pilafs or salads.
• Use it to stuff poultry and vegetables.
• Add it to soups and stews.

• Serve it alongside lamb, with which it blends particularly well.
• Mix it with rice for an interesting twist on plain rice.

   In addition to trying these basic uses, you can also look for barley that has been ground into flour. Use it instead of wheat in flatbreads or yeasted breads. Barley sprouts are the base for malt, too, and also for grain-based coffee substitutes.

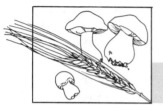

Barley with Mushrooms and Kale

3 tablespoons dried wild
   mushrooms such as
   porcini, cepes, or
   Chilean
2 cups cooked barley
2 shallots, minced
1 clove garlic, minced
2 tablespoons minced
   fresh chives
½ teaspoon dried thyme
1 tablespoon olive oil
2 tablespoons mild white
   vinegar such as
   champagne or rice
   vinegar
1 cup shredded cooked
   kale

   In a small bowl, in enough boiling water to cover, soak mushrooms until tender, about an hour. (If they float, weigh them down with a cup.)

   Meanwhile, in a large serving bowl or salad bowl, combine barley, shallots, garlic, chives, thyme, oil, vinegar, and kale.

   When mushrooms are ready, drain and mince them. Add to barley mixture and toss well. Serve at room temperature or slightly chilled with grilled or poached chicken or as an entrée accompanied by a quick sauté of seasonal vegetables.

   Note: The mushroom soaking water is quite tasty and can be added to soups or stews.

Makes 4 servings

BEANS, DRY

Cheap, but Rich in Health

Common beans: 215 calories per cup (cooked)
Lima beans: 260 calories per cup (cooked)

Forgive us, please, if you are a bean connoisseur who strongly prefers one type of dry bean over another. Nutritionally, differences between the various types are slight, so we've combined them into this single entry.

Whether red, white, pink, or brown, beans are now in the spotlight for their benefits to blood cholesterol and heart health. Although conventional wisdom holds that only a total diet—not the addition of a single food—can lower cholesterol, beans have a record that turns this notion on its head.

• James W. Anderson, M.D., and his co-workers at the University of Kentucky have documented a 19 percent reduction in blood cholesterol from adding about 100 grams of dry beans to the daily diet. That's equivalent to 1 cup of cooked dry beans.
• In their classic study that tested the effects of split peas, lima beans, and common beans (such as kidney beans) on blood cholesterol, Ancel Keys, Ph.D., and his colleagues at the University of Minnesota observed a 9 percent drop in blood cholesterol after replacing sugars, breads, and potatoes with beans.
• Dutch researcher R. Lukyen added beans (mostly brown ones) to the diets of staff members at the Netherlands Central Institute for Nutrition and Food Research. Blood cholesterol levels fell an average of 12 milligrams during the high-bean diet.

There's little doubt that the soluble fiber in beans is responsible for the striking effect on blood cholesterol. Nevertheless, beans contain generous amounts of insoluble fiber, too, making them just as useful for promoting digestive health. E. W. Hellendorn, Ph.D., also a researcher at the Netherlands Central Institute for Nutrition and Food Research, has shown that, like wheat bran, beans promote the passage of food through the digestive tract. That's a plus for those bothered by constipation and also for helping to prevent colon cancer.

Fiber Content of Beans

No matter what the type or color, beans are great sources of fiber. If you're a stickler for the details, here they are. Values are for a 1-cup portion of cooked beans, unless indicated otherwise.

Type of Bean	Fiber (g)
Pinto	20
Kidney	19
Lima	16
White	16
Butter	10
Mung, sprouted	8
Broad	5
String, raw	4

And beans have still more assets! In fact, few foods boast so much protein with so little fat, or so much potassium with so little sodium. (Unsalted beans are great for those watching their blood pressure.) They're also a good source of iron and thiamine.

Common Beans

At the Market: Dry beans should have a clear, bright, even color and uniform size. Regardless of variety, however, make sure that the beans have not shriveled.

If using canned beans, rest assured that plenty of protein, potassium, and iron is there. Unfortunately, salt will be added, too, sometimes in generous amounts. Rinse canned beans before using to wash away some of the salt. Check the label before buying if you are on a low-sodium diet.

Kitchen Tips: At home, keep dry beans in covered jars and store in a cool, dry place, such as the refrigerator.

When preparing beans, consider this advice from Alfred Olson, chemist at the U.S. Department of Agriculture's Western Regional Research Center in California. He has formulated this precooking procedure for removing many of the gas-forming factors.

- Rinse beans and sort out any foreign particles.
- Pour in boiling water to cover.
- Allow to soak for 4 hours or more (the time will vary with the type of bean).
- Drain so that beans are cooked in fresh water. (You should remove any beans that float to the top during soaking before you pour off the water.)

Now to cook them! Add water to the pot until it reaches 2 inches above the beans. If cooking over regular heat, cook until tender–about 1 to 3 hours, depending on variety. White beans tend to be toughest and need the most cooking. For the most tender result, wait until near the end of cooking to add salt, tomato juice, or acidic wines.

Is all this too time consuming? You can save time–and sometimes the need to soak–by preparing beans in a pressure cooker. Cooking times will vary with different models, so follow the manufacturer's directions for the pressure cooker you have. If you have not soaked the beans before pressure-cooking, add 5 minutes to the cooking time. (Incidentally, remember to never fill the pressure cooker more than three-quarters full of liquid.)

To test for doneness, set one or two beans on a spoon and blow on them. If the skins fly open, they are ready.

Accent on Enjoyment: Beans are delicious in so many different dishes. Because the flavor of red, pink, and white beans is uniformly mild, you can use them interchangeably in cooking. Whatever your preference, try beans in:

- Salads, croquettes, stews, soups, casseroles, sauces, and curries.
- Mexican and Cajun stews.
- Purees and dips.
- Dishes made with apples or other slightly sweet ingredients.

As your food bill will tell you, nothing stretches your budget like beans. A cup of dried beans will serve about four people when cooked–that's an awful lot from such a small investment.

Lima Beans

At the Market: The best fresh limas are available in spring and fall. If the pods feel firm and velvety, the beans inside should be good. If bean shapes are visible through the pods, try to choose evenly sized ones to help ensure even cooking. Fresh limas that look white and dryish are probably starchy and should not be fed to those who are picky about their lima beans.

Dried limas should be uniform in size and color. Sniff them; if they smell moldy, don't buy them.

Limas freeze well, so they are always available frozen. Check the label for purity.

Kitchen Tips: Keep fresh limas in their pods. Wrap in perforated plastic and refrigerate; they'll last for about a week. Fresh limas should always be cooked. Shell them first by snapping their pods open and nudging out the beans with your thumb. Then simmer in water or stock, loosely covered, un-

---

Test Your Bean

Okay, bean lovers, test your knowledge.
Which bean is lowest in calories?
Which bean is richest in calories?
Which beans have more than a gram of fat per ½ cup?

The answers are: lentils; soybeans; soybeans and chick-peas. If you answered them correctly, you're a nutrition wizard. If not, study this table so you'll do better next time. Values are for approximately ½ cup of cooked beans.

Type of Bean	Calories	Fat (g)
Black beans	132	less than 1
Chick-peas	171	2
Cowpeas	109	less than 1
Fava beans	110	less than 1
Kidney beans	127	less than 1
Lentils	106	less than 1
Lima beans	110	less than 1
Pinto beans	131	less than 1
Soybeans	173	9
White beans	143	less than 1

til tender–about 20 minutes. A pound of fresh limas in the pod makes two servings.

Frozen limas will keep for up to 12 months. To cook, simply simmer in water or stock, loosely covered, until tender, about 10 minutes.

Store dried limas in the refrigerator in a tightly covered glass jar. To cook, soak 1 cup of beans overnight in enough water to cover. Then simmer the soaked beans in 4 cups of water or stock, loosely covered, until tender–about 50 to 60 minutes.

Don't pressure-cook limas, because doing so ruins their texture.

Accent on Enjoyment: If you want to convert a lima bean hater, try one of these delicious ideas.

- Add to casseroles, soups, or stews.
- Substitute limas for favas.
- Combine limas with ingredients such as tomatoes, sweet corn, onions, mushrooms, chives, scallions, salsa picante, and most cheeses.
- Create a main dish salad with cooked limas and smoked turkey.

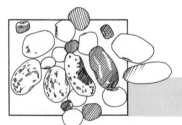

Black Beans with Sage and Garlic

2 teaspoons olive oil
2 cloves garlic, minced
1 green pepper, minced
1 bay leaf
2 cups cooked black beans
1 teaspoon dried sage
splash of hot pepper sauce, or to taste

In a large nonstick skillet, heat oil over medium heat. Then add garlic, peppers, and bay leaf and sauté until peppers have just begun to soften, about 4 minutes. (If garlic begins to brown and burn, reduce heat.)

Add beans, sage, and hot pepper sauce and sauté until heated through, about 3 minutes. Remove bay leaf and serve hot as an appetizer or side dish with garlic bread or warm, soft corn tortillas.

Makes 4 servings

Burritos with Pumpkin Seeds and Green Chilies

2 teaspoons olive oil
2 cloves garlic, minced
⅓ cup chopped onion
2 mild green chili
     peppers, minced
     (about ¼ cup)
1 jalapeño pepper,
     seeded and minced
¼ cup green pumpkin
     seeds (pepitas),
     chopped
½ teaspoon ground
     cumin
½ teaspoon ground
     coriander
1 teaspoon dried
     oregano
  splash of hot pepper
     sauce, or to taste
2 cups cooked pinto
     beans
4 large flour tortillas
½ cup grated Monterey
     Jack cheese
⅓ cup tomato juice

In a large nonstick skillet, heat the oil over medium-high heat. Add garlic, onions, chili and jalapeño peppers, pumpkin seeds, cumin, coriander, oregano, and hot pepper sauce. Sauté until vegetables have wilted and the mixture is fragrant, about 5 minutes.

In a large bowl, mix together chili mixture and beans, using a large rubber spatula to combine well.

Lay tortillas on a counter and divide bean mixture equally among them by placing it in log shapes on the edge of each tortilla. Sprinkle an equal amount of cheese on each bean log, then roll tortillas and use the back of a spoon to press in the filling on the sides.

Carefully set burritos in same nonstick skillet used to cook the filling (a long spatula is helpful here) and pour tomato juice over them. Simmer until burritos are soft and juice has evaporated, about 3 minutes. Occasionally use a spatula to square off the sides of the burritos to help keep the filling in.

Place burritos on a serving platter and serve hot, with additional hot pepper sauce on the side.

Makes 4 servings

BEANS, GREEN

Snap Up Some Iron

44 calories per cup (cooked)

The subject of green beans brings us to the Department of Pet Peeves. We all have our sore points, and among ours is the failure of nutritionists to even mention vegetables such as green beans as a source of a mineral that so many of us could use more of: iron.

Sure, some of the iron in flesh foods such as meats is the most absorbable heme form, and nonmeat sources don't have any heme iron. But nonheme iron is hardly worthless; it supplies a healthy percentage of the iron that we get. And this is our complaint: Nutritionists are so taken with the heme iron in meats that they forget to give fair credit to vegetable sources.

Green beans are a case in point; a small, ½-cup serving of fresh cooked green beans gives you a milligram of iron in only 20 calories. A food that packs this amount of iron into so few calories deserves some credit.

Of course, green beans have received their due on other counts; they are credited for their low fat and sodium content and as a source of potassium and fiber.

At the Market: Good green beans are a lively green and free of brown spots or discoloration. Small ones tend to be the most flavorful and tender, so as a general rule, leave behind those that are fatter than a pencil. Beans that bend rather than snap are not fresh.

Kitchen Tips: To keep beans at their best, rinse but don't dry them, then wrap them in perforated plastic bags and refrigerate. They will last up to two weeks with good care. If you want to keep them longer, blanch them for 3 minutes in boiling water, pat dry, wrap, and freeze—you may be able to keep them as long as a year. Frozen or fresh, 1 pound of green beans yields 4 cups of trimmed and chopped (or sliced) green beans.

Green beans take little time to cook; a pound will take about 4 minutes when simmered in water. They also can be steamed, sautéed, stir-fried, or microwaved. In fact, beans microwave beautifully, but to ensure even cooking, chop them before cooking.

Accent on Enjoyment: The flavor of green beans gets along famously with that of mushrooms, almonds, sweet peppers, or corn. To do something different:

• Chop raw green beans and add to tuna or pasta salads.
• Add chopped green beans to soups or stews.
• Flavor green beans with dill, tarragon, peanuts, garlic, or thyme. They will harmonize well with cheeses, fish, and poultry.
• Use broad beans (also called Italian beans) for a change of pace from common green beans. Use them just as you do common green beans, but be prepared for a slightly shorter cooking time.

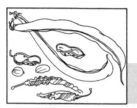

Chili Beans with Peanuts

1 pound green beans
2 tablespoons peanut oil
2 cloves garlic, slightly
    crushed
2 (2-inch) dried hot chili
    peppers
2 tablespoons raw
    blanched peanuts
1 teaspoon chili oil

Place beans in a strainer and pour boiling water over them for 5 seconds. Drain well, pat very dry, and set aside.

Heat a wok or large skillet over high heat until very hot, about 30 seconds. Pour in oil and heat for 20 seconds.

Add garlic and chili peppers and stir-fry for 10 seconds (do not let garlic burn). Add beans and peanuts and stir-fry for 30 seconds. Remove from heat. Toss with chili oil and serve immediately.

Makes 4 servings

Green Bean Soup with Chick-peas

1 tablespoon vegetable
 oil
½ cup minced celery
½ cup minced onion
½ cup minced carrot
1 clove garlic, minced
 bouquet garni (3
 sprigs parsley, 3
 sprigs chervil or 1
 teaspoon dried
 chervil, 3 sprigs
 thyme or ½ tea-
 spoon dried thyme,
 and 2 bay leaves,
 gathered together
 in a piece of
 cheesecloth and
 tied with string)
5 cups vegetable stock
2 cups cut green beans
 (1-inch pieces)
1½ cups cooked
 chick-peas
2 medium tomatoes,
 peeled, seeded, and
 chopped
 minced fresh parsley
 for garnish

Heat oil in a 4-quart saucepan over medium-low heat. Add celery, onion, carrot, and garlic and cook until vegetables are soft, about 5 minutes.

Add bouquet garni, stock, green beans, chick-peas and tomatoes. Bring to a boil. Reduce heat, cover and simmer until green beans are tender, about 15 to 20 minutes. Remove bouquet garni and serve, garnished with parsley.

Makes 4 to 6 servings

BEEF, LEAN

Staying in Tune with the Times

207 to 252 calories per 4 ounces (cooked)

Granted, beef has had its share of bad press. Not that we doubt that the hazards of high-fat beef and other red meats are real. But we also want to acknowledge that lean beef has its good points. We're particularly impressed with the way that small amounts of lean beef can bring out the best in the foods around it.

How does beef bring out the benefits of other foods? For some facts, let's turn to the nutritionist's bible, the handbook on Recommended Dietary Allowances (RDA). Updated every four to six years, this standard guide for evaluating nutritional adequacy is published by the National Research Council, a cousin of the government's National Academy of Sciences.

According to authors of the RDA handbook, small amounts of beef can boost the nutritional value of a diet in the following ways.

- It provides the so-called meat factor that helps us absorb more of the harder-to-assimilate nonheme iron in food and iron supplements. The RDA handbook cites this factor as one of the three most important influences on iron absorption.
- It supplies vitamin B_{12}. Just a little of this nutrient can help prevent the serious nerve damage that occasionally afflicts those who eat no meat for many years (only meat is proven to contain this important vitamin). But as the RDA committee notes, "it [is] unnecessary to consume vitamin B_{12} every day" because the vitamin is continually "recycled" by the body. So even small amounts of meat can go a long way toward keeping enough B_{12} on hand.
- It enhances the nutritional value of grain foods by making more of their protein useable–a help when the protein content of a diet is marginal. Less total protein is required, says the committee, when some high-quality protein such as that found in meat and dairy foods is included in the diet.
- It provides zinc in an easily absorbed form. Even though meat-free diets may contain large amounts of zinc, deficiencies sometimes occur because the zinc in nonmeat foods is harder to absorb. As the scientists say, diets that

64

include animal protein "usually contain adequate amounts of important trace nutrients," such as zinc, iron, and some vitamins.

Of course, those who don't eat meat are hardly doomed to develop nutrient deficiencies. In fact, we're long-time supporters of vegetarian diets. At the same time, however, we simply want to point out that the health problems of meat-eaters are more than anything the result of eating too much of the wrong kind of meat.

Portion Predicament

How can meat lovers have their beef and follow health recommendations, too? By eating sensible amounts of lean cuts. And how much beef is "sensible"? At a minimum, as little as a few bite-size pieces in a mixed dish such as a stir-fry will have nutritional benefits. For a maximum, we think of a 4-ounce serving as a reasonable limit.

If, like most of us, you wonder what 4 ounces looks like, here are some guidelines for common lean cuts of beef.

- Lean roast beef: three pieces, 4 inches by 2 inches by ¼ inch.
- Ground round: one 3-inch patty, about ¾ inch thick.
- Round steak: one steak, 4 inches by 3 inches by ½ inch.
- Flank steak: one piece, 4 inches by 2 inches by ¾ inch.

You also can think of 4 ounces of meat as slightly larger than the palm of your hand. Although an imprecise measure, this is an easy guideline.

In terms of choosing the leanest cuts, a good bet is simply to give your choices the "eyeball test." A piece of meat that looks fatty—with a lot of obvious fat in and around it—probably is. In addition, if the meat is graded, that will give you clues about its fat content. (See "Making the Grade," for more details.)

Of course, meat grades are but one influence on flavor and tenderness. Learning to select and prepare these meats for best taste is important, too. As guidelines for lean roasts differ from those for lean steaks, for instance, we've separated lean beef into three classes. You'll find recommendations for choosing, storing, and preparing each of them in the three sections that follow.

Making the Grade

Meat grading is an optional service provided by the U.S. Department of Agriculture. But because grading increases the cost of meat, some producers do without it. When used, however, grades do tell you this about flavor and fat content.

Prime. Meat that qualifies for this top grade comes from a young, mature animal, and as a result, it is flavorful, juicy and tender. Prime beef usually has a high degree of "marbling," that is, small flecks of fat within the muscle of the meat. As a result, its fat content tends to be high. Although supermarkets offer some prime beef, restaurants buy most of it.

Choice. The most common grade of beef in the supermarket, choice beef has less marbling (and therefore less fat) than prime. Nonetheless, it is still tender and juicy. If you are considering both taste and nutrition, choice grade beef is usually your best bet.

Good. Less tender than prime or choice, good (or "select") grade beef has the advantage of a lower fat content. By preparing it with methods recommended for lean meats, it can be as tasty and economical as it is nutritious.

Standard. Standard beef hails from a young, mature animal but contains little fat. Somewhat lacking in flavor and juiciness, standard beef is rarely sold in supermarkets.

Commercial. Commercial grade beef is neither tender nor lean. It is sold to the food industry for commercial use.

Lean Beef Roasts

At the Market: Beef roasts from the arm (foreshank), round, and rump are usually the leanest; rib, chuck, and brisket are fattier. Look for fine-textured, firm meats with a rich red color.

Kitchen Tips: Wrap fresh beef in waxed paper and store in the coldest part of the refrigerator for one to three days. For longer storage, freeze the meat after wrapping in aluminum foil or freezer paper. The meat will keep for as long as a year if properly frozen; lean meats keep longer than fatty ones. A strong odor, slimy texture, or gray-green color are signs of spoiled beef.

Beef round is especially flavorful, but lean round roasts tend to be tougher than fattier meats. As a result, they are best prepared with moist heat; we like to braise, simmer, or stew them, or use them for ground meat or hash. Cooking times for these roasts will depend on two things: size and your preferences for doneness.

Accent on Enjoyment: For excellent results, cook lean roasts in an oven cooking bag. This helps retain moisture and make the meat more tender. Lean roasts also are nice for a New England boiled dinner, served with potatoes, cabbage, and onions. Or poke slits in meat with a paring knife and fill each slit with a sliver of garlic. Then braise or simmer with onion and tomato.

Flank Steak

At the Market: Like lean roasts, flank steak should have a fine, firm texture and good, rich color. Cuts that are lighter in color often come from a younger animal and will yield more tender meat. A dark red color usually indicates that the meat came from an older animal. Store and judge freshness as you would beef roasts, discussed at left.

Kitchen Tips: To tenderize the meat before grilling, marinate well in your choice of seasonings. Soy sauce, garlic, ginger, and tomato are our favorites. Although moist heat usually is recommended for lean cuts of meat, flank steak should be broiled or grilled quickly, about 7 minutes on each side for rare meat. (Overcooking will make this meat tough.) Finally, slice flank steak thinly and against the grain for best results.

Ground Round

At the Market: Look for ground round as the lean alternative to hamburger. Some stores do not prepackage ground round but will grind any piece of lean meat for you on request. Of course, you can do this at preparation time with a meat grinder or food processor. This allows you to store whole meat longer than is possible with meat that is purchased ground.

Kitchen Tips: Wrap ground meat in waxed paper and keep it in the coldest part of the refrigerator. Because its fibers have been broken down by grinding, it doesn't last as long as chunks or large pieces of meat. Use it quickly.

Accent on Enjoyment: For a calorie-conscious alternative to the hamburger, form ground round into patties and fry in a nonstick pan, then add a bun and fixings. Ground round can also be microwaved or grilled; sautéed and added to soups, stews or chilies; or mixed with grains such as rice to make meatballs and meat loaf.

Thick, ripe tomato slices and sweet onions are classic accompaniments to ground round.

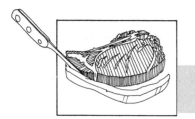

Sirloin Salad with Chunky Vinaigrette

1 pound sirloin, about ½ inch thick
1½ teaspoons Dijon mustard
3 cloves garlic, minced
freshly ground black pepper
1 yellow sweet pepper, chopped
1 red sweet pepper, chopped
2 medium ribs celery, chopped
3 tablespoons minced fresh parsley
1 tablespoon orange juice
1 tablespoon lemon juice
1 teaspoon balsamic vinegar
2 teaspoons peanut oil
splash of hot pepper sauce, or to taste

Rub sirloin all over with mustard, one-third of the garlic, and pepper. Then allow to marinate, at room temperature, if possible, for 30 minutes.

In a medium bowl, combine the remaining garlic, peppers, celery, parsley, juices, vinegar, oil, and hot pepper sauce.

Preheat the broiler or grill.

Broil or grill steak until cooked the way you like it, about 3 to 5 minutes on each side for medium-rare.

Place steak on a serving platter and let stand for about 5 minutes, then cut it into thin slices. Toss with dressing and serve warm.

Makes 4 servings

Meatballs with Blue Cheese Sauce

1 pound lean ground
   beef
1 egg, beaten
1 clove garlic, minced
¼ cup minced leeks
¼ cup minced fresh
   parsley
2 tablespoons bread
   crumbs
¼ cup milk
¼ cup crumbled blue
   cheese

In a large bowl, combine beef, egg, garlic, leeks, parsley, and bread crumbs. Use your hands to combine the mixture so that the ingredients are evenly mixed.

Wet your hands and form the mixture into about 40 walnut-size meatballs.

Heat a large nonstick skillet over medium-high heat and add as many meatballs as will fit without crowding. (If the pan is large enough, 20 may fit.) Sauté and stir the meatballs until cooked through and lightly browned, about 10 minutes.

Meanwhile, in a large bowl, combine milk and cheese.

When the first batch of meatballs is ready, remove them from the skillet and drain away any extra fat on paper towels. Add them to the bowl containing cheese mixture. The heat from the meatballs will melt the cheese and make a tasty sauce.

Continue cooking meatballs until all are cooked and added to sauce. Serve hot with rice or herbed pasta.

Makes 4 servings

BERRIES

Berry, Berry Good for You!

Blackberries: 74 calories per cup
Blueberries: 81 calories per cup
Raspberries: 60 calories per cup
Strawberries: 45 calories per cup

Watching your weight? If so, berries couldn't be better for you! Ideal as low-calorie sweets, they pack a bonus, too, by supplying fiber that apparently helps you absorb fewer of the calories that you do eat.

British researchers D. A. T. Southgate and J. V. G. A. Durnin report that the fiber in fruits, vegetables, and whole grain bread reduces absorption of the calories from food—enough to have a positive effect on weight without a negative effect on nutritional health.

When it's insoluble fiber that you want most, raspberries and blackberries are ideal. They taste nothing like bran or whole grain cereals, yet their insoluble fiber content is right up there with the best whole grain sources.

In addition, berries are just what experts such as Herbert Langford, M.D., suspect we need for better blood pressure. A professor at the University of Mississippi, Dr. Langford has done research that hints that our blood pressure woes may be due not simply to too much sodium, but also to a dietary pattern in which potassium (sodium's co-worker) is consumed in amounts too small to maintain a healthy balance between these two minerals. Because berries provide a healthy amount of potassium with almost no sodium, they can help restore a better balance between these two nutrients and help our blood pressure. Add their low fat content and you realize that they are truly a food to eat to your heart's content!

Blueberries and Blackberries

At the Market: Shop for berries that earn their name. Blackberries should have a jet black color; cultivated blueberries should be a powdery blue. All berries should be firm; soft, wet ones will not keep for long.

Kitchen Tips: Refrigerate berries as soon as possible, leaving them unwashed and uncovered. We prefer to transfer berries to a shallow plastic container to prevent them from crushing each other. (Separate crushed berries from the rest and use at once.) Even at their best and with ideal handling, berries may only last two to three days in the refrigerator.

Accent on Enjoyment: Firm berries can be enjoyed raw after removing any tiny stems. Some other options:

- Rather than discard overripe berries, cook them down with a bit of juice and use as a topping.
- Use berries in making pies, jams, preserves, puddings, syrups, crepes, ice cream, or yogurt.
- Add blueberries to muffin and pancake batters.
- Vary blueberry dishes with flavors of orange, cinnamon, and vanilla.

Raspberries

At the Market: Red raspberries dominate the marketplace because they're easiest to grow and ship. But from time to time, you'll find black raspberries available–and occasionally even yellow or white ones. Regardless of color, insist on berries that are plump and free of mold and feel dry and cool to a gentle touch. Attached stems should be a lively green with no discoloration.

Kitchen Tips: Beauty may only be skin deep, but make an exception for raspberries. For these delectable berries, beauty is the best sign of top quality. Buy for beauty, but recognize, of course, that every container is bound to contain a few crushed berries. Crushed berries are fine to eat as long as you do so right away; they won't keep long.

Store whole berries unwashed and uncovered in shallow containers in the refrigerator. They'll last for a few days if you can keep your hands off them that long. Beware of using tin, aluminum, or iron containers for red raspberries; if you do, you may find that their luscious red color has turned to blue.

Because raspberries are so delicate, always use the utmost care when washing them. Remove pieces of leaf and stem by hand.

Need to convert a pint of raspberries into weight or cups? A pint weighs in at about ½ pound, or about 3½ cups.

Accent on Enjoyment: Do you really need ideas for enjoying raspberries? We doubt it, but here are some ideas just in case.

- Use whole fresh raspberries in crepes, desserts, or omelettes, or to top frozen yogurt, cakes, or puddings.
- Puree raspberries, then taste for sweetness. Add a splash of honey if necessary, then fold in a bit of plain yogurt. Use as a dessert sauce.

Homemade Gourmet Raspberry Vinegar

Even a certified kitchen klutz can make raspberry vinegar fit for a gourmet. Simply toss about 1 cup of raspberries into a glass jar. Next, heat–don't boil–about 1½ cups of mild white vinegar. Pour over the berries, cover, and leave at room temperature overnight. In the morning, drain and refrigerate.

You'll love the sweet-and-sour sparkle that this adds to your salad dressings, marinades, and sauces. You can also use it to deglaze roasting pans.

- Add a splash of raspberry puree to sparkling mineral water or orange juice. Serve chilled, garnished with a twist of lime.
- Perk up green salads or chicken salad by tossing in a handful of raspberries. Season with a raspberry vinaigrette for a truly elegant dish.

Strawberries

At the Market: A perfectly ripe strawberry is bold red, shiny, firm, and has a little green cap attached. The berries should be dry to the touch and free of any traces of mold. If you have the luxury of choosing between varieties of strawberries, keep in mind that Midland, Fairfax, Earliglow, or Ozark Beauty rank best for taste. Suwanee, Redchief, and Redglow freeze best, however.

Because Mother Nature prevents many of us from enjoying fresh strawberries year-round, frozen berries are the only ones available during some months. Although strawberry connoisseurs may disagree, we find that frozen berries are fine for purees, sauces, and frozen desserts. Purchase them unsweetened, however, so you can add only as much sweetening as you prefer.

Kitchen Tips: Strawberries don't need elaborate storage at home. Leave them unwashed before storing; just place in an open paper bag and refrigerate them. They'll last a few days. Should you find yourself with underripe berries, set them on top of your refrigerator and cover loosely with plastic wrap. Let them sit there overnight, and they'll get sweeter. To prepare, wash first, then hull. That way you won't wash flavorful juices away.

Accent on Enjoyment: A good strawberry needs no embellishing. But strawberries mingle so well with other flavors that even the most ardent purist won't be able to pass up some of these ideas.

- Spread cinnamon toast with cream cheese and top with sliced strawberries.
- Toss small whole berries with chunks of avocado, orange sections, and walnuts. Dress with a clear vinaigrette and serve chilled.
- Puree strawberries, then add a bit of orange juice concentrate for sweetness if needed. Chill and use as a dessert sauce, drizzled over vanilla yogurt, lemon cake, or crepes.

There are many delicious ways to enjoy strawberries for dessert without lots of fat and refined sugar. Here are just a few ideas. Toss any of the following with 2 cups of berries.

- 1 tablespoon raspberry or blueberry vinegar.
- ¼ cup low-fat vanilla yogurt.
- 2 tablespoons unsweetened toasted coconut.
- ½ teaspoon minced gingerroot and ¼ teaspoon ground cinnamon.
- 1 tablespoon orange juice and ¼ teaspoon orange peel.

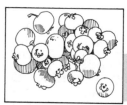

Blueberry Cocktail with Passion Fruit Cream

2 cups fresh or frozen
    blueberries
4 ripe passion fruits
¼ teaspoon orange peel
2 tablespoons plain
    low-fat yogurt

Rinse blueberries and if using fresh berries, remove any stems. Then set them in a colander to drain and dry.

Slice off the tops of passion fruits and use a teaspoon to scoop the pulp into a small bowl. Then press the pulp through a strainer to remove the seeds, catching the pulp in the same bowl. Fold in orange peel and yogurt.

To serve, place the blueberries in wine goblets or martini glasses and drizzle the passion fruit cream over them.

Note: If you can't find passion fruits, substitute 3 peeled kiwifruits pureed in a food processor or blender.

Makes 4 servings

Fresh Strawberries with Balsamic Vinegar

2 cups fresh strawberries
1 tablespoon balsamic
   vinegar

Rinse berries, then hull or use a sharp paring knife to remove the caps. Toss with vinegar and serve at room temperature or slightly chilled in wineglasses or tiny dessert bowls.

Makes 4 servings

Raspberry Tart

Crust
 2 tablespoons butter
 2 tablespoons maple
   syrup
 ¼ cup very ripe mashed
   banana
 1 egg, beaten
 ¼ teaspoon almond
   extract
 ½ cup plus 1 tablespoon
   flour
 ½ cup plus 1 tablespoon
   rolled oats
 ½ teaspoon baking
   powder
Filling
 1 cup plain low-fat
   yogurt
 1 tablespoon frozen
   orange juice
   concentrate
 1 pint fresh raspberries

Preheat the oven to 375° F.

To make the crust: In a large bowl, cream butter and maple syrup together. Add banana, egg, and almond extract and combine well. In a medium bowl, combine flour, oats, and baking powder. Add dry ingredients to wet ingredients and combine well.

Spray a 9-inch tart pan that has a removable bottom with vegetable cooking spray and press crust in evenly with slightly wet hands. Bake until crust is just beginning to brown and is dry to the touch, about 20 minutes. Let cool on a wire rack.

To make the filling: In a medium bowl, fold together yogurt and orange juice concentrate. Spread the mixture evenly in cooled tart crust, then arrange raspberries on top. Serve at room temperature or slightly chilled.

Makes 4 servings

BRAN, WHEAT

First in Fiber

60 calories per ¼ cup

If you're looking for a nutrient-rich food that alleviates digestive woes, wheat bran probably is what you want.

First, let's start with the basics. A quarter cup of bran is loaded with fiber, iron, and potassium; is low in sodium; and is a fine source of B vitamins. It even has a nice amount of protein.

Admittedly, you can find tastier sources of these nutrients. But bran is in the spotlight for some properties that no other food has yet to match. We're talking, of course, about its amazing ability to treat digestive disorders.

One of the most impressive successes has been in the treatment of diverticular disease, a digestive disorder that commonly occurs as we age. In a pioneering study, British scientist N. S. Painter and his co-workers prescribed 2 teaspoons of bran three times a day to patients suffering from diverticular disease. It's hard to imagine a simpler treatment than this one, yet 90 percent of the patients experienced "marked relief" of their symptoms! Rarely does treatment of any chronic disease deliver a success rate so high! Bran also has a remarkable success rate for alleviating constipation and works wonders for some patients with irritable bowel syndrome.

It's true that the fiber found in other foods, such as certain fruits and vegetables, also can help improve these disorders. But there are indications that unprocessed bran works the best. A study by S. N. Heller, Ph.D., and co-workers at Cornell University found that coarse bran better absorbs water in the digestive tract, a process that is believed to account for its beneficial effects.

At the Market: True, it resembles sawdust, but if you look closely enough you'll notice that the little flakes come in small, medium, and large sizes. All three are interchangeable in recipes, so take your choice. Wheat bran is usually sold in plastic bags or in bulk; smell it for freshness before you buy. It should smell nutty with no mustiness.

Kitchen Tips: Store wheat bran tightly covered in the refrigerator and it will last for up to a year. Note that 1 cup of small-flake wheat bran will weigh more than 1 cup of large-flake wheat bran. This may prove important in baking, and adjustments to the recipe may be needed for best results. Also, when replacing some of the flour with bran in baking, add a bit more liquid. Bran absorbs more than flour.

Accent on Enjoyment: Although rarely eaten by itself, wheat bran adds desirable nuttiness to many foods. For example:

- Add a handful of wheat bran to the batter for corn bread, fruited quick breads, pancakes, waffles, and muffins.
- Replace some of the meat in meatballs, meat loaves, or stuffings for vegetables with wheat bran.
- Add wheat bran to oats and oat bran before cooking.

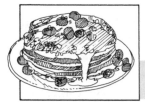

Blueberry-Bran Pancakes

½ cup wheat bran
¾ cup whole wheat
    pastry flour
1 teaspoon baking
    powder
½ teaspoon baking soda
½ cup fresh or unthawed
    frozen blueberries
2 tablespoons frozen
    orange juice
    concentrate
¾ cup buttermilk
1 egg, beaten
2 teaspoons canola oil

In a medium bowl, combine bran, flour, baking powder, and baking soda. Add berries and stir to combine.

In another medium bowl, whisk together orange juice concentrate, buttermilk, and egg. Add wet ingredients to dry ingredients and use a large spatula to combine. (Don't overmix; about 10 strokes should be sufficient.)

Meanwhile, heat a well-seasoned cast-iron skillet over medium heat. (If you don't have a cast-iron skillet, use a nonstick one.) When the skillet is hot, rub a small amount of oil on the bottom. Then add scoops of batter (about 2 tablespoons per scoop).

Cook pancakes until they are bubbly on top, then turn them. (The cooking time will be about 3 minutes on each side, but it will vary, depending on the type of skillet used.) As each batch of finished pancakes is done, place it in a warm oven while you prepare the rest. Remember to rub the skillet with oil between batches.

These pancakes are delicious topped with blueberry yogurt.

Makes 4 servings

BREAD

On the Rise

Rye bread: 61 calories per slice
Whole wheat bread: 67 calories per slice

Bread is back, and this time it's here to stay. Its days as a much-maligned "fattening food" are over, enough so that most diets include rather than eliminate it. In fact, high-fiber bread has even been used as the basis for a weight-loss program. (See the entry on overweight, beginning on page 322, for details.)

Now that it's lived down its bad reputation among dieters, bread is gaining attention for other attributes, too. We're not talking about its long-granted virtues–B vitamins, iron, and the like. Rather, we want to focus on more contemporary issues related to bread consumption.

Happier hearts. Noting that heart health is best where diets are rich in complex carbohydrates, Virgil Brown, M.D., of the Mount Sinai School of Medicine in New York City, and dietitian Wahida Karmally point to a report that blood cholesterol fell 12 to 20 percent on a diet in which bread supplied half the calories. We don't expect you to eat that much bread, of course–but don't avoid it either.

Easier digestion. Just substituting whole wheat bread for white can make a difference. In a study conducted by Scottish researcher Martin Eastwood and his colleagues, couples who normally ate white bread switched to whole wheat bread. As a result of this single change, they reported better digestive health.

Better protection from cancer. Fiber-rich breads are recommended by virtually every cancer-prevention expert around. They suspect that the insoluble fiber helps reduce our exposure to cancer-causing chemicals–a theory put forward in the 1970s by famed British researcher Denis Burkitt, M.D. While visiting Africa, Dr. Burkitt noticed the rarity of colon cancer and the commonness of high fiber intakes. He put two and two together for what has now become conventional wisdom in preventive health circles.

With benefits like these, it's no surprise that a survey by Dutch researcher Maarten Nube and co-workers linked consumption of brown bread (along with other factors, of course) to longer life span among men (but not women). Studies such as this one don't absolutely prove a link between the staff of life and long life, but they certainly are points in favor of eating more whole grain bread.

Rye Bread

At the Market: Try to choose a rye bread that lives up to its name by looking for one that lists rye flour first. Coloring is sometimes added to breads containing mostly white flour to give the appearance of rye.

Of course, making your own rye bread lets you control the amount of rye flour that's used. Before you buy, give rye flour the smell test. Though rye flour is a bit sour by its nature, it should smell fresh and not musty. For quick breads made with rye, consider flaked rye. It resembles rolled oats but is grayer. Again, a good batch smells fresh and grainy, not musty. Ditto for rye berries–they are long, deep brown, and thin, and you boil or sprout them like other grains. Sprouted rye bread, anyone?

Kitchen Tips: Rye bread will keep at room temperature for a few days. You can refrigerate it for slightly longer storage–about ten days–but you may find that if you do, it only tastes good toasted. Unlike some breads, rye freezes well–for as long as a year.

If you make your own rye bread, be sure to keep rye flour, flaked rye, and rye berries in tightly covered jars. Store these raw ingredients in the refrigerator and they will last for about six months.

Should you tire of rye bread, you can cook flaked rye much like old-fashioned rolled oats and enjoy as a hot cereal. To cook rye berries, combine 1 cup of berries with about 4 cups of water and simmer, loosely covered, until tender, about an hour. You'll then have about 2¾ cups to use as you like. (We like to use them in poultry stuffing.)

Accent on Enjoyment: Rye is a favorite grain in Scandinavian countries, where no one who bakes would be without it. Once you begin to explore rye's tastes and textures, you'll agree.

Start the creative process with some of these ideas.

- Combine rye flour half-and-half with wheat flour in yeast bread recipes. It will contribute flavor, moistness, and a crisp crust.
- If your taste buds demand that you sweeten rye batter, try molasses. It blends perfectly.
- Spice rye-containing dishes with dill, caraway, fennel, anise, mustard, horseradish, onion, and garlic; all harmonize well with its distinctive taste.

• If your homemade rye bread is too heavy for your taste, add a teaspoon of baking powder to the dry ingredients for each loaf.

Whole Wheat Bread

At the Market: Buyer beware: "Wheat" bread often contains little whole wheat flour. If you want the real thing, be sure the package is labeled "whole wheat." If a bread that contains part white flour and part whole wheat will do, check the ingredient panel to see if whole wheat flour is listed first. That way, you can be assured of a substantial whole grain content. Then let your senses take over; look for a toasty warm color, springy crust, moist, tight crumbs, and fresh aroma.

Do-it-yourselfers are encouraged to buy whole wheat flour and make their own breads. If you're new to bread baking, keep in mind that your best bet is whole wheat *bread* flour. Another type of flour—whole wheat pastry flour—is also sold. Because it has less gluten than the bread flour, it isn't nearly as well suited for this purpose. Nutritionally, stone-ground whole wheat flour is a fine choice, too, but its texture affects the rising of the dough, and not everyone is pleased with the results.

Kitchen Tips: Keep whole wheat bread in its original wrapper, or wrap it yourself in foil or plastic wrap. Store at room temperature; it will keep for about a week. For longer storage—up to three months—freeze it. Don't opt for refrigeration, though, or the bread will dry out. Whole wheat flour is another story, however; you should keep it tightly covered in the refrigerator. It will keep for about three months.

Accent on Enjoyment: Fresh or toasted whole wheat bread makes a great sandwich, but why stop there? Consider these suggestions.

• Create your own croutons. Cut whole wheat bread into cubes and toss lightly in olive oil. Then sauté until brown and toasty.
• Use whole wheat bread instead of white for poultry stuffing.
• Make fresh whole wheat bread crumbs. Tear a couple of pieces of whole wheat bread into four pieces each. Then place them into a food processor or blender and process until you have crumbs. Use as is, store in a jar and refrigerate, or toast in a dry skillet.

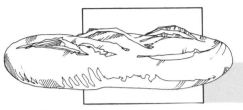

Easy Four-Grain Bread

1 package active dry
    yeast
1 cup buttermilk,
    warmed to 110°F
2 tablespoons honey
2 tablespoons safflower
    oil
½ cup whole wheat
    bread flour
2 cups unbleached white
    flour
¼ cup rye flour
½ cup masa harina
¼ cup rolled oats
½ teaspoon salt

Pour yeast into a small bowl and stir in buttermilk, honey, and oil. Cover with plastic wrap and let stand until it swells and bubbles, about 10 minutes.

Meanwhile, in a large bowl, combine flours, masa harina, oats, and salt. When yeast mixture is ready, pour it into flour mixture and use a large rubber spatula to combine. When it gets too sticky, begin to use your hands to combine and gradually work the dough into a ball. Knead for 10 minutes.

Set dough in an oiled bowl and turn so its surface is lightly covered with oil. Cover the bowl with plastic wrap and allow dough to rise until doubled in size, about 30 to 45 minutes.

Oil an 8½ × 4½-inch loaf pan.

Punch dough down with your fist, then form it into a loaf and set it in the loaf pan. Let dough rise again for about 30 minutes.

Preheat the oven to 350° F.

Spray the top of dough with water, then bake for about 35 minutes. Remove bread from the pan and set it directly on the oven rack. Spray again with water and continue to bake until done, about another 5 minutes.

Makes 1 loaf

Garlicky Quick Bread

1 cup whole wheat
    bread flour
1 cup unbleached white
    flour
1 tablespoon baking
    powder
½ teaspoon salt
3 cloves garlic, minced
⅓ cup grated cheddar
    cheese
2 tablespoons sweet
    butter, melted
1 egg, beaten
¾ cup buttermilk

Preheat the oven to 375° F.

Sift together flours, baking powder, and salt into a large bowl. Add garlic and cheese and combine well.

In a medium bowl, whisk together butter, egg, and buttermilk.

Add wet ingredients to dry ingredients and mix, using a large rubber spatula. When dough becomes too stiff, use your hands and continue to mix, forming dough into a ball.

Oil an 8½-inch round cake pan.

Press dough into the cake pan and use a sharp knife to make eight wedge-shaped cuts about ¼-inch deep.

Bake until light brown, about 35 to 40 minutes. Let cool on a wire rack, then serve in wedges.

Variation: One delicious way to serve this bread is to slice each wedge horizontally, then spread the crumbly side with a bit of sweet butter and sprinkle with freshly grated Parmesan cheese. Broil until golden and serve with grilled steak.

Makes 1 loaf

Corn Muffins with Jalapeño

1 cup flour
1 cup yellow cornmeal
1 tablespoon baking
    powder
½ teaspoon salt
1 egg, beaten
1 cup buttermilk
2 tablespoons honey
¼ cup cooked corn
    kernels
1 jalapeño pepper,
    seeded and minced

Preheat the oven to 375°F.

In a large bowl, combine flour, cornmeal, baking powder, and salt.

In a medium bowl, whisk together egg, buttermilk, and honey, then add corn and jalapeño pepper.

Add wet ingredients to dry ingredients and use a large rubber spatula to combine them well.

Lightly oil a 12-cup muffin tin.

Pour batter into the muffin tin and bake for about 20 to 25 minutes. Let cool on a wire rack, then serve, perhaps spread with a bit of ricotta cheese.

Makes 1 dozen

BROCCOLI

King of the Cabbage Clan

24 calories per cup (raw)
46 calories per cup (cooked)

It's official! Broccoli is America's favorite vegetable! According to a poll by the EPCOT Center, the team of broccoli and cauliflower ranked first for "favorite veggie." Fully 40 percent of the voters named broccoli and cauliflower as number one with them.

In our opinion, three health facts about broccoli stand out.

Broccoli is the number one anticancer vegetable. Saxon Graham, Ph.D., and his co-workers at the State University of New York at Buffalo studied food habits and cancer risk in more than 1,000 men. Eating broccoli was linked to lower risk of colon cancer–a finding that has been confirmed in more recent work.

How does broccoli help prevent cancer?

- One: It belongs to the cabbage family of anticancer vegetables.
- Two: It is rich in carotene, a nutrient that is believed to help prevent cancer.
- Three: A cup of fresh cooked broccoli tops the scales with 2½ times the Recommended Dietary Allowance for vitamin C.
- Four: Broccoli is one of the best vegetable sources of calcium–another nutrient that looks like it has cancer-preventing properties.
- Five: It contains almost no fat–the best news for those concerned about cancers of the breast, colon, prostate, and other organs.

Broccoli is all heart. With almost no fat and some soluble fiber, it couldn't be kinder to your blood cholesterol level. And your blood pressure will love all the potassium that broccoli gives you–and all the sodium that it doesn't give you.

Bones love broccoli. As mentioned above, broccoli is one of the few calcium-containing vegetables–with a cup providing about 140 milligrams. And broccoli gives its calcium without high levels of protein that are now suspected of promoting loss of calcium from the body.

At the Market: Choose heads of broccoli with small, closed, compact buds and firm stems. Color is a clue also; the stems should be dark and the entire head should be free of yellowing. A purplish tint on the buds is a sign of freshness in some varieties. Reject broccoli that is limp, has buds that have begun to open, or has any yellowing flowers.

Kitchen Tips: Wrap broccoli in perforated plastic and refrigerate as soon as possible. It will last about three days. If you want to keep fresh broccoli longer, blanch it until it is bright green. You can then refrigerate it for about five days.

To prepare, separate the head into spears and florets if desired. The spears require more cooking time, so if preparing both, you might prefer to start them before the florets. Peel tough stalks so you can cook them along with the leaves and buds.

Accent on Enjoyment: Broccoli is excellent even when prepared simply. Steam it until tender—about 7 minutes. It also can be:

- Microwaved, poached, stir-fried, or sautéed.
- Added to soups, stews, fried rice, and pasta dishes.
- Topped with just a sprinkling of a sharp herb such as fresh thyme or freshly cracked pepper for a low-calorie delight.

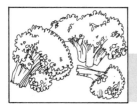

Broccoli Soup with Potato and Cheddar

1 tablespoon olive oil
¾ pound broccoli, chopped
1 large potato, chopped
1 leek, chopped
2 shallots, chopped
2 cups chicken stock
1 teaspoon dried thyme
1 teaspoon dried oregano
½ teaspoon curry powder
2 teaspoons Dijon mustard
1 cup milk
⅓ cup shredded cheddar cheese

Heat oil in a large heavy-bottom pot. Add broccoli, potato, leek, and shallots and sauté, stirring frequently, over medium-high heat for about 5 minutes.

Add 1 cup of stock, along with thyme, oregano, and curry, then cover and simmer until vegetables are very tender, about 30 minutes. Stir occasionally.

Let the soup cool, then pour it into a food processor or blender along with mustard and process until it's a smooth puree. (Don't over-process or the potato will become gummy.)

Pour the puree back into the pot and add remaining stock, milk and cheese and heat slowly, stirring to blend well. When cheese has just about melted, it's ready. Serve hot.

Makes about 1 quart

BRUSSELS SPROUTS

The Cabbage Family Queen

55 calories per cup (cooked)

There's no middle ground, we find, when it comes to brussels sprouts. Either you love 'em or you hate 'em. But to the nutritionist, there's another issue: How healthful are these tiny nuggets that look like minicabbages?

Probably no one has pondered the question more than Lee Wattenberg, M.D., professor at the University of Minnesota School of Medicine. Dr. Wattenberg has pioneered the study of "cancer inhibitors" in food. Cancer inhibitors are substances that appear to detoxify harmful chemicals so their ill effects are less likely to occur. Following up on reports that those free of cancer eat more cabbage family vegetables such as brussels sprouts, Dr. Wattenberg has isolated substances called indoles in cabbage family foods that probably explain their beneficial effects.

One piece of Dr. Wattenberg's research is especially heartening for brussels sprouts lovers. He and his co-workers designed a diet rich in brussels sprouts and cabbage, which was then given to healthy young people. And sure enough, the diet improved the functioning of a metabolic system that deals with certain cancer agents.

The fact is, however, that brussels sprouts would draw rave reviews from nutritionists even without findings such as these. They are, in a word, ultra-nutritious. A 1-cup serving is:

- Extremely high in vitamin C.
- Richer in protein than most vegetables.
- Very low in sodium and fat.
- Moderate in vitamin A, riboflavin, and iron.
- Moderately high in potassium and fiber.

At the Market: Look for brussels sprouts that have firm, tight heads that are heavy for their weight. The core end should be clean and white. Sprouts that are small, green, and firm will have the best flavor. Avoid sprouts that are yellow or brown.

Kitchen Tips: Store brussels sprouts, unwashed, in perforated plastic bags in the refrigerator. They will last up to a week. At cooking time, remove any yellowed or withered leaves. If the cores are tough, draw an *X* in them with a sharp knife to allow for better results from cooking. Cook sprouts until tender by steaming, simmering, blanching, boiling, baking, braising, or microwaving.

Accent on Enjoyment: Here are some other cooking and serving ideas.

- Add brussels sprouts to sautés and stir-fries.
- Toss with a dill vinaigrette after cooling.
- Season with mustard, caraway, dill, garlic, or sage.
- For a change of pace, try them raw. Trim off the core and slice sprouts thinly. Then toss into salads and enjoy.

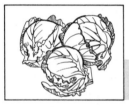

Brussels Sprouts in Packets

3 teaspoons sweet butter, melted
2 shallots, minced
1 tomato, chopped
½ teaspoon caraway seeds
½ teaspoon dill
1 pound brussels sprouts

In a large bowl, combine butter, shallots, tomato, caraway seeds, and dill.

Rinse brussels sprouts well and remove any brown or damaged leaves. Cut off the stem ends, then cut each sprout into slices, cutting from top to stem end. Add sprouts to tomato mixture and stir well to combine.

Preheat the oven to 375° F.

Lay out six 12 × 12-inch aluminum foil squares and divide sprout mixture equally among them, making a small mound on half of each square. Then fold each square over to cover the mound and crimp all the edges closed.

Arrange the packets on a baking sheet and bake until sprouts are tender, about 30 minutes. Use a kitchen shears to cut the packets open, then serve hot.

Makes 6 servings

BUCKWHEAT

Kasha, Anyone?

335 calories per cup (raw)

This nutty-flavored grain can be put to countless uses–from simple side dishes to elaborate breads and desserts. In India, for instance, buckwheat is typically made into flatbread (chapati), pancakes, or soup.

In a minute, some kitchen talk. But first a word about buckwheat and good health. In a recent study, R. J. Bijlani, of the All-India Institute of Medical Sciences in New Delhi, and his co-workers demonstrated a beneficial effect of buckwheat on glucose tolerance. They tested how well healthy students metabolized sugar before and during a diet that contained buckwheat chapatis stuffed with potato. After several months on the buckwheat diet, the students showed healthier responses on the sugar test.

The improvement in glucose tolerance wasn't the only impressive finding. In three-quarters of the students, blood cholesterol levels fell, too (although the cooking oil used in preparing the buckwheat might have played a role here). Buckwheat is also low in fat and sodium.

At the Market: Unroasted buckwheat is pale in color. Roasting causes it to take on a brown coloring, and the roasted form is commonly called kasha.

Kitchen Tips: Store buckwheat in an airtight container and keep it in the refrigerator. Its shelf life is long–up to a year under good conditions. If stored too long or improperly, the grains will have a rancid odor.

Unroasted grains should be pan roasted briefly in a dry skillet until brown. Traditionally a beaten egg is then added, followed by 1½ to 3 cups of water for each cup of raw kasha (the lesser amount of water is for pilafs and side dishes; the greater amount will yield a creamy breakfast cereal). Bring the water to a boil, then reduce the heat. Cover and simmer the kasha for about 20 minutes, or until all the water has been absorbed.

Accent on Enjoyment: For delicious results, try these suggestions.

• Toss cooked kasha with shredded spinach and freshly grated Parmesan cheese.

87

- Serve it with its traditional Russian accompaniment, bow-tie pasta.
- Buy buckwheat that has been ground into flour and use it to make delicious pancakes and crepes.

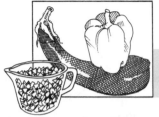

Buckwheat with Roasted Eggplant and Pepper

1 small eggplant (about
   ¾ lb)
1 sweet red pepper,
   cored and cut in half
   vertically
2 teaspoons olive oil
1 cup buckwheat
2 cloves garlic, minced
2 cups chicken stock
1 bay leaf
   juice and pulp of
    1 lemon
2 teaspoons sweet butter
1 teaspoon dried sage
1 teaspoon dried thyme
¼ cup minced fresh basil

Cut eggplant in half vertically, then blanch in boiling water until tender, about 10 minutes. Preheat the broiler.

When eggplant is ready, set it cut side down on a baking sheet, along with pepper halves. Broil until charred, about 6 to 7 minutes, then put vegetables into a brown paper bag, fold to seal and set aside.

In a large nonstick skillet, heat oil over medium heat. Add buckwheat and sauté until fragrant and roasted, about 5 minutes. Add garlic, stock, and bay leaf, then cover and simmer until all the liquid is absorbed, about 7 to 8 minutes.

Add lemon juice and pulp, butter, sage, thyme, and basil to buckwheat and stir well.

Remove pepper and eggplant from the bag and use your fingers to remove the charred skins. Chop vegetables, add them to buckwheat, and stir well. Remove bay leaf, then place the mixture in a serving dish and serve warm or at room temperature as an appetizer or side dish.

Makes 4 servings

BULGUR

Wheat of the Middle East

About 240 calories per cup (prepared)

Although a stranger to some, bulgur is simply wheat that has been parboiled, dried, and cracked. It's another food that has more than its share of good stuff–such as protein, niacin, and iron–and none of the bad stuff–such as fat and sodium. The bottom line is that bulgur is ideal for a range of healthy diets–whether they are designed to benefit heart health, digestion, diabetes, or even body weight.

At the Market: Bulgur comes in three "cracks": coarse, medium, and firm. Coarse is best for stuffings; fine is preferable for salads. Regardless of the crack, bulgur should smell clean and nutty.

Kitchen Tips: Store bulgur in a tightly covered glass jar in the refrigerator. It will last for about eight months.

To cook, pour enough boiling water over the bulgur to cover it. Let stand for about 20 minutes, or until the grains are soft. Drain off any liquid.

Accent on Enjoyment: You can use cooked bulgur in the following ways:

• Add to cold salads.
• Add to bread dough before kneading.
• Add to pancake and waffle batters.
• Substitute bulgur for rice in pilafs.

Would you believe bulgur is for breakfast, too? If you have some prepared bulgur from the night before, you can make a quick breakfast. Just scoop a serving into a microwave-safe bowl, cover with plastic wrap and microwave on full power until heated through–about a minute. Top with vanilla yogurt and enjoy.

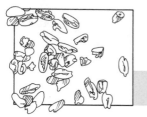

Apple-Bulgur Stuffing

2 teaspoons olive oil
2 shallots, minced
⅔ cup applesauce
½ cup milk
½ teaspoon thyme
   dash of freshly grated
     nutmeg
1½ cups cooked bulgur

In a nonstick skillet, heat oil over medium-high heat. Add shallots and sauté until soft, about 4 minutes.

Add applesauce and milk and simmer, stirring frequently, until the mixture has thickened and is reduced by half, about 5 minutes. Remove the skillet from the heat and add thyme, nutmeg, and bulgur.

Use to stuff a roasting chicken, four boneless breasts, four fish fillets or four Cornish game hens.

Makes 4 servings

CABBAGE

The Cabbage Patch Diet Makes News

Green: 16 calories per cup (shredded, raw)
32 calories per cup (shredded, cooked)
Red: 18 calories per cup (shredded, raw)
32 calories per cup (shredded, cooked)

If you're ready to adopt a new vegetable, let us suggest cabbage. Of all foods now believed to have cancer-preventing effects, few rate as high as cabbage.

A good example of its power is a study conducted by Saxon Graham, Ph.D., and his colleagues in Buffalo, New York. Dr. Graham's research team interviewed colon cancer patients and those free of the disease about their food habits. It turned out that participants who never ate cabbage were three times as likely to develop colon cancer as those who ate it at least once a week. Of course, experts now recommend not only cabbage, but other members of this family of foods.

Naturally, the idea that cabbage contains compounds that can help combat the ill effects of cancer-causing agents has attracted a lot of attention. Let's not forget, though, that there are plenty of other reasons to enjoy cabbage. It's low in calories, has almost no sodium or fat and as you might expect, also has its share of fiber. (Red cabbage comes in slightly ahead of other types on this count.) And a cup of red cabbage gives you two-thirds of the recommended allowance of vitamin C.

At the Market: The best cabbages are heavy for their size and have leaves that look crisp and colorful. Avoid cabbages that have wilted or blemished outer leaves. If, however, you find a head that has crinkled outer leaves—similar in texture to the normal appearance of inside leaves—take note. The cabbage may be old, with the wilted outer leaves removed to give a fresh appearance.

Wrap cabbage in plastic and refrigerate; the crisper drawer is a good place. Cabbage is one of our hardier fresh vegetables; properly stored, it will keep for two to three weeks. A medium head will yield about 2 pounds or 7 to 8 cups of shredded cabbage.

Getting the Odor Out

If you love cabbage but not the odor it emits during cooking, here are two tips for you.

While you are cooking cabbage, add a whole English walnut (in its shell) or a celery stalk to the water. Or choose brief, healthful methods for cooking cabbage–such as microwaving or stir-frying.

Either way, you will minimize that characteristic odor.

Be prepared for cabbage to play chameleon. If stored for a long time, green cabbage may lose its color and turn white. (Some varieties of cabbage, however, are naturally white; these are used mostly for sauerkraut.) Also expect red cabbage to bleed when cut or cooked, causing surrounding ingredients to turn bluish red.

Kitchen Tips: Cabbage should be washed and the outer leaves trimmed at preparation time. Cut the stem even with the bottom of the head. If you see a yellow ring around the core, that part will be hot and bitter; eat only the outside of the head.

Grate or shred cabbage raw to use in salads or coleslaw–even the core can be used. If using a food processor, use the slicing blade to shred cabbage. The shredding blade will chop it too finely.

We like cabbage steamed. It's easy; just cut the head into wedges, then steam for 10 to 15 minutes. It can also be braised, sautéed, or cooked in the microwave.

Accent on Enjoyment: Try sautéing shredded red cabbage with red cooking apples and a pinch of freshly grated nutmeg, then serve with grilled chicken.

A scooped-out head of green cabbage makes an attractive container for dips. Afterward, chop and toss it and add it to salads. Use dill, caraway, fennel, onion, curry, citrus, parsnips, or carrots to complement its flavor.

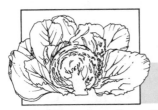

Sautéed Cabbage with Fennel

1 tablespoon olive oil
2 cloves garlic, minced
1 tablespoon fennel seeds
3 scallions, minced
4 cups shredded cabbage
2 tablespoons freshly
   grated Parmesan
   cheese

In a very large skillet, heat oil on medium-high heat. (If the skillet is too small, the cabbage will be mushy.) Add garlic, fennel, scallions, and cabbage and sauté until cabbage is cooked through but still crunchy, about 5 minutes.

Place cabbage mixture in a large serving bowl, sprinkle with Parmesan and serve hot.

Makes 4 servings

CANCER

Betting on Better News Ahead

Cancer experts are more optimistic than ever. Several decades ago, they declared a "war on cancer," and sure enough, the battles are starting to pay off. But who would have expected that nutrients found in fruits, vegetables, grains, and other foods would prove to be our best preventive weapons?

The case for preventing cancer through nutrition is impressive, and getting more so as research intensifies. In fact, the American Cancer Society, the National Academy of Sciences, and the National Cancer Institute (NCI) have all issued nutritional guidelines for preventing cancer. And the NCI has put its money where its mouth is. Today, this federal research institute has more than a dozen studies under way that are seeking answers about the role of key nutrients in cancer prevention.

Of course, nutritional strategies look promising for some, not all, forms of cancer. Let's start by looking at the forms that good nutrition is most likely to help prevent.

The Link with Lifestyle

One thing is certain: Lifestyle, not heredity, most influences our chances of avoiding some common forms of cancer. How can we be so sure? For 30 years now, researchers have been documenting that cancer patterns change—often dramatically–as people migrate from one place to another. That's as good a proof as any that the world around us–not the genes within us–is what matters most. From the dozens of studies now complete, the link is clear between our environment (including the food we eat) and at least ten forms of cancer. For instance:

- In his pioneering studies of Japanese who left their homeland for the United States, the NCI's William Haenszel, Ph.D., found that these immigrants also left behind the high risk of stomach cancer characteristic of their native land. After settling in the United States, however, they were more likely to develop cancers of the breast, colon, uterus, prostate, and ovary –all uncommon among their friends and relatives in Japan.
- Later, an NCI research group headed by Joseph Fraumeni, M.D., showed that Florida residents are less likely to develop colon cancer than northerners.

Countless Floridians are retirees who lived most of their lives in the Northeast. Somehow, moving south late in life clearly reduced their risk.
• Most recently, Australian nutritionist A. J. McMichael found that European migrants to Australia developed less cancer of the pancreas or stomach than citizens who remained in one of the European countries where they originally lived.

The message is loud and clear: If where we live is such a strong influence, something in the environment must play the key role. And the signals tell us that often this "something" is one or more nutritional factors. Read on for more evidence of nutrition's protective role.

Digging Deeper for Clues

The changing cancer patterns of migrants aroused the curiosity of researchers. The next step was to investigate food habits among those who remained free of cancer and those who did not. The results were just as revealing as the migrant studies.

• Richard Shekelle, M.D., and his co-workers found that smokers who ate lots of carotene-rich fruits and vegetables were far less likely to develop lung cancer than smokers who ate few of these foods. In fact, the high-carotene group was only one-seventh as likely to contract the disease as the low-carotene group.
• The NCI's Dr. Haenszel interviewed people who had colon cancer and those who did not, and found that those free of the disease reported eating more cabbage.
• Researchers at the Roswell Park Memorial Institute in Buffalo, New York, confirmed that people who did not have lung cancer took in more vitamin A than patients with the disease. Following up on their findings, they linked higher intakes of vitamin A to better protection from cancers of the esophagus, bladder, and larynx.

In a nutshell, the research strongly links beneficial nutritional factors to less chance of cancers that begin in the skin or in the lining of the mouth and other organs. As a group, these types of cancer are called carcinomas. By contrast, cancers that originate in muscle and bone (sarcomas), in blood-forming organs (leukemias), or in the lymph system (lymphomas) seem to be influenced by very different factors—viruses, radiation, and toxic chemicals, to name a few.

An Expert Opinion

Now let's hear what the boss has to say about all of this. Peter Greenwald, M.D., directs the NCI's Division of Cancer Prevention and Control, and he clearly is impressed. Recently, he commented on several of the nutrients now in the spotlight.

Taking Supplements Safely

Does the nutritional advice connecting certain foods to cancer prevention sound too complicated? Too much to think about every day? Is your lifestyle too hectic to allow for careful meal planning? Or are the recommended foods that you like best just too expensive?

If your answer to any of these questions is yes, supplementation may be for you. After all, supplements offer a simple alternative, one that many consumers prefer. And in some cases, supplementation with a nutrient is less expensive than obtaining it solely through food.

To us, supplementation is one of the easiest things you can do to protect your health. Every now and then, however, supplementation causes trouble for someone who decides that if some is good, more is better. So taking supplements sensibly and safely is the key to reaping their benefits. And that need not be difficult. Just keep in mind some basic facts about safe doses and signs of overuse. If signs of excessive intake are recognized early, the chances for full and rapid recovery are excellent.

Here's a rundown of the six nutrients that we consider good bets for cancer prevention, along with tips on taking them safely. These guidelines, of course, assume that you are an adult in good health.

Carotene. The plant form of vitamin A is nontoxic. Large amounts may cause a yellowing of the skin that will subside with a reduced intake, but the condition is not harmful. Don't confuse nontoxic carotene with synthetic vitamin A or vitamin A in fish-liver oils, however, which may cause headache, skin problems, fatigue, and other problems at daily doses above 25,000 international units. And during pregnancy, women should take vitamin A only as prescribed by a doctor.

Vitamin C. This is one of the safest vitamins. At doses in the four-figure range, some people experience diarrhea or sour stomach. Daily doses greater than 1,500 milligrams may reduce absorption of other

According to Dr. Greenwald, the carotene-vitamin A factor alone could help lower the chances of certain forms of cancer by 30 to 50 percent. He counts "about 20 studies" supporting the role of carotene, vitamin A, or both.

To these he adds the potential benefits of vitamins C and E. Like carotene, these two vitamins have antioxidant properties now believed to help in preventing formation of cancer-causing substances. Dr. Greenwald points to

nutrients, but at doses in the 250- to 1,000-milligram range, problems are extremely rare.

Vitamin E. Most of us also tolerate vitamin E very well, especially at doses up to 400 international units daily. Some people experience digestive upset at higher doses, but again, this occurs only rarely.

Selenium. This mineral can be toxic at high doses, but its danger has been exaggerated. Problems have not occurred with total intakes as high as 350 to 500 micrograms per day, and 100 to 200 micrograms seems like a sensible supplementary range. At 1,000 micrograms or more, signs of excess may occur: dry hair, streaked fingernails, and garlic odor on the breath are the most common. Should these occur, by all means stop supplementation until the symptoms disappear. If you want to start again, resume at a lower dose and be alert for symptoms.

Calcium. In order to overdose on calcium, it usually requires far higher daily doses than the 1,000 to 1,500 milligrams recommended for maintaining bone health. We believe that staying within this safe range is also suitable for cancer prevention. Some forms of calcium may cause digestive upset and constipation, though. If so, take the supplement with meals or switch to another form of calcium. Don't take supplemental calcium without your doctor's approval if you have heart or kidney disease, cancer, high blood calcium from any cause, or the chronic organ condition known as sarcoidosis.

Vitamin D. Because ill effects may occur at intakes only a few times the recommended allowance, vitamin D is often called the most toxic vitamin. No harm from supplementation with 400 international units per day–the amount found in a multivitamin pill–is known. Because vitamin D helps with calcium absorption, however, you should consult your doctor before taking it if you have any of the conditions mentioned above that call for careful use of calcium.

studies in northern Iran and China that link diets low in vitamin C-rich fruits and vegetables to extraordinarily high rates of cancer of the esophagus.

Although far less cancer research has been done with vitamin E, Dr. Greenwald notes supplementation with both vitamins E and C helps to reduce the formation of gene-altering mutagens in the intestinal tract. He, like many of his fellow scientists, suspects that by keeping those mutagens at bay, the cancer process can be discouraged.

Of course, no discussion of nutrition would be complete without mentioning selenium. Like the three vitamins, this mineral also wears the antioxidant hat. Dr. Greenwald feels that the anticancer effect of selenium deserves serious study, particularly because adding the mineral to drinking water helps protect test animals from cancer-causing chemicals.

He says, though, that it's not just these vitamins and minerals that help. He's also sold on the benefits of reducing fat and increasing fiber. Cancer experts recommend cutting back on all fats, but for fiber, the story is more complicated. Only the insoluble form of fiber that abounds in whole grain foods, beans, and some fruits and vegetables is now believed to offer a protective effect. (See the entry on constipation, beginning on page 151, for more details.)

In 1985, the NCI took the issue out of the laboratory and into the kitchen with the following set of recommendations for reducing cancer risk.

- Double fiber intake to a total of 25 to 35 grams daily.
- Lower fat intake to 30 percent of daily calories.
- Eat more "cruciferous" vegetables—brussels sprouts, cabbage, broccoli, cauliflower, rutabagas, and turnips.
- Eat foods high in vitamins A and C.
- Reduce your exposure to aflatoxins, which are naturally occurring molds that can grow on improperly stored nuts, grains, and seeds and are potent carcinogens.
- If you drink alcohol at all, drink only in moderation (two or fewer drinks a day), especially if you smoke.
- Whenever possible, bake, oven-broil or microwave meats instead of barbecuing or frying at high temperatures. This will reduce the formation of possibly harmful substances.

The Calcium Connection

We're so impressed with the value of fiber, low-fat foods, and antioxidant nutrients that additional favorable evidence won't surprise us. We were surprised, however, when scientists recently reported a link between two more nutrients and reduced cancer risk.

In the spotlight now are calcium and vitamin D. Long recognized for building bone, this duo looks as though it helps prevent cancer, too. In a ground-breaking study published in 1985, Dr. Shekelle and his co-workers reported a strong link between ample calcium intake and low risk of developing colon cancer.

These findings broke new ground not only for calcium but also for vitamin D. Earlier, we mentioned a riddle that scientists had yet to solve: why New Yorkers who retire to Florida are less likely to develop colon cancer than those who remain in the north. But with these new findings, we're starting to get the picture. Florida residents no doubt make more vitamin D—it's produced when the body is exposed to sunlight—because they are outdoors so much more than northerners. The vitamin D, of course, promotes calcium absorption, which in turn shores up our cancer-prevention defenses.

Our best guess? We're predicting that someday, calcium will be considered as important to cancer prevention as to bone health.

Putting Prevention on the Menu

This week's worth of meal plans provides key cancer-preventing nutrients without large amounts of fat.

Day 1

Breakfast
1 ounce spoon-size shredded wheat
1 orange
1 cup plain low-fat yogurt
1 cup skim milk
   coffee

Lunch
3 ounces water-packed tuna
1 tablespoon reduced-calorie mayonnaise
Salad (¼ cup loose-leaf lettuce, 5 radishes, ¾ cup celery, 2 tablespoons
   oil-free salad dressing)
   iced tea

Snack
1 cup skim milk
4 graham crackers

Dinner
4 ounces flank steak (London broil)
1 baked potato
¾ cup peas
¾ cup fruit salad

Day 2

Breakfast
½ cup 100% natural cereal, plain
1 cup skim milk
½ pink or red grapefruit
1 slice cinnamon toast
1 tablespoon apple butter
   coffee

Lunch
Salad (¾ cup crisphead lettuce, ½ cup fresh spinach, ½ fresh tomato,
   8 cucumber slices, ½ cup celery, 1 tablespoon low-calorie Italian
   dressing)

1 apple
3 rye crackers
1 cup low-fat cottage cheese
½ cup orange juice

Snack
1 cup low-fat vanilla yogurt
¼ cup blueberries

Dinner
3 ounces white meat turkey
2 pieces Italian bread
¾ cup green beans
1 ear corn
1 teaspoon margarine

Day 3

Breakfast
2 rice cakes
1 cup low-fat vanilla yogurt
¾ cup toasted wheat germ
½ cup fresh strawberries
1 teaspoon margarine
½ cup skim milk
coffee

Lunch
Crispy turkey sandwich (3 ounces turkey breast, 2 slices whole wheat
toast, 2 tablespoons plain low-fat yogurt, ½ cup green pepper, 1 carrot)
iced tea

Snack
1 banana

Dinner
4 ounces steamed lemon sole
½ acorn squash with ⅓ cup applesauce
1 cup asparagus
1 piece whole grain bread with jam
1 cup skim milk

(continued)

Day 4

Breakfast
1 ounce spoon-size shredded wheat
1 cup skim milk
¾ cup juice-packed peaches
1 cup low-fat cottage cheese
  coffee

Lunch
3 ounces water-packed tuna mixed with 1 tablespoon reduced-calorie
    mayonnaise
2 whole wheat crackers
¾ cup tossed salad with oil-free dressing
1 cup apple juice

Snack
½ cup sherbet
½ cup strawberries

Dinner
3 ounces lean roast beef
2 slices whole grain bread
1 teaspoon ketchup
1 teaspoon prepared mustard
1 teaspoon onions
¾ cup chopped celery
1 carrot
1 ear corn
1 cup skim milk

Day 5

Breakfast
¾ cup instant oatmeal, plain
½ pink or red grapefruit
1 cup low-fat fruit yogurt
1 cup skim milk
  coffee

Lunch
Garden pita (1 pita bread filled with ¼ cup crisphead lettuce, 3 slices
    turkey breast, 2 tablespoons chopped onions, 3 radishes, ½ cup celery,
    ½ cup green pepper, 1 tablespoon low-calorie Italian dressing)

1 banana
1 cup iced tea

Snack
1 baked apple
½ cup skim milk
   tea

Dinner
4 ounces steamed scallops
Vegetable medley (¾ cup brown rice, ¾ cup carrots, ¾ cup broccoli,
   ¼ cup ginger sauce)
1 piece whole grain bread
1 teaspoon margarine

Day 6

Breakfast
⅓ cup Grape-Nuts, plain
1 cup skim milk
1 slice whole wheat toast
1 tablespoon jam
1 orange
   coffee

Lunch
Chicken 'n' pasta salad (1 ounce chicken breast, without skin, 1 cup
   cooked, cooled pasta, 1½ tablespoons reduced-calorie mayonnaise,
   ½ cup green pepper, ½ cup red pepper, ⅛ cup onions)
1 papaya
   iced tea

Snack
1 cup low-fat lemon yogurt

Dinner
3 ounces lean sirloin steak, trimmed of fat
1 baked sweet potato
¾ cup broccoli
1 teaspoon margarine
½ cup fruit salad with ½ cup sherbet

(continued)

Putting Prevention on the Menu–Continued

Day 7

Breakfast

1 bagel with 2 tablespoons apple butter
1 cup low-fat yogurt drink
   coffee

Lunch

Salad (½ cup crisphead lettuce, ¾ cup fresh spinach, 1 carrot, ½ cup
   celery, ½ cup green pepper, 1 tablespoon low-calorie Italian dressing)
1 piece whole grain bread
1 teaspoon margarine
1 cup low-fat cottage cheese
1 cup orange juice

Snack

½ cantaloupe filled with ½ cup fresh strawberries

Dinner

6 oysters
¾ cup green beans
1 cup onion soup
1 piece whole grain bread
1 teaspoon margarine
1 baked potato
¾ cup cauliflower
¼ cup low-fat yogurt

CARROTS

The Rabbits Are Right!

48 calories per cup (shredded, raw)
70 calories per cup (sliced, cooked)

Carrots are one of the most flavorful, economical, and widely available sources of carotene. And carotene–the plant form of vitamin A–has impressed us with the potential for preventing cancer.

That fact has caught the attention of the National Cancer Institute, which now is sponsoring about a dozen cancer-prevention studies of carotene. These, of course, come on the heels of many others that have linked carotene-rich foods to reduced risk of cancer. In a comprehensive review of several dozen studies, internationally known cancer expert Richard Peto, Ph.D., and his colleagues list cancers of the lung, esophagus, stomach, intestines, mouth, throat, bladder, and prostate as forms of cancer that a high carotene intake has shown potential to prevent.

But current Recommended Dietary Allowances (RDAs) don't consider the cancer-prevention issue. In fact, we have no RDA for carotene itself; the only relevant RDA is for total vitamin A, which is 5,000 international units daily–whether in the form of carotene from plants or as preformed vitamin A from animal foods or synthetic sources.

We're confident that this will change, but until then we prefer the "Watson recommendation." Ronald Ross Watson, Ph.D., is a cancer researcher at the University of Arizona. In a paper published in the *Journal of the American Dietetic Association,* Dr. Watson and his colleague Tina Leonard suggest that an intake of 12,500 international units of carotene–2½ times the current RDA–would be desirable for preventing cancer.

If 12,500 international units daily sounds like a lot, consider how much carotene you can get in a single serving of carrots. A cup of raw, shredded carrots provides 31,000 international units. Because carrots become denser with cooking, cooked carrots have slightly more vitamin A: 38,000 international units per cup. And the carotene in cooked carrots is actually better absorbed than that in raw carrots.

Carrots have other pluses, too. Consider, for instance, that fresh carrots are a good source of potassium, whether raw or cooked; are virtually fat free; are high in soluble fiber; and are a modest source of vitamin C when raw.

At the Market: For best taste, choose smooth carrots that are small to medium in size and tapered at the tips. (Baby carrots—about 2 inches in length—are almost always tender but can be tasteless.) Carrots should have a bright orange-red color and a firm texture. Limpness, sprouts on the carrots, or signs of decay at the tips indicate carrots that have passed their prime. By contrast, greens at the top of carrots are a sign of freshness.

Kitchen Tips: Before storing carrots, remove any tops that are present. Store the carrots in plastic in the refrigerator; a good batch will keep two to three weeks. Carrot greens, however, are fussier and will last only about five days. For best taste, store carrots away from apples to prevent bitterness.

Before serving carrots, wash them well and scrape the skin if it looks tough and old. A swivel-bladed peeler makes for easiest peeling. Expect a pound of raw carrots to yield about 4 cups shredded.

You may prefer cooked carrots to raw. For fast cooking, cut carrots into coin-shaped pieces and steam until tender, about 10 minutes. For boldest taste, cut the carrots on a diagonal; this exposes more surface and enhances flavor. Raw carrots, of course, are standard for snacking and salads.

Accent on Enjoyment: Carrots blend well with countless healthy foods. We suggest that you:

- Toss them with pasta, marinated vegetables, or your favorite stir-fry.
- Combine them with one or more of these tasty foods: parsnips, oranges, raisins, chicken, potatoes, broccoli, or lamb.
- Spice them with tarragon, dill, cinnamon, nutmeg, and allspice to vary the flavor.
- Save carrot greens; chop and add to salads and soups to boost taste and nutritional value.
- Use as a natural sweetener: Add chopped carrot to soups, stews, and tomato sauce for a full, natural sweetness without refined sugar.

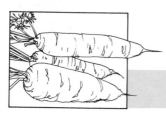

Marinated Chunky Carrots

1 pound carrots, cut into
    chunks on the
    diagonal
1 tablespoon olive oil
2 tablespoons cider
    vinegar
1 teaspoon Dijon
    mustard
  pinch of dry mustard
1 tablespoon minced
    fresh mint
1 tablespoon minced
    fresh dill or
    1 teaspoon dried dill
1 teaspoon capers,
    drained and minced

Steam carrots over boiling water until just tender, about 7 to 10 minutes.

Meanwhile, in a small bowl, whisk together oil, vinegar, and mustards. Then stir in mint, dill, and capers.

In a large bowl, toss together carrots and dressing. Cover and refrigerate for at least an hour or overnight. Serve chilled.

Makes 4 servings

CAULIFLOWER

Good Health in Every Bite

24 calories per cup (raw)
30 calories per cup (cooked)

Sure it's pricey, but nutritionally, cauliflower is worth it. It's among the vegetables recognized by the Committee on Diet, Nutrition, and Cancer of the National Academy of Sciences as one of the best bets for preventing cancer.

The committee made its comments after reviewing research that "suggests that certain vegetables, especially cruciferous [cabbage family] ones, have a possible protective effect against cancer at several sites." But at the time of its 1984 report, the committee felt that "the responsible constituent or constituents cannot be identified on the basis of present information."

In other words, there's something good in vegetables like this one, but they aren't sure what that something is. We know that some people won't be convinced until its exact identity is known, and to those folks, we simply want to point out that other attributes of cauliflower are already on the books and reason enough to credit it as a healthy food. It is:

- Low in calories, fat, and sodium.
- Endowed with enough vitamin C so that a 1-cup serving provides 100 percent of the Recommended Dietary Allowance.
- A fine source of the mineral potassium.
- A source of fiber.

At the Market: Size, weight, and color are the keys to choosing cauliflower. A good head is firm and compact, yet heavy; white to ivory in color; and surrounded by leaves that look tender and green. Brown spots on the head or florets that have started to open are signs that the cauliflower is past peak freshness.

Purple cauliflower is becoming more available. Although this type should have a nice purple-green color, you can use the same guidelines for choosing it as you use for the white variety.

Kitchen Tips: Wrap cauliflower in perforated plastic bags and store, unwashed, in the refrigerator. It will last there about seven days. By storing it

108

unwashed and using it as soon as you can, you can help minimize brown spots.

Some love their cauliflower raw, but when you prefer it cooked, we suggest steaming. Simply wash and trim the head, cut into florets, and steam for about 10 minutes.

Accent on Enjoyment: Here are just some of the many ways to use cauliflower, as well as some facts for the cook who is new to this vegetable.

- For a quick yet elegant side dish, season just-cooled florets with a splash of olive oil and minced fresh dill.
- For a fancier presentation, blanch cauliflower–don't overcook–and marinate in lemon juice, a splash of olive oil, and caraway seeds.
- If your area has hard water, you can help prevent cauliflower from yellowing during cooking by adding about a teaspoon of lemon juice to the cooking water. And don't be surprised if you encounter pink cauliflower; some varieties turn pink when canned or pickled. But experts say the color change has no effect on taste.

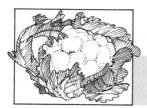

Cauliflower with Mustard Sauce and Dill

1½ cups chicken stock
1 teaspoon dill seeds
3 bay leaves
1 pound cauliflower, cut into bite-size pieces
2 teaspoons Dijon mustard
1 teaspoon minced fresh dill

Pour stock into a 10-inch skillet and add dill seeds and bay leaves. Cover and bring to a simmer. Add cauliflower, cover, and continue to simmer until cauliflower is tender, about 7 to 8 minutes.

Uncover the skillet and place it in the refrigerator. Let cauliflower chill in its stock for about 30 minutes.

Drain cauliflower, reserving stock, and place it in a serving dish. Strain stock and combine ¼ cup of it with mustard. Drizzle sauce over cauliflower, sprinkle with minced dill, and serve.

Makes 4 servings

CELIAC DISEASE

One Man's Wheat Is Another Man's Poison

For some, the troubles begin as early as infancy. The luckier ones are spared symptoms until their teen or adult years. But no matter when things first go wrong, typical symptoms will be these telltale signs of celiac disease.

• Loss of weight and appetite.
• Anemia.
• Tiredness.
• Bulky, light-colored, fatty stools.

Hopefully, symptoms like these will lead to prompt testing—and better still, to successful treatment. But if left unchecked, complications such as nerve or bone pain—and even broken bones—can be the result.

Fortunately, however, celiac disease is no longer the mystery that it once was. Research has caught the culprit red-handed. No, it's not stress or anyone's imagination that's to blame. To the contrary, celiac disease comes from the inability to tolerate gluten, a protein found in common grains—wheat, rye, barley, and oats. Although the staff of life for many, these grains spell trouble for those with celiac disease. Eating them not only causes unpleasant symptoms but also damages the intestinal tract.

Celiac disease is far more common in some countries than in the United States, where only about 1 of every 5,000 citizens is affected. Its relative rarity here can leave you feeling a bit at sea when first diagnosed, as if no one else can understand your symptoms. Actually, you needn't feel that way. Celiac disease is but one of a family of disorders known as malabsorption syndromes. Count up those affected by these related conditions and you will realize that you have plenty of company.

What causes celiac disease? Three facts stand out.

• A defect in the immune system is the leading suspect, but the jury is still out on this belief.
• Disorders that damage the small intestine can bring celiac disease with them, even in older individuals who never experienced the symptoms before.

110

• Celiac disease is a family affair, which is most likely to strike those whose relatives also have the condition. Obviously, this means that genetic factors are at work.

Coping with the Condition

The first order of business, of course, is to be sure that the symptoms are signs of celiac disease. (By the way, you may also hear the disorder referred to as nontropical sprue, gluten-induced sprue, idiopathic steatorrhea, or gluten enteropathy.)

No matter how strongly doctors suspect celiac disease, they will want a biopsy of the small intestine to be sure. If their suspicions are confirmed by a positive result, you'll be asked to follow a special diet that eliminates gluten. You may also be advised to limit lactose–an enzyme found in milk products–in your diet at first. Sometimes those with severe symptoms have a problem handling lactose, but this generally goes away once the celiac symptoms are brought under control.

To help cope with your new restrictions, you'll want to take the following measures.

• Write to food companies for a list of their products that are gluten free. Most have such a list ready to send.
• Visit health food stores for special products made without gluten.
• Contact Ener-G Foods, a mail-order source of gluten-free (and lactose-free) breads, pastas, cereals, and baking mixes. You can write to them at 6901 Fox Avenue South, Seattle, Washington 98124-0723.

The Long View

As anyone who has suffered through an attack of celiac disease can tell you, your long-term health is the last thing on your mind when the symptoms strike. But once these are under control, you will want to discuss a few other issues with your doctor. Some of these issues are:

• Supplementing your diet with vitamins and minerals to compensate for reduced absorption of nutrients from food.

- Ensuring that complications of celiac disease—such as rickets in young children—are ruled out (and promptly treated if found).
- Staying alert for any signs of the abdominal cancers that are more common among those who have had celiac disease for many years.

The Gluten Getaway

A gluten-free diet is a two-step mission. First and foremost, you'll need to ferret out gluten-containing foods in your diet. That accomplished, you'll be free to concentrate on the foods that you can eat without worry. Here are details on both counts.

Foods to Avoid

- Bread, biscuits, cakes, cookies, crackers, crispbreads, doughnuts, flour (white or whole grain), muffins, pancakes, pastry, pies, pretzels, rolls, toast, and waffles.
- Breakfast cereals made with wheat or oatmeal, such as All-Bran, wheat flakes, puffed wheat, shredded wheat, Sugar Smacks, Grape-Nuts, oatmeal, and wheat germ.
- Macaroni, noodles, spaghetti, semolina, vermicelli, and other pasta.
- Meat pies, luncheon meat, canned meat, meat loaf, commercial hamburgers, sausages, bologna, and frankfurters.
- Canned soups and soup mixes.
- Vegetables with cream sauces or crumbs, such as baked beans.
- Commercial sauces and ketchups, gravies and salad dressings.
- Packet and pudding mixtures, pastry mixtures.
- Malted milk, Ovaltine, Postum, beer, and commercial milk flavoring.
- Baking powder.
- Cheese spreads.
- Most ice creams (except those specifically approved).
- Commercial chocolates and licorice sweets.

Now just when you're thinking this leaves you with a *no*-foods diet, you'll be pleased to know you're actually left with plenty of options.

Foods to Use Freely

- Milk, all kinds, and yogurt (although you may be told to eliminate these initially); homemade syrup or unprocessed cocoa may be added for flavoring.

You may also want to join a support group for people in your area who have celiac disease or other malabsorption syndromes. There's no substitute for talking things over with others who have faced the same problem and overcome it.

- Fresh meats, poultry, and bacon, fish (fresh or canned), shellfish, and organ meats.
- Gravies made with cornstarch or rice flour.
- Cheese and eggs (boiled, poached, scrambled, in omelets and mixed dishes).
- Vegetables (fresh, frozen, canned), raw or cooked.
- Potatoes and rice.
- Nuts.
- All fruits and fruit juices.
- Bread and flour made from wheat starch, arrowroot, cornmeal, soybean, rice, or potato flour.
- Breakfast cereals made from rice and corn only.
- Cream, butter, margarine, peanut butter, cooking fats, and oils.
- Sugar, jam, jelly, marmalade, honey, syrup, boiled sweets, hard candies, homemade candy, and plain chocolate.
- Desserts and puddings made with gelatin, tapioca, sago, rice, and cornstarch.
- Cakes and cookies made with gluten-free flour.
- Coffee, tea, and carbonated beverages.
- Salt, pepper, mustard, spices, garlic, and vinegar.
- Specifically approved ice creams.

The key to keeping symptoms at bay is avoiding wheat starch containing more than 0.3 percent protein, a very small amount. Unfortunately for celiac sufferers, many mixed and manufactured foods contain small amounts of wheat flour, but they aren't small enough. You'll want to check ingredient lists regularly and update your list of forbidden and permissible foods. Remember, the effort will pay off every time you catch a potential troublemaker and keep it off your plate.

Gluten-Free Meal Plans

To be sure, restricting gluten in your diet–as these plans do–is no easy feat. But you'll quickly find that the effort is well worth the trouble.

If you are advised at first to limit lactose as well as gluten, you will need to adapt these meal plans to exclude lactose-containing foods. (See the entry on lactose intolerance, beginning on page 276, for more information.)

Day 1

Breakfast

    1 ounce crisped rice cereal
    1 apple
1 ⅓ cups skim milk
    coffee

Lunch

    1 cup tuna salad
    ¾ cup crisphead lettuce
    1 fresh tomato
    1 cup seedless raisins
    1 cup skim milk

Snack

    ½ cup tapioca pudding

Dinner

    3 ounces chicken breast (without skin)
    ½ cup brown rice
    ¾ cup French-cut green beans
    ½ tablespoon margarine
    1 cup skim milk
    1 orange

Day 2

Breakfast

    1 ounce corn flakes
    1 cup fresh strawberries
1 ⅓ cups skim milk
    coffee

Lunch
Salad (several leaves of fresh spinach, ¼ cup mushrooms,
    1 sliced, hard-cooked egg, 1 cup onions, ½ cup shredded cheese,
    2 ounces shredded turkey breast, 4 radishes, ½ cup green pepper,
    2 tablespoons low-calorie salad dressing)
    1 cup iced tea

Snack
    1 ounce peanuts

Dinner
    3 ounces lean sirloin steak (trimmed of fat)
    1 baked potato
    ¾ cup carrots
    ½ tablespoon margarine
    3 fresh apricots with ½ cup low-fat fruit yogurt

Day 3

Breakfast
    1 cup cream of rice cereal
    1 banana
    1 cup skim milk
      coffee

Lunch
    3 ounces white meat turkey
    ½ cup brown rice
    ½ cup wax beans
    1 teaspoon margarine
    ¼ cup cranberry sauce
    1 cup iced tea

Snack
    1 cup low-fat fruit yogurt

(continued)

Gluten-Free Meal Plans–Continued

Dinner
2 corn tortillas
2 ounces lean ground beef
¼ cup grated carrots
1 fresh tomato
1 ounce Swiss cheese
½ cup corn
1 cup fresh raspberries

Day 4

Breakfast
1 ounce puffed rice cereal
½ white grapefruit
1⅓ cups skim milk
    coffee

Lunch
6 oysters
1 carrot
½ cup cauliflower
1 cup skim milk
1 cup nectarines

Snack
½ cup chopped dates

Dinner
2½ ounces lean sirloin steak (trimmed of fat)
½ cup cooked eggplant
½ cup raw broccoli
½ cup peas
½ tablespoon margarine
⅓ cup raw sliced mushrooms
1 cup skim milk
½ cantaloupe

Day 5

Breakfast
1 cup Corn Chex cereal
1 banana

¾ cup skim milk
½ cup pineapple juice
coffee

Lunch
1 cup fresh spinach
½ cup raw cauliflower
1½ ounces Swiss cheese
1 fresh tomato
¼ cup onions
2 tablespoons low-calorie salad dressing
1 cup skim milk

Snack
2 plain rice cakes with 2 tablespoons peanut butter

Dinner
6 to 8 oysters
½ cup peas
1 small baked potato with ½ cup plain low-fat yogurt
1 tablespoon margarine
1 cup melon salad (cantaloupe, honeydew, watermelon)

Day 6

Breakfast
1 rice cake
1 scrambled egg with grated Swiss cheese
1 cup fresh berries
1⅓ cups skim milk
coffee

Lunch
Salmon salad plate (½ cup pink salmon, ½ tablespoon reduced-calorie
mayonnaise, ½ cup loose-leaf lettuce, 6 cucumber slices, 1 cup celery,
1 cup mushrooms)
1 cup skim milk

Snack
1 cup low-fat fruit yogurt

(continued)

Gluten-Free Meal Plans–Continued

Dinner
   3 ounces chicken breast (without skin)
   ½ cup brown rice
   1 ear corn
   ¾ cup brussels sprouts
   1 tablespoon margarine
   1 cup skim milk
   1 cup cantaloupe

Snack
   1 fresh pear
   1 ounce reduced-fat cream cheese

Day 7

Breakfast
   1 homemade banana smoothie (skim milk, banana, honey, ice
      cubes)
   1 cup fresh strawberries
   2 rice cakes
      coffee

Lunch
   3 ounces white meat turkey
   ½ cup broccoli
   1 pat margarine
   1 cup skim milk
   ½ cup rice pudding (homemade, not packaged)

Snack
   1 apple
   1 ounce feta cheese

Dinner
   3 ounces veal cutlet
   ¾ cup green beans
   1 ear corn
   2 pats butter
   1 cup skim milk
   1 cup fresh orange sections

CEREALS, HOT

Warming Up to Wheat

Cream of wheat: 133 calories per cup (cooked)
Whole wheat cereal: 150 calories per cup (cooked)

Some people think that the term "hot breakfast" means bacon and eggs. But you can have a hot breakfast with a lot less effort–and much less fat and cholesterol, too. Just reach for a hot wheat cereal.

Hot wheat cereals are a great way for sodium watchers to start the morning. They contain almost no sodium–or fat for that matter–unless it's added in preparation. You also get some protein and B vitamins.

Now for some differences between whole wheat and cream types. Whole wheat cereals contain all three parts of the grain–the bran, the germ, and the endosperm. Because the bran remains, these cereals have more potassium, zinc, and fiber than cream of wheat, which retains the germ of the wheat but not the bran. Cream of wheat has a lighter texture and is often fortified with enough iron to put it way ahead of the whole wheat cereal on this count.

Cream of Wheat

Kitchen Tips: Store cream of wheat tightly covered in a cool, dry place.

Accent on Enjoyment: You can save on cooking time by preparing cream of wheat in a 9-inch nonstick skillet rather than in the usual saucepan. Serve with sliced fresh apples or pears, or with chopped dried fruit such as apricots and pineapples. For a low-fat, low-sodium way to thicken soups, add about 2 tablespoons of cream of wheat to soup to serve four. Let it bubble for about 5 minutes, stirring frequently.

Whole Wheat Cereal

At the Market: First check for purity of ingredients, then read the package for preparation time, which varies among brands. Many wheat cereals include other grains, such as barley, and these make tasty alternatives.

Kitchen Tips: Store unopened packages in a cool, dry place. After the package has been opened, transfer the cereal to a jar with a tight-fitting lid and refrigerate. Many people cut the preparation instructions off the box and tuck them into the jar.

Accent on Enjoyment: Is hot, creamy, whole wheat cereal drizzled with maple syrup and sprinkled with walnuts and chopped apples your kind of breakfast? Then you'll love exploring these ideas.

• Cook whole wheat cereal with apricot nectar instead of water.
• Keep a container of whole wheat cereal handy and add a handful to quick breads, muffins, pancakes, and waffles.
• Sprinkle a bit of whole wheat cereal into soups and stews as a low-fat thickener.
• Keep in mind that many spices that are used in baking are perfect companions to whole wheat cereal. Try vanilla, cinnamon, nutmeg, allspice, mace, ginger, and almond.

CEREALS, READY-TO-EAT

And Better Than Ever

(See also *Bran, Wheat*)

All-Bran: 71 calories per ounce

Bran Buds: 73 calories per ounce

Bran Chex: 91 calories per ounce

Crunchy Bran: 98 calories per ounce

Grape-Nuts: 102 calories per ounce (regular or flakes)

Nutri·Grain: 102 to 108 calories per ounce

Shredded wheat: 102 calories per ounce

Wheat Chex: 104 calories per ounce

You can't watch television for long without being reminded that ready-to-eat bran and whole grain cereals give you health-promoting fiber. But fiber is just one of the good things in these cereals. Here we'd like to focus on another, less-talked-about attribute in these cereals: minerals.

Nature puts some of the minerals there. But manufacturers often fortify their products with extra amounts to boost their nutritional value. As a result, these packaged cereals often provide more minerals than unprocessed bran. Some examples:

- Bran Buds are a good source of iron, manganese and zinc.
- All-Bran is a remarkably good source of iron, zinc, copper, and manganese.
- Corn Bran contributes a healthy dose of iron and zinc.
- Grape-Nuts Flakes best the bunch for iron with a whopping 5 milligrams per 1-ounce serving. (They are fortified with extra iron, of course.) Regular Grape-Nuts also have a respectable 1 milligram of iron per serving. In addition to their iron, Grape-Nuts also provide zinc, copper, and manganese.

So why don't advertisers emphasize the minerals in cereal as they do their fiber? Probably the biggest factor is the long-held fear by nutritional experts that the fiber in these foods binds up minerals and interferes with their absorption.

Where's the Fiber?

Is fiber what you're looking for when it comes to breakfast cereals?

If so, this table can be your guide for choosing ready-to-eat cereals at the supermarket. For your convenience, they are arranged from high to low according to their fiber content. Values are for 1 ounce of cereal.

Cereal	Fiber (g)
All-Bran	8
100% Bran	8
Bran Buds	7
Oat bran, dry	7
Corn Bran	6
Raisin Bran	6
Bran Chex	5
Bran Flakes	5
Cracklin' Bran	5
Puffed wheat	5
Corn Chex	4
Grape-Nuts Flakes	4
Most	4
Oats, regular, dry	4
Shredded Wheat	4

The fact is, however, that we have yet to find a report of mineral inadequacy caused by substituting bran or whole grain cereal for a refined grain cereal in a varied diet. Consider these reassuring findings:

• James W. Anderson, M.D., of the University of Kentucky School of Medicine, has treated diabetics with diets containing 50 grams of fiber a day (that's more than twice our current intake). Some of his patients have been on

Cereal	Fiber (g)
Wheaties	4
C. W. Post, Plain	3
Corn Flakes	3
Country Morning	3
Grits, dry	3
Life	3
Natural cereal	3
Oatmeal, instant, dry	3
Oatflakes	3
100% Natural	3
Post Toasties	3
Ralston, dry	3
Total	3
Wheat Chex	3
Cheerios	2
Rice Krispies	2
Cream of Wheat	1
Farina, dry	1
Rice Chex	1

SOURCE: Fiber content based on values compiled by James W. Anderson, M.D., Wen-Ju Chin, and Beverly Sielig, HCF Research Foundation. Inc., Lexington, KY 40502.

his high-fiber diet for years without developing any signs of inadequate mineral nutrition. To play it safe, Dr. Anderson has them take a multimineral supplement—a policy that we believe makes more sense than avoiding these foods for fear of their effect on mineral nutrition.

- Swedish researcher Brittmarie Sandstrom treated elderly patients with bran in amounts similar to that found in a serving of All-Bran cereal. The bran did not reduce the amount of calcium, magnesium, zinc, or iron in the patients' blood.
- Another test of bran fiber on elderly patients—this one using a crispbread made of whole wheat and rye—also found the high-fiber treatment to be free of ill effects on four minerals: iron, calcium, phosphorus, and potassium.

Based on findings such as these, we feel that increasing fiber *in a varied diet* is more likely to help than hurt. Obviously, eating a diet composed almost exclusively of whole grain foods is another matter. In those parts of the world where whole grains dominate the diet, people are truly at risk of poor mineral nutrition.

At the Market: Choosing ready-to-eat cereals requires no special knowledge. To ensure freshness, though, you may want to check the expiration date. If you have a good nose, sniff the package; the aroma should be fresh and nutty—not musty.

Kitchen Tips: Keep packages of whole grain cereal tightly closed. Especially during humid weather, transferring the contents to a covered container is a good idea. Store in a dry, well-ventilated area.

Accent on Enjoyment: Of course, ready-to-eat cereals are designed to give us a no-fuss option that at most requires the addition or milk or fruit. But creative cooks have found many other ways to use and enhance their flavor.

- Add bran cereal—crushed or whole—to muffin, pancake, and waffle batters. If you prefer a lighter texture, let the batter soften for a few minutes before cooking.
- Crush bran cereal with a rolling pin or in a food processor or blender. Use in place of bread crumbs or chopped nuts in casseroles, to bread tender foods such as scallops and veal, to replace up to one-third of the flour in a recipe, or to extend meat loaf and other ground-meat dishes.
- Top frozen desserts, hot cereals, or yogurt with bran cereal.
- Add "chunky" whole grain cereals such as Bran Chex, Wheat Chex, and Corn Bran to trail mixes for super nutrition during hikes. At home they're perfect for snack mixes.
- Toast crunchy whole grain cereals such as Bran Chex in the oven, then crumble with a rolling pin and sprinkle on vegetables, casseroles, and

Sizing Up a Cereal's Sodium

Manufacturers add sought-after minerals to their cereals for the sake of better health (and maybe even better sales, too!). But many also add a not-so-sought-after mineral to their cereals for the sake of better taste. That mineral? Sodium.

Typically, ready-to-eat cereals contain 100 to 350 milligrams of sodium per ounce. How does this range stack up? We consider it moderate – that is, okay for most, but not all of us. If you're on a strict low-sodium diet, stick with the stand-out selection below – shredded wheat – or a similar sodium-free alternative.

Despite the added sodium, you don't have to worry about fat in most cereals. In fact, we suspect that more and more of us are choosing cereal for breakfast because it is the perfect low-fat way to start the day. Values given are per 1-ounce serving.

Cereal	Sodium (mg)
Shredded wheat, plain	3
Bran Buds	174
Nutri·Grain	187-193
Wheat Chex	190
Grape-Nuts	200
Corn Bran	244
Bran Chex	264
All-Bran	320

stir-fries as a lower-calorie alternative to nuts.
- Use sturdier cereals such as Chex as a crispy garnish for soup. Toss on right before serving.
- Make ultranutritious pie crusts by crushing a slightly sweetened whole grain cereal such as Wheat Chex and pressing into a pie plate. (This is a great substitute for a graham cracker crust.)
- Fold nugget-shaped cereals such as regular grape-nuts into vanilla ice cream before serving, or sprinkle them on fruit salads.

No matter how rushed you are, you have enough time to enliven your morning bowl of cereal with different combinations of fruit and nuts. For example, corn-based cereals such as Corn Bran and Nutri·Grain corn are delicious with chopped pecans and fresh peaches.

Tastier Brans

When it comes to breakfast cereals, All-Bran, 100% Bran, and Fiber One are the fiber champs. But let's face it–coarse bran cereals aren't the favorite ingredient of Cordon Bleu chefs. Or to be more blunt–as one cereal box puts it–"Most people would like more fiber in their diet ...but not if it means having to eat bran cereals that taste like twigs and gravel."

Well, not all bran cereals are guilty on this count. Even the most adamant bran haters are likely to find that these newer choices can make increasing your bran intake a pleasure. Corn Bran, for instance, has a more delicate texture than coarse wheat bran and a nice sweet and nutty flavor. Bran Chex and Wheat Chex are also a far cry from "twigs" when it comes to taste.

For the record, here is a list of ready-to-eat cereals to choose from when you are looking for the goodness of whole grain or bran.

- All-Bran
- Bran Buds
- Bran Chex
- Crunchy Bran
- Fiber One
- Bran Flakes
- 100% Bran
- Raisin Bran
- Wheat germ

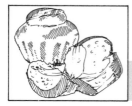

Tender Bran and Molasses Muffins

1½ cups Bran Buds
½ cup apple juice
⅓ cup raisins
1 cup flour
1½ teaspoons baking soda
1 egg, beaten
1 cup lemon yogurt
¼ cup molasses
¼ cup safflower oil

Preheat the oven to 400° F.

In a medium bowl, combine cereal, juice, and raisins and let stand for about 10 minutes.

Sift together flour and baking soda into a medium bowl.

In another medium bowl, combine egg, yogurt, molasses, and oil.

Oil a 12-cup muffin tin.

When cereal is ready, stir in dry ingredients, then wet ingredients. Use a large rubber spatula to combine ingredients, using about 20 strong strokes. Spoon batter into the muffin tin, filling the cups three-quarters full, and bake for about 20 minutes. Let cool on a wire rack before serving.

Makes 1 dozen

CHERRIES

Answering That Snack Attack

Sour red: 52 calories per cup (with pits)
Sweet red: 82 calories per cup (with pits)

On a diet? Have some cherries.

You may not think of cherries as a diet food, but we do–and we have good reason. For one, fresh cherries can fill the bill for dieters who enjoy sweets. They also allow you to follow the golden rule of "behavior modification" that the experts extol: that is, eat *slowly.*

If you grab a candy bar in response to a snack attack, you can gobble down 300 calories in no time at all. Bet you can't eat 300 calories worth of cherries nearly as fast. And research by obesity expert Henry Jordan, M.D., has suggested that foods that are easily wolfed down are more likely to cause trouble because the body doesn't have the time it needs to let the feeling of fullness take over.

Cherries have other benefits, too. A cup of sour cherries provides almost 25 percent of the Recommended Dietary Allowance of vitamin A. In fact, cherries are a good plant source of vitamin A for those who turn up their noses at vegetables.

Cherries also earn honors as a sodium watcher's best friend. A cup provides a mere 2 milligrams of sodium. And your heart will also appreciate their modest fiber content–as well as the virtual absence of fat.

At the Market: Select sweet cherries that are dark red to black, with a smooth, firm texture. Sour cherries should be clear red, or yellow with a blush. The stem should be green and firmly attached to the cherry. Size and quality are closely related, with large cherries (about an inch in diameter) generally having the best texture and flavor.

One bad cherry can spoil the barrel, so to speak, so it's best to pick them carefully to ensure that a few that have gone bad don't encourage the rest to do likewise.

Kitchen Tips: Cherries should be refrigerated immediately, without washing or covering. Storage time will vary, but may be up to two weeks. Some cherry lovers insist that a hair barrette makes the best cherry-pitting utensil because its metal tip is just the right size for easy pitting. They simply buy a new one and keep it in the kitchen with their other utensils, to be used whenever cherry season rolls around.

Accent on Enjoyment: Sweet cherries are great eaten plain and are also a traditional ingredient in clafouti, a tasty baked fruit custard. They can also be incorporated into desserts, salads, mousses, and sorbets. Sour cherries are best when used in jams, preserves, and compotes, or cooked and served as an accompaniment to grilled or curried chicken.

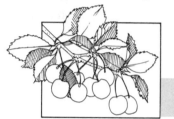

Curried Cherries

juice and pulp of 1
  lime
1 teaspoon honey
½ teaspoon ground
  ginger
½ teaspoon ground
  cinnamon
1 teaspoon curry powder
2 bay leaves
2 cups fresh sweet
  cherries

In a small saucepan, combine lime juice and pulp, honey, ginger, cinnamon, curry, and bay leaves. Heat over low heat until honey becomes liquid, then stir well to combine. Remove from heat.

Rinse and pit cherries and add them, still wet, to the saucepan. Simmer over medium heat, stirring frequently, until cherries are slightly wilted and are well coated with curry mixture, about 5 minutes. Serve warm with roasted meats or poultry.

Makes about 2 cups

CHICKEN

Putting Poultry Power to Work!

White meat: 245 calories per 4 ounces
Dark meat: 285 calories per 4 ounces

It used to be that a chicken in every pot was the symbol of prosperity. Today, it's the symbol of health.

It's hard to think of a health-conscious diet where chicken doesn't fit in. Nutritionally, chicken is high in protein, iron, niacin, and zinc. If it's your heart that concerns you most, chicken has a fat and sodium profile that is favorable for both blood cholesterol and blood pressure. (Of course, those on very strict low-sodium diets need to consider the 100 or so milligrams of sodium in a 4-ounce serving.)

Best of all, chicken is ideal for a low-calorie diet. In fact, chicken breast has the distinction of being the lowest in fat and calories of any chicken part. And it's the best-tasting part of the chicken, too. (Its premium price will attest to that!)

You don't have to pass up the rest of the chicken, though, if you're concerned with fat and calories. These two gremlins lurk primarily in the skin and in pads of fat located just below it. Remove them and you're cooking with a lean and nutritious food.

At the Market: At peak freshness, chicken is plump and firm. The skin looks moist and has a creamy white color. Fresh chicken should have no coarse pinfeathers and no odor.

Kitchen Tips: Store chicken in the coldest part of the refrigerator, wrapped in waxed paper, for one to two days. To freeze, wrap as airtight as you can with freezer paper; you can then freeze it for up to six months. If you also have the giblets, store them separately from the rest of the chicken.

Although skinned chicken is healthiest, we suggest that you wait until after cooking to remove the skin. This helps to keep the flesh moist. And after

---

What a Difference the Skin Makes!

If you forgo the chicken skin, you will save on fat and calories. And you can't use the vitamins and minerals as an excuse for eating it, either. The amount of certain key nutrients is about the same whether you eat your chicken skinned or unskinned.

	Broiler-Fryer (roasted with skin; 4 oz.)	Broiler-Fryer (roasted without skin; 4 oz.)
Calories	270	214
Fat (g)	15	8
Protein (g)	31	32
Niacin (mg)	10	10
Iron (mg)	1.4	1.3
Zinc (mg)	2.2	2.4

---

handling chicken, make sure you take a minute to wash the knife, cutting board, and your hands with hot, soapy water to get rid of any bacteria that have been present in the meat.

Accent on Enjoyment: Boneless, skinless breasts (chicken cutlets) are the lowest in fat and calories. They can be poached, sautéed, stir-fried, or microwaved. We like to marinate them in olive oil, lemon juice, and oregano, then grill or broil them and serve with hot pasta.

Here are some pointers.

- You can't beat boneless breasts for convenience. They can be microwaved (1 pound for about 5 minutes at high), then kept in the refrigerator for sandwiches, salads, or snacks.
- Roasting is ideal for cooking chicken without added fat. Use a raised roasting rack set with a drip pan so the bird doesn't sit in fat. For maximum juiciness with minimum fat, preheat the oven to 450° F. Then set the bird

in the oven and immediately reduce the temperature to 350° F. Continue to roast for about 20 minutes per pound. Skip the stuffing, by the way, or it too, can absorb lots of fat.
- If you have an old bird, cook it with moist heat to preserve tenderness. Put the chicken in a heavy pot, cover with a cup or more of liquid, and simmer over low heat until meat is tender and cooked to the bone. Let cool, remove skin, and shred the meat for sandwiches and casseroles.

If your family says "beef" when you say "chicken," try this compromise. Grind skinned chicken and substitute it for ground beef in your family's favorite recipes. The result is a lean alternative that tastes too good to complain about.

Comparing White Meat to Dark

Sooner or later, every nutrition-conscious chicken lover wonders whether white meat and dark meat differ in any major way. White meat has less in the fat and calorie departments, whereas dark meat takes the lead on certain minerals. Here is more about how the two stack up nutritionally.

	White Meat (3 oz.)	Dark Meat (3 oz.)
Calories	185	215
Fat (g)	9	13
Protein (g)	25	22
Niacin (mg)	10	5
Vitamin B_6 (mg)	0.44	0.26
Iron (mg)	1.0	1.2
Potassium (mg)	193	187
Magnesium (mg)	21	19
Sodium (mg)	64	74
Zinc (mg)	1.0	2.1

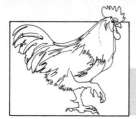

Chicken and Ziti with Two Tomatoes

1 tablespoon flour
½ teaspoon dried oregano
½ teaspoon dried thyme
1 teaspoon dried basil
1 pound chicken cutlets, sliced into ½-inch ribbons
2 teaspoons olive oil
8 Italian tomatoes, peeled and chopped
5 dried tomatoes, cut into slivers
3 cloves garlic, sliced
2 bay leaves
⅓ cup chicken stock
1½ cups cooked ziti freshly grated Parmesan cheese

In a large bowl, combine flour, oregano, thyme, and basil. Add chicken and coat well with flour mixture.

In a large nonstick skillet, heat oil over medium heat.

Add chicken to the skillet and sauté until cooked through, about 8 minutes. Remove chicken and set aside.

Add Italian tomatoes, with their juice, to the skillet, along with dried tomatoes, garlic, bay leaves, and stock. Bring to a boil, then continue to boil for about 2 minutes. Reduce heat to medium, add chicken and ziti, and heat until they are warm and dried tomatoes have softened, about 2 minutes. Remove bay leaves and serve hot in shallow bowls, sprinkled with Parmesan.

Makes 4 servings

Chili-Roast Chicken

½ cup plain low-fat yogurt
1 teaspoon ground cinnamon
1 teaspoon chili powder
1 teaspoon hot pepper sauce, or to taste
2 cloves garlic, minced
1 roasting chicken (about 3 to 3½ pounds), quartered

In a large glass baking dish, mix together yogurt, cinnamon, chili powder, hot pepper sauce, and garlic. Then add chicken and coat with marinade. Cover the dish tightly and marinate in the refrigerator, overnight.

Preheat the oven to 500°F.

Place chicken skin side up on a raised broiler rack and place it in the oven. Immediately reduce the temperature to 350°F and roast for about 1¼ hours. Serve hot or cold. (If you're cutting fat and counting calories, remove the skin before eating.)

Makes 4 servings

The Name Game

If you've ever wondered how a roaster differs from a stewing chicken, here are some answers.

Name	Description	Weight
Broiler-fryer	The most common type of chicken; 9-12 weeks old	1½ to 3½ pounds
Capon	A large desexed rooster; all white meat; 12-18 weeks old	About 7 pounds
Roaster	A widely available chicken, larger than a broiler-fryer but also with tender meat; 12-18 weeks old	3½ to 5 pounds
Rock Cornish game hen	A unique-tasting bird; 5-7 weeks old	2 pounds or less
Stewing chicken	A mature hen that is fattier and less tender than other chickens	2½ to 5 pounds

CHICK-PEAS

Chock-Full of Good Things

About 216 calories per cup (cooked)

They look funny and their name is even funnier. But when it comes to nutrition, chick-peas are nothing to laugh at. Also known as garbanzo beans (snicker, snicker) in the United States and as Bengal gram (come on now, stop laughing) in Eastern countries such as India, chick-peas are getting some serious attention from Western nutritionists.

Americans are a little behind the times, we must admit. Twenty-five years ago, when lots of supermarkets in this country didn't even stock chick-peas, researchers overseas were on the trail of their special health benefits. Their interest was piqued when a survey showed that poor residents of northern India had far lower blood cholesterol levels than higher-income residents. Suspecting that the chick-pea-rich diet eaten by the poor people was the reason, researchers proceeded to put this hunch to the test. In a pioneering study, wheat and cereals in the diet of the rich were replaced with chick-peas. Cholesterol levels fell dramatically—an average of 56 milligrams—during the chick-pea splurge.

Even if your cholesterol level needs no improvement, chick-peas have much to offer you. A cup of cooked chick-peas provides lots of protein, fiber, iron, and potassium, as well as substantial amounts of the B vitamins thiamine and niacin. All delivered, of course, without high levels of fat or sodium.

Want numbers? If so, figure 3 grams of fat and 16 milligrams of sodium per cup of cooked, unsalted chick-peas.

At the Market: Chick-peas are available cooked, in cans, or as dried beans. The latter are sometimes sold in bulk. When buying them, look for whole, unbroken beans with an even khaki color, no odor, and uniform size. Don't be concerned by the wrinkly surface of the beans; it's normal.

Kitchen Tips: Store chick-peas in an airtight container and keep in the refrigerator. Plan for each cup of dried chick-peas to yield about 3¼ cups when cooked.

To start the cooking process, wash dried beans thoroughly. Cover with water and allow to soak overnight. Next, simmer over low heat for about 2½ hours or pressure-cook according to manufacturer's directions (usually about 15 to 20 minutes). Canned beans, of course, are time-savers, because they are already cooked, but they often contain added salt. Rinse them first to wash some of it away.

If you want to cook your own but are short on time, here's an option that you may not be aware of. Chick-peas freeze fairly well. Next time you make some, cook more than you can use and freeze the extras. They'll keep for about four months.

Accent on Enjoyment: Chick-peas are perfect for turning a green salad into a substantial meal. They add a nutty taste and new texture and are particularly good with minced onion and marinated artichoke hearts. Don't forget to try chick-pea dip; it's a snap to make in the food processor or blender. Just puree the beans and add olive oil; tahini, or nut butter; and garlic. Serve with pita bread or raw vegetables.

If you are faced with a die-hard meat fan, how about this compromise. Make meat loaf or meatballs, substituting finely chopped chick-peas for some of the ground meat.

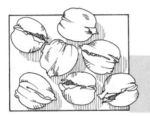

Chick-pea, Pepper, and Pine Nut Salad with Creamy Basil Dressing

1½ cups cooked chick-peas
1 sweet red pepper, cored and cut into julienne strips
1 tomato, seeded, juiced, and chopped
2 scallions, cut into julienne strips
2 tablespoons buttermilk
1 tablespoon lemon juice and pulp
1 tablespoon wine vinegar
1 tablespoon olive oil
1 clove garlic
2 tablespoons steamed fresh basil leaves
1 tablespoon pine nuts red lettuce leaves for serving

In a medium bowl, combine chick-peas, pepper, tomato, and scallions.

Pour buttermilk, lemon juice and pulp, vinegar, oil, and garlic into an electric spice grinder and process until thick. Then add basil and process again until leaves are minced. (If you don't have a spice grinder, whisk liquid ingredients together and mince basil and garlic by hand. It will taste good but won't be as creamy.)

To toast pine nuts, heat a dry, nonstick skillet over medium heat. Add pine nuts and sauté until toasted, about 2 minutes. Be careful not to let them burn.

Pour dressing over chick-pea mixture and toss well to combine. Spoon onto lettuce leaves and sprinkle with pine nuts. Serve as a first course, a light lunch, or an accompaniment to roast lamb.

Makes 4 servings

CHOLESTEROL

The Infamous Fat

Food is the best medicine for a healthy heart, and nowhere does this statement ring more true than when it comes to conquering cholesterol.

Some 30 years ago the National Health Education Committee became the first official organization to endorse cholesterol-lowering diets. Just a few years ago, the National Heart, Lung, and Blood Institute joined them. In between, dozens of expert committees signed on as endorsers.

What amazes us most is not the sheer number of believers but how similar the recommendations are no matter whom you consult. In fact, today's advice for controlling cholesterol differs little from what was advocated decades ago.

- Eat more fruits and vegetables.
- Substitute fish, chicken, beans, and grains for some of the meat on your menu.
- Choose only lean red meats (round, rump, flank steak) and trim them well.
- Replace whole milk and dairy products made from whole milk (ice cream, most hard cheeses, some yogurts) with reduced-fat or skimmed varieties (such as part-skim or low-fat cheeses, nonfat yogurt, ice milk).
- Use margarine or liquid vegetable oil (soy, corn, sunflower, and safflower are good) instead of butter and hard shortenings, but remember that these, too, are rich in calories and should be used sparingly.

And now we can add another: Eat two or three helpings a week of fish high in omega-3 fatty acids. If you've been paying attention to the headlines over the last few years, you know that omega-3's ability to fight cholesterol is the biggest news to come from the science of protective nutrition in years.

The Fish Fix

Fish, of course, is not exactly a newcomer when it comes to nutritional integrity. It has always been welcome on cholesterol-lowering diets because it contains so little saturated fat—and as a bonus also has some of the polyunsaturated fat that helps lower blood cholesterol. What's new, though, is the finding that the unsaturated fat in fish packs more cholesterol-lowering punch than previously thought.

It was long believed that the polyunsaturated fat in fish was as good as but no better than the kind in vegetable oils when it came to lowering cholesterol levels. Yet research at the Oregon Health Sciences University, for instance, found that fish oil even outranks vegetable oil when it comes to lowering cholesterol and triglycerides. These findings, published in the *New England Journal of Medicine* in 1985, showered attention on fish as never before.

There was other good news about fish at the same time. New research also was proving that the fat in certain fish had a heart-helping power apart from its ability to lower blood cholesterol. Heart researchers trying to understand why Eskimos rarely suffered heart attacks found that the omega-3 fats in their fish-rich diet made their blood less prone to clotting. And although normal clotting is essential for survival, abnormal clotting can be deadly, especially to hardened arteries that are already clogged and narrowed. It's all too frequent that a clot will lodge in such an artery, blocking the flow of blood to the heart.

With findings like these, fish has gained more fans than ever among heart researchers. But if it doesn't rate high on your list of favorite foods, don't despair. You have an alternative: fish-oil capsules. Just keep in mind, however, that a single capsule of fish oil does not provide as much omega-3 oil as a serving of fatty fish.

Roll with the Oats

So you say you just can't stand fish? Well, there are still other dietary choices that you may find more pleasing to the palate: oat bran and beans.

Nutritionists at one time believed that no one food could significantly reduce blood cholesterol. Then along came James W. Anderson, M.D., and his co-workers at the University of Kentucky, who showed otherwise. In a series of studies, the Anderson team found:

• Oat bran muffins (about two large ones per day) lowered blood cholesterol among healthy college students by almost 10 percent.

(continued on page 140)

Fish Oil Facts

Here's everything you ever wanted to know about the omega-3 content of fish. The table gives you the omega-3 content for a modest-size 3½-ounce portion.

As you can see, the best sources contain at least 1 gram (that is, 1,000 milligrams) of omega-3. By contrast, a single capsule of fish oil typically contains 0.3 grams (300 milligrams). That means that you would need 3⅓ capsules to supply 1 gram of omega-3.

Estimating the number of 300-milligram fish-oil capsules that would provide as much omega-3 as fish is simple. Just find the value for the fish of your choice, drop the decimal point, and divide by 3. If the fish contains 1.5 grams, for example, drop the decimal point so that 1.5 becomes 15, then divide by 3. In this case, you would need five fish oil capsules to equal the omega-3 content of the real thing.

Prefer to get your omega-3 from fish? If so, the experts recommend at least two servings a week. If your risk for heart disease is above average, however, we'd recommend even more.

Food (3½ oz. raw unless otherwise indicated)	Omega-3 Fatty Acids (g)
Finfish	
Mackerel, Atlantic	2.5
Anchovies, canned	2.1
Salmon, Atlantic	1.7
Salmon, pink, canned	1.7
Herring, Atlantic	1.7
Sablefish	1.5
Whitefish	1.4
Tuna, bluefin, fresh	1.2
Shark	0.9
Bass, striped	0.8
Bluefish	0.8
Swordfish	0.8

Food	Omega-3 Fatty Acids (g)
Bass, freshwater	0.7
Trout, rainbow	0.7
Eel	0.6
Halibut, Atlantic and Pacific	0.4
Pollack, Atlantic	0.4
Sea trout	0.4
Perch	0.3
Pike, walleye	0.3
Snapper	0.3
Whiting (Hake)	0.3
Cod, Atlantic	0.2
Flatfish (flounder and sole)	0.2
Haddock	0.2
Pike, Northern	0.1
Crustaceans and Mollusks	
Mussels, blue	0.5
Oysters, eastern	0.5
Shrimp	0.5
Squid	0.5
Crab, blue	0.3
Crayfish	0.2
Scallops	0.2
Clams	0.1

SOURCE: Information courtesy of Nutrition Action, September 1984.

- When larger amounts of oat bran–slightly more than 1 cup daily, as hot cereal or muffins–were taken by men with high blood cholesterol levels, their readings were reduced by an impressive 20 percent.
- In these same men with high cholesterol, ½ cup of dry beans, cooked and incorporated into a soup or side dish, also reduced cholesterol by about 20 percent. Most often, cooked kidney or pinto beans were used.

So, you're probably wondering, what gives oat bran and beans the power to bring cholesterol down? It's their fiber, or more specifically, their *soluble* fiber. Soluble fiber and cholesterol bind together and are eliminated from the body.

The Soluble Fiber Solution

How do oat bran and beans benefit blood cholesterol? Scientists think that the fat-busting factor is the soluble fiber they contain.

Although beans and oat bran are the foods that researchers have found to work, we are optimistic that other foods rich in soluble fiber may also help lower cholesterol. Remember, of course, that you need fairly large amounts–more than a single serving a day–to reap the benefits you're looking for. We suggest about four servings a day from the following list.

- Apples (2 medium)
- Apricots (2 raw)
- Bananas (1½ medium)
- Beans, kidney or pinto (⅓ cup cooked)
- Beans, lima (¼ cup cooked)
- Beans, white (½ cup cooked)
- Broccoli (¾ cup cooked)
- Cauliflower (¾ cup raw)
- Chick-peas (½ cup cooked)
- Crunchy Bran cereal (¾ cup)

As a result of the success of these studies, the Anderson team recommends 50 grams daily of oat bran or dry beans. That's the equivalent of ⅔ cup of uncooked oat bran or ½ cup of raw beans. They each represent about two good-size servings a day.

This is great news, of course, for anyone who wants a simple way to lower cholesterol. At the same time, we aren't saying that you can eat all of the high-fat foods you want. If your cholesterol remains too high after a trial of oat bran or beans, you'll have to cut down on saturated fat and cholesterol, too. And of course, adding oat bran or beans to a low-fat diet is an even better bet. You'll find lots of ideas for cooking with beans and oat bran—and some great recipes—beginning on pages 55 and 305.

- Corn (½ cup)
- Eggplant (1 cup cooked)
- Figs (2 medium)
- Greens, collard, kale, mustard, or turnip (1 cup cooked)
- Lettuce, dark green or loose-leaf (1 cup)
- Oat bran (⅓ cup dry)
- Oatmeal (¾ cup cooked)
- Okra (¾ cup)
- Peas, cowpeas (¼ cup cooked)
- Peas, green (½ cup)
- Peas, split (½ cup cooked)
- Post Toasties cereal (1 cup)
- Potato (¾ medium baked)
- Prunes (5)
- Zucchini (¾ cup)

NOTE: Other plant foods usually contain at least some soluble fiber, but not as much as the items listed above. We've kept this list to unusually good sources in the interest of simplicity, but we do realize that the soluble fiber in foods not mentioned here can also contribute to cholesterol control.

Conquering Cholesterol

When it comes to lowering cholesterol, cutting back on saturated fat is key. Limiting cholesterol-rich foods is also part of the plan. We've put the approaches together here, with these meal plans emphasizing cholesterol-friendly foods such as fruits, vegetables, fish, beans, and oats. The results should make your heart glad!

Day 1

Breakfast
   1 cup cooked rolled oats
   1 banana
   1 slice Italian bread
   1 teaspoon high-polyunsaturated margarine
   1 cup orange juice
      coffee

Lunch
   3 ounces turkey breast
   1 slice whole wheat bread
   ¼ cup loose-leaf lettuce
   1 fresh tomato
   ½ tablespoon reduced-calorie mayonnaise
   1 cup fresh strawberries
   1 cup skim milk

Snack
   1 cup skim milk
   1 papaya
   2 rye crackers

Dinner
   3 ounces fillet of sole, steamed, with lemon
   ¼ cup slivered almonds
   ½ cup asparagus
   ½ cup cauliflower
   1 baked potato
   3 pats high-polyunsaturated margarine
   1 cup skim milk

Day 2

Breakfast
   1 ounce oat bran cereal
   1 apple
1⅓ cup skim milk
   1 slice rye bread
   1 teaspoon margarine
      coffee or tea

Lunch
Salad medley (1 cup fresh spinach, ¼ cup celery, ¼ cup croutons or dry
   bread cubes, 3 large, ripe, pitted olives, 6 cucumber slices with peel,
   ½ cup grated carrots, 4 radishes, olive oil to taste)
½ baked chicken breast

Snack
   1 cup cantaloupe

Dinner
   3 ounces broiled or baked salmon
   ½ cup brown rice
   ½ cup brussels sprouts
   ½ cup sliced mushrooms
   2 pats high-polyunsaturated margarine
   1 slice angel food cake
   1 cup strawberries
   ¼ cup blackberries

Day 3

Breakfast
   2 oat bran muffins
   1 teaspoon high-polyunsaturated margarine
   ½ white grapefruit
   1 teaspoon honey
   1 cup skim milk
      coffee

(continued)

Conquering Cholesterol–Continued

Lunch
    2 slices whole wheat bread
    1 tablespoon jelly
    2 tablespoons peanut butter
    1 raw carrot
    1 cup tossed salad
    1 cup skim milk

Snack
  1½ cups iced tea
    ½ cup chopped dried dates

Dinner
    3 ounces baked veal cutlet
    1 baked potato
    ⅔ cup baked winter squash
    ½ cup peas
    3 pats high-polyunsaturated margarine
    1 cup skim milk

Day 4

Breakfast
    2 oat bran muffins with prune butter
    ½ cup orange juice
    1 cup cocoa made from skim milk

Lunch
    1 pita bread
    ¼ cup crisphead lettuce
    ½ cup fresh spinach
    1 slice low-fat cheese
    ½ cup chick-peas
    ½ fresh tomato
    2 onion slices
    ¼ cup sweet green pepper
    ¼ cup croutons or dry bread cubes
    2 tablespoons low-calorie dressing
    1 cup skim milk

Snack
　1 kiwifruit
　½ cup vanilla low-fat yogurt

Dinner
　3 ounces flank steak (London broil)
　1 cup peas and carrots with onions
　½ cup potato salad (no eggs)
　½ tablespoon margarine
　1 cup skim milk
　1 piece watermelon

Day 5

Breakfast
　1 ounce shredded wheat cereal
　1 orange
　1 slice rye bread
　1 teaspoon high-polyunsaturated margarine
　¾ tablespoon jelly
　1 cup skim milk
　　coffee

Lunch
　2 tablespoons chopped walnuts
　¼ cup chopped apple
　3 ounces water-packed tuna
　½ tablespoon reduced-calorie mayonnaise
　½ cup butterhead lettuce
　2 oat bran muffins
　4 pineapple rings (juice-packed)
　1 cup skim milk

Snack
　1 cup skim milk
　1 piece oatmeal-carrot cake (made with oil)

(continued)

Conquering Cholesterol–Continued

Dinner

3 ounces baked chicken breast
¾ cup cooked spinach
¾ cup brown rice
3 pats high-polyunsaturated margarine
½ cup pinto beans
1 cup fresh strawberries
1 cup iced tea

Day 6

Breakfast

1 ounce oat bran cereal
1 apple
1 cup skim milk
   coffee or tea

Lunch

Tofu griller (1 slice rye bread, 1 pat high-polyunsaturated margarine,
   1 piece tofu, 1 slice low-fat cheese)
½ cup green beans
5 vanilla wafers
1 cup skim milk
1 banana

Snack

1 cup apple juice
1 ounce peanuts

Dinner

1 cup oysters
Simple salad (½ cup broccoli, 1 carrot, ½ tomato, 2 teaspoons oil and
   vinegar to taste)
½ cup cooked kale
1 baked sweet potato
½ tablespoon high-polyunsaturated margarine
1 cup skim milk
½ cup raspberry sherbet
½ cup cantaloupe

Day 7

Breakfast
  2 oat bran muffins
  2 pats high-polyunsaturated margarine
  1 tablespoon jam or preserves
  1 cup cantaloupe
  1 cup skim milk
    coffee

Lunch
Fruit 'n' tuna plate (1 papaya, 3 ounces water-packed tuna,
  1 tablespoon reduced-calorie mayonnaise)
  1 slice whole wheat bread
  ½ cup butterhead lettuce
  1 medium tomato
  2 teaspoons salad oil with vinegar and herbs to taste
  1 cup iced tea

Snack
  4 fig bars
  ¾ cup skim milk

Dinner
  3 ounces baked chicken breast
  ¾ cup broccoli
  1 bagel
  1 pat high-polyunsaturated margarine
  1 baked apple with ½ cup vanilla ice milk and 1 tablespoon chopped
    walnuts
  1 cup skim milk

COLDS

Feed Them with Nutrition Power

Whoever first offered the advice to "feed a cold, starve a fever," sure knew what he was talking about.

Today's science of protective nutrition makes clear that the question is not *whether* to feed a cold, but *what* to feed it. No one food or nutrient has earned the distinction of being "the best," but three in particular deserve mention. One is in the headlines regularly, another is a recent discovery that may be news to many, and the third is "Grandma's advice."

Kudos for Vitamin C

Vitamin C's ability to beat the common cold has been a subject of debate for years. But it wasn't until 1987 that vitamin C's uphill battle for scientific respect turned a corner. Elliot Dick, Ph.D., professor of preventive medicine at the University of Wisconsin in Madison, surprised scientists at the International Symposium on Medical Virology with impressive findings about vitamin C and the common cold. It's dirty work by viruses, of course, that brings on a cold and its misery.

With the willing participation of 16 healthy student volunteers, Dr. Dick set the stage for a confrontation between C and the cold virus. Half of the 16 received 2,000 milligrams of vitamin C daily, taken in four doses of 500 milligrams each. The others received a blank pill, but no one knew who took what.

After about a month of taking the pills, all volunteers spent a week living among cold sufferers. Not surprisingly, 13 of the 16 picked up a cold in no time. However, those who had been primed for the hostile environment with the extra vitamin C had much milder symptoms. The average sick time for the vitamin C-takers was only 7 days, compared to 12 days among those who had been on the placebo.

Dr. Dick's findings confirm a series of university studies done in Toronto during the 1970s. In this series involving more than 1,000 students, Terrence W. Anderson, Ph.D., also found a trend toward less severe cold symptoms among those taking supplemental C. In one test, for instance, the number of days "home sick" with a cold was 30 percent lower for vitamin C users than for nonusers.

Our favorite among the latest in vitamin C research is a study of identical twins done by Alan B. Carr of the University of Sydney, Australia. Dr. Carr ingeniously tested vitamin C in pairs of twins, giving 1,000 milligrams of the vitamin to one member of each pair and placebos to the other. Three months of this treatment produced no evidence that vitamin C affected whether or not colds developed. But it, too, turned up a benefit of C once a cold had struck. According to Dr. Carr, vitamin C shortened the life of colds by an average of about 20 percent. Now that's nothing to sneeze at!

The Zinc Link

You don't have to be a professor to leave your mark in science history. Just ask George Eby, an urban planner from Texas.

One day when Eby gave his three-year-old daughter her daily zinc supplement, she refused to swallow it because she was suffering from cold symptoms that made swallowing too painful. So she sucked on the pill instead. A few hours later, her observant father noticed that her symptoms seemed to have disappeared. Too impressed to turn away, he sought out William Halcomb, M.D., and nutrition scientist Donald R. Davis, Ph.D., who helped him mount a state-of-the-art scientific study of zinc.

The research team prepared two sets of lozenges—one containing 23 milligrams of zinc in the form of zinc gluconate, the other a blank look-alike. During the study, volunteers with colds were asked to suck on two tablets of the test medicine every 2 hours while awake. The results showed that the volunteers who had been using zinc recovered from their colds an average of seven days sooner than those who had been sucking on the fake lozenges. A few, however, complained about the taste of the lozenges, and about one-quarter experienced digestive upsets that, happily, proved avoidable if the lozenge was taken with food.

Although the research team cautions that their findings need confirmation, zinc gluconate lozenges have made their way onto drugstore shelves. Whether they will stand the test of time remains to be seen.

Kitchen Cures

Score another one for folk wisdom. The winner this time is chicken soup. The age-old cold remedy now has some science behind it, says Mike Oppenheim,

M.D., who practices medicine in Los Angeles.

Dr. Oppenheim cites the work done at the Mount Sinai Medical Center in New York City that credited hot chicken soup–but not hot water–with increasing the flow of mucus, thereby helping to relieve congestion. Exactly which ingredient in the soup does the job remains a mystery. Speculation centers on its smell or taste as having some property that plain hot water lacks.

Needless to say, plenty of doctors will tell you that more evidence is needed before chicken soup can be recommended to combat congestion. Yet chances are that the same doctors already advise their patients to "force fluids" during a cold–that is, to get plenty of liquids to replace what the body loses to fever and sweating. Soup is certainly suitable in this regard, so it can be recommended even if one isn't sold on its potential to combat congestion.

We suspect that soup is not alone in helping to break up congestion. Until the scientific studies evaluate a longer list of liquids, we have to settle for word-of-mouth reports that other hot liquids–as well as juices–also help.

CONSTIPATION

Easy Answers That Work

No, it isn't life threatening, nor is it a sure sign of failing health, but constipation can nonetheless be a nuisance and a cause of discomfort. It's one of those symptoms that–in theory–can strike anyone at any time. In reality, though, it's most common among the elderly and pregnant women, or when one of the following factors is present:

• Low intake of fiber or fluids.
• Sedentary lifestyle or long-term bed rest.
• Diseases of the glands, such as hypothyroidism.
• Use of certain drugs or mineral supplements.
• Long-term use of enemas.

Before getting into the nutritional side, we'd like to mention some of the tried-and-true measures that deserve consideration whenever constipation becomes too annoying to ignore:

• Getting more exercise, which speeds the movement of food through the digestive tract, easing constipation.
• Drinking more fluids (water is great), which helps control the symptoms.
• Using laxatives (bulk-forming agents such as Metamucil are the safest and your best bet), but only within reason and when other measures won't do the job.
• Seeking emotional support, if needed, to help cope with symptoms that are disabling.

Some Remarkable Results

Although nutritionists like to think in terms of total diet, the simple fact is that adding just one food to your menu may be enough to keep constipation at bay. That food, of course, is bran–or one of its fiber-rich cousins.

For preventing or treating constipation, you want to eat the richest

(continued on page 154)

Fiber Facts at Your Fingertips

No doubt about it, a daily dose of bran is one of the best ways to avoid constipation. But not everyone likes it, and some people just won't eat it at all.

This list of other foods that are good sources of insoluble fiber is designed to bring a little variety into your life. Hopefully, it won't take you long to determine how many servings you'll need per day to feel your best.

Each food that follows contains about 3 grams (or more) of insoluble fiber in the serving size shown.

Food	Portion
Breads and Cereals	
All-Bran cereal	⅓ cup
Bran Buds cereal	⅓ cup
Bran Chex cereal	⅔ cup
Bread, pumpernickel	1 slice
Bread, whole wheat	2 slices
Cracklin' Oat Bran cereal	½ cup
Crunchy Bran cereal	¾ cup
Kellogg's Bran Flakes cereal	1 cup
Most cereal	⅔ cup
100% Bran cereal	⅓ cup
Post's 40% Bran cereal	1 cup
Ralston cereal, dry	⅔ cup
Ralston's 40% Bran cereal	1 cup
Wheat germ, plain	¼ cup
Fruit	
Blackberries, fresh	½ cup
Boysenberries, canned	½ cup
Cranberries, fresh	1 cup

Food	Portion
Currants, Europe, black, fresh	½ cup
Pears, canned	½ cup
Prunes, canned	⅓ cup
Raspberries, red, canned	½ cup
Raspberries, red, fresh	¾ cup

Vegetables

Artichoke, fresh, cooked	½ globe
Asparagus, frozen spears, cooked	¾ cup
Asparagus, white, canned	¾ cup
Peas, green, young, canned	½ cup
Peas, green, young, cooked, fresh	½ cup
Squash, winter, cooked	½ cup

Dry Beans and Peas

Beans, butter, cooked	½ cup
Beans, kidney, canned	½ cup
Beans, kidney, cooked	½ cup
Beans, lima, baby, frozen	½ cup
Beans, lima, canned	½ cup
Beans, pinto, cooked	½ cup
Beans, pinto, raw	⅙ cup
Cowpeas, cooked	½ cup
Peas, split, mature, cooked	½ cup

sources of insoluble fiber—wheat bran and certain fruits and vegetables—that have the ability to "bulk up" and start mobility in the intestines. To make the selection process easy for you, we've compiled "Fiber Facts at Your Fingertips," which tells you which foods are your best sources.

We also want to tell you about some proven programs for alleviating constipation simply and inexpensively. You can choose whichever of the following sounds (or tastes) best to you. Or you can modify these programs to your own tastes by adding some of the other food sources of insoluble fiber shown in the table.

Success Story Number One

Our first success story comes from Sweden. In a remarkably simple yet effective study, P. O. Sandman, R.N., and her co-workers at the University of Umea added a fiber-rich crispbread (Wasa Fiber) to the diets of elderly patients. Made from whole rye meal and wheat bran, this product can often be found in specialty stores.

As a result of eating only 2½ to 6 pieces of this small crispbread each day (the average patient took 5 pieces daily), the men and women in this study:

- Decreased their laxative consumption by 93 percent.
- Seemed to get better relief from their symptoms than they did when using laxatives.
- Maintained their normal levels of minerals in the blood, contrary to fears that the high fiber intake would interfere with mineral nutrition.

Success Story Number Two

If the taste of rye or whole wheat leaves you cold, don't be discouraged. Here's an option for you. Consider these results from J. C. Valle-Jones, M.D., who practices medicine in Burgess Hill, England. He treated constipated patients with two oat bran biscuits daily, sold in the United Kingdom under the brand name Lejfibre. And once again, the results were excellent.

- Symptoms of constipation responded dramatically to the oat bran product.
- Not one of the 50 patients complained of any side effects or inconvenience from using the fiber biscuits.

• As an added bonus, the patients lost an average of 2 pounds during the 12-week treatment.

Success Story Number Three

Want to keep things as plain, simple, and inexpensive as you can? Then take the hint from Swedish researcher Brittmarie Sandstrom and co-workers. Their patients on a geriatric ward found that 3 to 4 tablespoons of simple wheat bran daily was an easily tolerated treatment for their constipation. And the bran had no ill effects on their calcium, magnesium, zinc, or iron nutrition.

Try It!

Impressed with these success stories? There are countless more that, like these, show that nutritional approaches are ideal for treating symptoms of constipation.

The first step is finding the food or foods that work best for you. The second is to try the food in different amounts to determine your optimal intake. Of course, this will vary from one person to another and takes time to figure out. Once you have done so, however, you may not have to do anything else to keep your symptoms under control.

Now how often do you hear news that's this good?

Filling Up on Fiber

A high-fiber diet can do a lot more than curb constipation. It can promote overall digestive health and weight control, and it may even help prevent cancer. These multiple health benefits alone should be enough to get you interested in a fiber-filled diet. Here's a plan rich in insoluble fiber to help get you started.

Day 1

Breakfast
1½ ounces All-Bran cereal
  1 orange
  1 slice whole grain raisin bread
  1 teaspoon margarine
  1 cup skim milk
    coffee

Lunch
Garden sandwich (1 piece whole grain pita bread, ½ avocado, ¼ cup
  celery, 4 radishes, ¼ cup grated carrots, ½ cup green pepper, ¼ cup
  onions)
  1 apple
  1 cup skim milk

Dinner
2½ ounces lean sirloin steak (trimmed of fat)
  1 baked potato
  ½ cup broccoli
  ½ cup cauliflower
  1 tablespoon margarine
    tea of your choice

Day 2

Breakfast
1½ ounces granola cereal
  1 plum
  1 cup skim milk
    coffee

Lunch
  2 slices whole wheat bread
  ¾ cup tuna salad
  ¼ cup butterhead lettuce
  1 fresh pear
  1 cup celery
  1 cup skim milk

Snack
  3 graham crackers

Dinner
  3 ounces chicken breast (without skin)
  ½ cup brown rice
  ½ cup peas
  1 whole grain roll
  1 tablespoon apple butter
  1 tablespoon margarine
  1 cup fresh raspberries with ½ cup vanilla low-fat yogurt

Day 3

Breakfast
  1 cup cooked corn grits
  ¾ cup chopped dried dates
  1 cup 1% milk
    coffee

Lunch
  3 ounces white meat turkey
  1 slice Swiss cheese
  2 slices whole wheat bread
  ½ tablespoon reduced-calorie mayonnaise
  ¼ cup alfalfa sprouts
  1 orange
  1 cup 1% milk

Snack
  ¾ cup fresh strawberries   *(continued)*

Filling Up on Fiber–Continued

Dinner

2½ ounces lean pork chop (trimmed of fat)
  ¾ cup cooked eggplant
  1 fresh tomato with Italian dressing
  1 slice whole wheat bread
  1 teaspoon margarine
  1 cup 1% milk
  3 fresh apricots

Day 4

Breakfast

  1 ounce spoon-size shredded wheat
  1 banana
1⅓ cups skim milk
    coffee

Lunch

  2 slices whole wheat bread
  1 piece tofu (soybean curd)
  1 slice tomato
  ½ cup fresh bean sprouts
  2 tablespoons shredded cheese
  1 ounce reduced-calorie cream cheese
  1 cup skim milk

Snack

  2 plums

Dinner

  4 ounces baked flounder
Easy salad (¼ cup celery, 6 cucumber slices, ¼ cup onions, ½ tomato,
  1 tablespoon low-calorie salad dressing)
  1 ear corn
  ½ cup baked winter squash
  1 tablespoon margarine
  1 whole grain roll
  1 cup skim milk

Day 5

Breakfast
  1 cup cooked corn grits
  1 slice whole wheat bread
  1 teaspoon margarine
  1 cup fresh raspberries
  1 cup skim milk

Lunch
  ¾ cup fresh spinach
  1 tomato
  4 radishes
  ¼ cup onions
  6 cucumber slices
  1 hard-cooked egg
  2 rye crackers
  ½ cup chopped dates
    tea of your choice

Snack
  3 cups popcorn

Dinner
  3 ounces turkey breast (without skin)
  ⅓ cup canned cranberry sauce
  1 baked sweet potato
  1 slice 7-grain bread
  1 tablespoon margarine
  ½ cup peas
  1 cup skim milk

Day 6

Breakfast
  1 ounce All-Bran cereal
  ¾ cup fresh strawberries
  1 cup skim milk
    coffee

(continued)

Filling Up on Fiber–Continued

Lunch
  3 ounces chicken breast (without skin)
  1 teaspoon reduced-calorie mayonnaise
  2 slices whole wheat bread
  1 cup black bean soup
  1 cup celery
  1 cup skim milk

Snack
  ½ cup seedless raisins

Dinner
  6 oysters
  ½ cup brown rice
  ½ cup green beans
  1 tablespoon margarine
  1 cup skim milk
  ½ cup blackberries

Day 7

Breakfast
  ¾ cup orange juice
  1 slice whole wheat toast
  1 cup cooked kasha
  1 scrambled egg
  ½ cup skim milk
    coffee

Lunch
   1 cup fresh spinach
   1 tomato
   4 radishes
   ¼ cup onions
   6 cucumber slices
   2 tablespoons low-calorie Italian dressing
   1 cup skim milk
   1 cup three-bean chili

Snack
   1 baked apple
      tea of your choice

Dinner
   3 ounces chicken (without skin)
   ½ cup peas
   ¾ cup zucchini
   1 cup skim milk
   1 tablespoon margarine
   1 cup fresh raspberries

CORN

A Cornucopia of Good Things

178 calories per cup (cooked)

It's just not fair. Years ago corn got a bum rap as the food responsible for pellagra, a once-epidemic deficiency disease that results from poor niacin nutrition. As research progressed, however, it became clear that corn alone was not the direct cause of the disease. Still, the idea persists that corn has little nutrition to offer. It just isn't so.

Consider the Tarahumara Indians of Mexico: They eat corn, beans, and little else, and according to W. Virgil Brown, M.D., high blood cholesterol and hardening of the arteries are about as common there as the Tarahumara diet is here–in other words, almost nonexistent.

While we're giving corn its due, we should also mention that it is a respectable source of iron and zinc, a fine source of potassium, and very low in sodium (28 milligrams per cup). Moreover, research at the University of Nebraska has shown its protein quality is better than nutritionists originally assumed. So don't feel guilty if it's the only vegetable that your kids will eat.

At the Market: When choosing corn, insist on green husks. If the kernels are visible, make sure that they are plump and unblemished. Corn that feels hot may be old.

Kitchen Tips: Freshly picked corn has the best flavor, but, often we have to settle for whatever the supermarket has. When you bring it home, refrigerate the unhusked corn as soon you can to delay the inevitable conversion of its sugars to starch. Even under the best conditions, however, refrigerated corn may last only a day or two.

To prepare corn, husk the ears and remove silk by rubbing it away under water or with a dry vegetable brush. Bring water to a boil, immerse the ears in the pot, and boil until tender–about 7 to 10 minutes. Corn may also be steamed over water or microwaved in wet husks. You can also remove the kernels from the cob and steam them for about 5 to 8 minutes. Two medium ears of corn will yield about a cup of kernels.

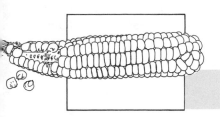

Roasted Sweet Corn Soup

8 ears roasted sweet
   corn
1 tablespoon sweet
   butter
1 medium onion,
   chopped
1 bay leaf
1 teaspoon dried thyme
2 cups milk
   sweet red and green
   pepper slivers for
   garnish

Remove corn from cobs. (One easy way is to hold the ear vertically with the bottom end resting on a cutting board. Then, starting from the top, use a sharp paring knife to shave off the kernels.)

In a large nonstick skillet, melt butter over medium heat. Add onion, bay leaf, and thyme and sauté until onion is fragrant and wilted, about 5 minutes.

Place onion in a food processor or blender. (Discard the bay leaf.) Add corn and ½ cup of milk and process until the mixture is very smooth.

Pour the mixture into a large saucepan and add remaining milk. Heat very gently for about 5 minutes; don't boil. Serve hot, garnished with pepper slivers.

Note: To roast the corn, strip off leaves and wrap in foil. Bake in a preheated 375°F oven for 30 to 40 minutes, or until tender.

Makes 4 servings

Fresh baby corn can be grilled right in the husk. It needs little cooking time, yet turns out delicious.

Accent on Enjoyment: Want to do something different with this familiar vegetable? Here are some ideas.

- Stuff green peppers with corn kernels, mild cheese, and sweet onions.
- Toss corn kernels into a green salad, marinated vegetable salad, or chicken salad.
- Sprinkle corn on the cob with crushed tarragon or basil instead of plain old salt.

Ideas for Flavoring Popcorn

- Toss popcorn with a mixture of Worcestershire sauce and curry powder. Use just enough to lightly moisten the kernels. Then add some raisins and peanuts and bake at 300°F until dry, about 45 minutes, stirring several times. Serve warm or at room temperature.
- Spread popcorn out on a baking sheet and sprinkle with some grated cheddar cheese. (You will need about ⅓ cup of cheese for 4 cups of corn.) Bake at 350°F until the cheese melts, about 10 minutes. Serve hot.
- Toss popcorn with chopped dried fruits such as dates, apricots, and currants or seeds such as sunflower and sesame.

COTTAGE CHEESE, LOW-FAT

The Ladies' Choice

205 calories per cup (2% fat)

If you spend much time analyzing food habits, it becomes obvious that gender plays a role in food choices. We don't know why, but some foods clearly appeal to men more than to women, and vice versa.

Cottage cheese is a case in point. Women are much more likely to eat it regularly. And in our view, it serves them well. Women are far more vulnerable to osteoporosis than men are. And low-fat cottage cheese is good for bone health—especially for the many women who can't drink milk or prefer not to.

If you're up on the calcium content of food, describing cottage cheese as "good" may sound odd to you. It's true that cottage cheese contains substantially less calcium than milk, yogurt, or hard cheeses. But in our view, 150 milligrams per cup is respectable—especially because it comes with less fat than the calcium in whole milk and hard cheeses. Nutritionists have long believed that high fat intake can impair calcium absorption.

We rate low-fat cottage cheese as favorable for bone health for another reason. Many high-protein foods, especially meats, contain large amounts of the mineral phosphorus. Although phosphorus is an essential mineral, diets that contain far more phosphorus than calcium are suspected of encouraging osteoporosis. As Morris Notelovitz, M.D., noted bone expert, points out, Eskimos seem especially prone to osteoporosis and often develop it at an unusually young age. Their diet—which contains far more phosphorus than calcium—is suspect.

Unlike flesh foods, however, cottage cheese contains a fairly favorable balance between phosphorus and calcium. At the same time, it's admirably low in fat and calories, yet rich in riboflavin—a B vitamin.

At the Market: Check the expiration date before buying cottage cheese. If you want calcium, choose a brand that is partially creamed—the label will indicate a milk fat content of 1 to 2 percent. If you don't want salt, look for an unsalted brand.

Kitchen Tips: Cottage cheese, of course, requires refrigeration. To make it into the smoothest puree for dips and spreads, press it through a sieve with the back of a spoon. To vary the flavor, try dill, chives, scallions, or tomatoes—or a combination of these.

Accent on Enjoyment: Few people think of cottage cheese as sinfully delicious, but once you learn how to use it in cooking, you'd be amazed how great foods made with it can taste. Some of our favorite uses are to make reduced-fat cheesecakes, tender pancakes, and creamy dips. We regularly substitute it for some of the cream cheese in recipes and also like to puree it and add fresh crushed herbs for a calorie-conscious dip.

We also use low-fat cottage cheese in casseroles and fillings—but rarely by itself. Because of its low fat content, cottage cheese breaks or curdles when heated. To ensure good texture—as well as taste—we mix low-fat cottage cheese with an equal amount of a higher-fat cheese such as part-skim ricotta. The results are excellent.

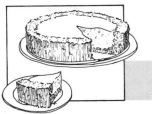

Maple-Pumpkin Cheesecake

1 pound low-fat cottage
    cheese
½ cup plain low-fat
    yogurt
¾ cup pumpkin puree
¼ cup flour
3 eggs
1 teaspoon vanilla extract
¼ cup maple syrup
½ teaspoon pumpkin-pie
    spice
1 8-inch prepared
    graham cracker
    crust

Preheat the oven to 325° F.

Place cottage cheese, yogurt, pumpkin, flour, eggs, vanilla, maple syrup, and spice into a food processor while the motor is running. (Do this through the feed tube, allowing time for each ingredient to combine before adding the next.) Process until smooth, then pour the mixture into the crust, using a rubber spatula to spread it evenly.

Place the pie in the middle of the oven and bake for about 50 minutes. Let it cool before serving. Store any leftovers in the refrigerator.

Makes 10 to 12 servings

COWPEAS

A Southern Delight

190 calories per cup (cooked)

Tasty, economical, and nutritious–that's what cowpeas are. You may know them by their other name, of course–black-eyed peas. If you're like the many southerners who have been eating them for years, you've done well. Each serving is rich in fiber, protein, potassium, and iron, yet low in fat and sodium (20 milligrams per cup).

At the Market: Good cowpeas are evenly sized, creamy white, and oval shaped, with a small black eye.

Kitchen Tips: Store cowpeas in the refrigerator in a tightly covered container. A cup of dry peas yields about 2½ cups when cooked.

To prepare, use 4 cups of water per cup of peas. Cook on the stove for about an hour or pressure-cook for about 10 minutes.

Accent on Enjoyment: Cowpeas are good:

- Added to soups and ragouts.
- In marinated bean or vegetable salads.
- Tossed with shredded spinach, garlic, and olive oil.

In some parts of the United States, it's considered good luck to eat cowpeas on New Year's Day. Considering their health benefits, we think it's a fine idea *any* day of the year.

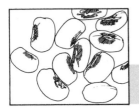

Pea and Spinach Toss

2 cups cooked cowpeas
1 cup minced fresh
    spinach or kale
1 carrot, minced
¼ cup minced leeks
    juice and pulp of
        ½ lemon
1 teaspoon red wine
    vinegar
½ teaspoon dried basil
½ teaspoon dried sage
2 teaspoons olive oil
    pinch of dry mustard

If you use canned cowpeas, rinse them, then pat dry. Place them in a large bowl along with spinach or kale, carrot, and leeks.

In a small bowl, whisk lemon juice and pulp, vinegar, basil, sage, oil, and mustard. Pour over pea mixture and toss to combine.

Makes 4 servings

DENTAL PROBLEMS

The Right Food Each Day Keeps the Dentist Away

Is there anyone who is unaware that sugar promotes tooth decay? Certainly, the connection is nothing new, although more recent research shows that the amount of sugar eaten is not what matters most. The consistency of sugar-rich foods appears to be the biggest factor: Sticky, sugary foods that adhere readily to teeth are by far the most notable troublemakers.

In this book, though, we promised to accentuate the positive. So rather than repeat what you already know about the damage done by sticky, sugary foods, we'd like to focus on some foods that have won attention as having protective, or at least low decay-producing, potential.

Setting a Trap for Decay

For the story, let's turn to a British authority on dental health, R. J. Andlaw, Ph.D. After reviewing the many scientific reports regarding food and tooth decay, Dr. Andlaw concluded that several have little or no decay-producing potential. They are cheese, meats, nuts, carrots, and fruits.

Of these foods cited by Dr. Andlaw, apples and cheese have had the most attention. In the entry on apples, beginning on page 37, we've already mentioned the possibility that apples clean debris away from teeth, protecting dental health in the process. As for cheese, William Bowen, D.D.S., of the University of Rochester, says that it appears to help neutralize the harm done by decay-producing acids in the mouth.

Of course, hard cheeses are usually high in fat and calories, and nutritionists advise cutting back on them. Is this another dilemma, where eating a food helps one problem but causes another? We have our doubts. According to research at the University of Glasgow and University of Newcastle upon Tyne, the amount of cheese needed to promote dental health may be modest—as little as a ½-ounce serving. That's not excessive in a normal diet.

And, of course, keep in mind that fruits that are processed in a way that makes them stickier than fruit off the tree are an exception to the rule. As far as your teeth are concerned, there's a big difference between raisins and fresh fruit.

Great Gums

According to some, there's nothing good to be said about aging. But your teeth know that this pessimistic attitude is wrong. Under normal conditions, teeth actually become more resistant to decay with age.

A process called mineralization is the key. As we age, our bodies deposit more and more mineral in our teeth, making them better able to fend off the decay-producing acids that cause cavities. That's why most of us need fewer fillings in adult life than during childhood.

Despite better resistance to decay, adults are not home free. They simply have a different set of dental problems than children do. Far and away the most common is periodontal disease. Swollen gums that bleed easily are a frequent symptom. Worse is loss of bone from the jaw, which can ultimately lead to loss of teeth. Obviously, if teeth aren't firmly anchored, you're in for trouble. Tens of millions of Americans have learned this the hard way: They've already lost their teeth to periodontal disease.

Like so many age-related problems, periodontal disease has more than one cause, and nutrition is but one of them. And of course, there is disagreement as to how big a role nutrition plays. Authorities agree, however, that at the very least, nutrition does have an indirect part in the story, and some consider it to have a lead role.

Part Consensus, Part Controversy

The first recommendation for healthy gums is to get your fair share of vitamins and minerals. According to the American Dental Association's *Guide to Dental Health,* poor nutrition alone will not cause periodontal disease, but it is suspected of speeding up the course of the disease and making symptoms more severe. That's reason enough, say the authors, to ensure good intake of foods rich in vitamins and minerals. Vitamin C, in particular, has been cited as especially important for keeping gums healthy.

What's controversial among the experts is the role of calcium in periodontal health. Some believe that periodontal disease is related to osteoporosis –that loss of bone from the jaw is part of the same process that later shows up as stooped posture or wrist or hip fractures.

While working at the Veterans Administration Hospital in Sepulveda, California, Leo Lutwak, M.D., Ph.D., put this idea to the test. He and his co-workers supplemented some of their periodontal disease patients with calcium–at a dose of 1,000 milligrams per day. Other patients received a blank pill that contained no calcium. After a year of treatment, the calcium group showed significant improvement in periodontal health. Those who had taken the placebo, however, showed no such improvement.

To us, these are impressive results. We know that others consider them speculative. But think about the big picture. Calcium benefits health in so many ways that even if it proves to be without value for dental problems, you can still come out ahead. We're concerned that waiting for definitive results might mean losing valuable time.

The same nutritional strategy recommended for preventing osteoporosis can be used to promote periodontal health. This approach–a healthy intake of vitamin D and calcium as well as a good balance between the minerals calcium and phosphorus–is detailed in the entry on osteoporosis. A week's worth of meal plans constructed around these goals is presented in "A Week of Bone-Building Meals," beginning on page 316.

Eroded Enamel

Periodontal disease is far more likely to land you in the dentist's chair than another food-related problem called dental erosion. But both are worth trying to avoid, because treatment can be time-consuming and expensive.

Dental erosion refers to a wearing away of the tooth enamel. However, it is not the same as the garden-variety tooth decay that we all know so well. The tooth decay process depends heavily on sugar and refined carbohydrates. By contrast, the list of nutritional factors linked to dental erosion bears little resemblance to the list of "most wanted" decay-producing foods. In addition, nonnutritional factors–certain medicines or occupational exposure–can also be the cause.

Very acidic foods and beverages such as citrus juices and soft drinks are most frequently linked to dental erosion. Yet not everyone reacts the same way to these foods; consuming a lot of these foods does not guarantee that the teeth will suffer. But should you have this trouble, the list in "Putting Beverages to the Acid Test," will give you an idea of the beverages that are most acidic.

A related factor that deserves mention is vitamin C. This popular vitamin is known for promoting dental health–and it deserves the credit. A few dentists have warned that in chewable form, however, supplements of the vitamin may actually promote erosion. The most dramatic case was reported by John Guinta, D.D.S., professor of dentistry at Tufts University in Medford, Massachusetts.

Dr. Guinta reported the story of a 30-year-old woman diagnosed as having severe dental erosion that would require 12 crowns to repair. A second opinion confirmed the diagnosis. The concerned patient naturally wanted to

Putting Beverages to the Acid Test

Want to cut back on acidic beverages? Here's a list that divides them into three categories, based on the degree of acidity. Although these beverages are most frequently mentioned as dietary causes of dental erosion, remember that citrus fruits, pickled foods, sourballs, and mints have also been cited as possible contributors.

Most Acidic	Moderately Acidic	Slightly Acidic
Apple juice	Apricot nectar	Cocoa (instant)
Cola soft drink	Club soda	Half-and-half
Cranberry juice	Coffee (brewed)	Skim milk
Diet cola	Peach nectar	Tea (instant)
Ginger ale	Pear nectar	Whole milk
Grapefruit juice	Prune juice	
Grape juice	Sanka (instant)	
Orange drink	Tomato juice	
Orange juice		
Orange soda		
Pineapple juice		
7-Up		

know the cause of her woes. It took some detective work, but Dr. Guinta was able to pinpoint her long-term use of large amounts of chewable vitamin C as the most likely cause. To convince her, he had to expose a human tooth to vitamin C in his laboratory; on seeing the damage it did to the enamel, she decided to stop using chewable C.

Although we know of no other reports quite like this one, we're hesitant to dismiss this issue. We take heart that modest intakes of chewable C–100 or 200 milligrams, for instance–have never been linked to problems. But if you want to play it safe, we suggest that you choose a C supplement that is swallowed, not chewed. The higher your dose, the more strongly we'd advise against taking chewable vitamin C.

DIABETES

Fiber to the Rescue

To a doctor, *diabetes* is a general term that means two things: extreme thirst and excessive urination. In a comprehensive medical dictionary, you will find about a dozen different conditions listed under diabetes. In common usage, though, diabetes is shorthand for the most common form: diabetes mellitus, or DM.

DM–as the doctors like to call it–is a disorder of carbohydrate metabolism. It's this form of diabetes that calls for a sound nutritional strategy. So from here on, when we say diabetes, we're referring to the DM form of the disease.

The Two Types

The DM form of diabetes has two types: Type I and Type II. Some experts refer to Type I as juvenile-onset diabetes or insulin-dependent diabetes. The corresponding terms for Type II are maturity-onset diabetes or noninsulin-dependent diabetes. As these terms imply, Type I diabetes is usually a childhood disease, while Type II affects mostly adults. Nonetheless, both Type I and Type II result from problems with the all-important hormone called insulin.

Type I diabetes is marked by *deficiency* of insulin–a problem that usually requires that insulin injections be taken to make up for the shortage. Type II diabetes is marked by an *excess* of insulin–but it is insulin that doesn't work as it should. Apparently, Type II diabetics have become resistant to the action of their own insulin.

Type I diabetes is relatively rare compared to Type II. Of the more than five million Americans who have diabetes, fewer than 10 percent have Type I. The diabetes epidemic is the result of the widespread Type II form–the one that looks easiest to prevent and treat.

Cornering the Culprit

What causes diabetes? We don't know for sure, and as with most chronic diseases, no one factor is likely to explain all cases. Experts do have their suspicions, though, about the probable causes. The following are highest on their list.

Genes. Family history strongly influences the chances of developing diabetes.

Obesity. The vast majority of Type II diabetics are overweight, and weight loss often dramatically improves control of their diabetes.

Viruses. Researchers are pursuing leads that viral factors may set the stage for diabetes to develop later.

Medication or other diseases. Sometimes diabetes develops as a result of other pancreatic diseases, liver disease, or long-term use of certain prescription drugs.

Sugar Blues: The Telltale Signs

Treatment of diabetes is better than ever. Before anyone can take advantage of the new advances, however, a firm diagnosis is a must.

Naturally, laboratory testing is needed to confirm the presence of diabetes. Nevertheless, there are signs that no laboratory can document as well as you can. Be alert for:

Excessive urination. When too much sugar accumulates in the blood, this is usually the first sign.

Thirst, hunger, and weight loss. If diabetes is not diagnosed and treated when the earliest sign appears, this trio of symptoms will often follow.

Recurrent yeast infections in women. Vaginal yeasts thrive on the sugary urine of female diabetics. A stubborn yeast infection, or one that keeps coming back, calls for a test to rule out diabetes.

Vomiting, hunger for air, and coma. These three symptoms are signs of Type I diabetes that is worsening. The key to preventing them? Seeking treatment when the first signs of illness appear. We may not be able to prevent Type I diabetes yet, but preventing symptoms such as these is an important first step.

Dr. Anderson's Amazing Diet

For decades, the low-carbohydrate diet was the standard prescribed for virtually all diabetics. It seemed to make good sense: If you couldn't process carbohydrates normally, avoiding them seemed like the thing to do. Well, what sounded great in theory turned out to have its shortcomings. Although the low-carbohydrate diet seemed to help keep the blood sugar in better control than typical diets, diabetics also were experiencing far higher rates of heart attack than nondiabetics.

Enter James W. Anderson, M.D., a professor at the University of Kentucky School of Medicine. Alarmed by the poor heart health of his (and everyone else's) diabetic patients, Dr. Anderson began experimenting with a different nutritional approach. Instead of limiting all carbohydrates, Dr. Anderson's diet restricted sugars but not the complex carbohydrates in beans, grains, and vegetables.

The results were remarkable. Although designed to protect the heart health of diabetics, the fiber-rich, high-carbohydrate diet proved to be the most important advance since insulin injections! Dr. Anderson and others have now tested the diet many times, but we'd like to cite just one study that we think says it all.

The study dates back to the early 1970s, when the reigning diabetic diet was restricted in carbohydrates. Dr. Anderson and his co-workers compared the effects of this traditional diabetic diet to a high-carbohydrate, high-fiber (HCF) diet in 13 diabetic patients. Here are their exciting results.

- Average blood sugar dropped from 179 on the standard diet to 119 on the high-carbohydrate diet.
- Five of the men needed pills to control their condition while on the standard diet but were able to stop taking this medication after a few weeks on the HCF diet.
- The eight remaining men needed insulin injections on the standard diet, but five of them were able to reduce or eliminate their need with the HCF diet.
- Blood cholesterol levels improved dramatically with the HCF diet, and blood triglyceride levels dropped about 15 percent.

And what about taste? In a follow-up study, dietitian Linda Story from Dr. Anderson's group looked at the acceptability of the HCF diet. She rated the adherence of subjects who followed the diet for four years as "good to excellent" in a full 80 percent of the patients.

What Makes It Work?

Some people only care about *what* works. But others want to know *why* things work. If you're in this latter category, this section is for you.

Diabetes experts have spent years trying to understand how low-fat diets and fiber-rich diets work their wonders. At this point, it looks like there are several explanations.

- Diets high in starches (not sugars) help the body process glucose more efficiently.
- Foods rich in soluble fiber slow the absorption of food into the blood. This helps to prevent sharp swings in blood sugar levels.
- Burning sugar is easier when the diet is low in fat because the body doesn't have to channel as much effort into metabolizing fats. So there is more freedom to concentrate on processing carbohydrates.
- High-fiber, low-fat diets generally promote weight loss, which in turn lessens the severity of Type II diabetes.

Diet and Diabetes: One Man's Victory

If you're diabetic and could use an upbeat story to lift your spirits, here it is. This inspiring tale, written by James W. Anderson, M.D., was published in *Diabetes and Nutrition News*. No one knows how to turn diabetes around with nutrition as Dr. Anderson. His patient's story speaks for itself!

In 1974 John Moore, a 38-year-old man with Type I (insulin-dependent) diabetes of 14 years' duration, entered the new research unit at the Lexington Veterans Administration Medical Center. On a traditional American Diabetes Association-type diabetes diet in the hospital he needed about 55 units of insulin daily for good blood glucose control. He was the first individual we treated with our new high-carbohydrate and high-fiber (HCF) diet. This diet provided substantially more carbohydrate, one-fourth as much fat, and four times as much fiber as his traditional American Diabetes Association-type diet.

His insulin dose decreased by 16 percent to 46 units daily and his blood glucose values were improved with the HCF diet. His cholesterol decreased from 180 to 131 mg/dl with the HCF diet.

Designing a Diet

Diabetic diets need to be customized to individual calorie and nutritional needs. That's why we haven't listed meal plans here. If you want the general flavor of a low-fat, high-fiber diet, however, take a look at the meal plans in "Putting Prevention on the Menu," beginning on page 100, accompanying the cancer entry; these are fairly low in fat and fairly rich in sugar-controlling soluble fiber.

You'll also find a very low-fat meal plan in "Diet for a Picky Gallbladder," beginning on page 210, accompanying the entry on gallbladder disease. These menu plans are moderately high in fiber and can be made more so by substituting whole grain foods for refined grain products. Why add whole grains, rich in insoluble fiber, when it's the soluble form that helps control blood

Because his diabetes was better managed and his blood lipids [such as cholesterol and triglycerides] were lower, we developed a high-fiber diet for him to use at home; this diet provided 55 percent of energy as carbohydrate, 20 percent as protein, and 25 percent as fat, with about 50 grams of dietary fiber per day (compared to an average American fiber intake of 15 grams per day). With this diet his diabetes was well managed and his blood lipids were lower. Currently his diabetes is well-controlled on 36 units of insulin daily.

Not only did the high-fiber diet improve his diabetes control, it also made him feel better. He had fewer insulin reactions and had more energy. Lowering fat intake and blood fat levels often produce this "feeling better" state.

Diabetes and Nutrition News is a newsletter for anyone interested in nutritional treatment of diabetes. To subscribe, contact HCF Diabetes Foundation, P.O. Box 22124, Lexington, Kentucky 40522. The foundation also publishes excellent handbooks on diabetes management for patients and professionals. For a list of current publications, send your request to the foundation along with a self-addressed, stamped envelope.

sugar? Actually, insoluble fibers show benefits to diabetics, too, even though they don't directly affect blood sugar as does soluble fiber in fruits, vegetables, beans, and oats.

Early Efforts Pay Off

No matter how you look at it, learning to follow a diabetic diet takes effort. Is it worth the trouble? Consider the facts and decide for yourself!

Good control of diabetes brings two kinds of benefits. First and foremost, it keeps "acute complications" at bay. These are the life-threatening reactions that occur when the blood sugar surges out of control.

Chronic complications of diabetes–those that develop slowly and gradually over the course of many years–affect far more people, however. And they can be especially troublesome. Now we ask you, does knowing that following a diet that helps prevent problems such as heart attack, kidney failure, gangrene, and blindness give you the motivation that you need to keep at it?

And while you're at it, we have one final request. Don't go it alone. Diabetes doesn't go away like a cold does; it's a chronic condition. You may start to feel much better as you bring your condition into better control, but do yourself a favor and resist the temptation to make any changes in your medication by yourself. The new nutritional breakthroughs are enormously important. But they're not a cure, or a substitute for medical follow-up.

DIVERTICULAR DISEASE

Bran Scores Again

Diverticulosis and diverticulitis are related conditions known collectively as diverticular disease. (Say that three times fast!) Diverticulosis always comes first; when it does, the object is to keep it from progressing to the more troublesome condition called diverticulitis.

First, some definitions are in order. In diverticulosis, small, saclike swellings develop in the wall of the large intestine. Imagine them as little pouches that have pushed out of the intestinal wall. Now imagine these small sacs becoming extremely irritated. This more severe stage–inflammation of the saclike areas–is diverticulitis.

The Who, What, and Why

How common is diverticular disease? That depends on where you live. In the United States, for instance, about 30 to 40 percent of adults aged 50 or older are affected.

The symptoms of diverticulosis vary from one person to the next. In fact, some of those affected have no symptoms at all. Others, however, suffer with cramping, pain, constipation, and/or diarrhea. However troublesome these symptoms may be, the condition is neither contagious nor related to cancer.

For years, diverticular disease was accepted as an inevitable part of aging. But that idea, like so many others about aging, has been turned on its head–probably for good. Consider these recent findings from Dr. O. Manousus and co-workers at Athens Medical School, who compared food habits between patients with and without diverticulosis.

- Diverticulosis patients said they ate less brown bread, vegetables, potatoes, and fruit than the subjects free of the disorder.
- Those with diverticulosis also used meat and dairy products more frequently than the others.
- Respondents who rarely ate vegetables and frequently consumed meat were as much as 50 percent more likely to develop diverticulosis as those who ate vegetables often and meat infrequently.

Findings such as these tell us that diverticulosis isn't simply an inescapable part of aging; rather, the way we live affects our chances of developing the condition. These results also tell us that carbohydrate-rich diets probably help prevent diverticulosis. And not surprisingly, a similar kind of diet has also proven to be one of the best treatments. We'll look at the details next.

The Fiber Factor

It's just one of those things. Sometimes the very food suspected of aggravating a disease proves to be helpful rather than harmful. And nutritional treatment of diverticulosis is a case in point. For years, a low-fiber diet was a standard part of treatment. But along came skeptics such as Denis Burkitt, M.D., the British physician who pointed out that digestive diseases like this one are less common where diets are high in fiber.

A few doctors decided to put Dr. Burkitt's theory to the test. Sure enough, they found:

• Adding about an ounce of bran daily to the usual diet of 40 patients with diverticular disease resulted in notable improvement. The 40 patients were studied by British researchers A. J. M. Brodribb and D. M. Hymphreys, and they followed the diet for an average of eight months.
• Supplementing normal diets with bran tablets that provided the equivalent of about 3 tablespoons of bran daily brought at least partial relief to each of 20 diverticular disease patients studied by British researchers Dr. I. Taylor and Dr. H. L. Duthie.
• Replacing the bran tablets used by Dr. Taylor and Dr. Duthie with a high-fiber diet that included supplemental bran was also a successful treatment that improved the condition of all patients.

Great, you say, but what about all of the people who don't like bran? As an alternative, other foods rich in insoluble fiber can be tried; these, too, may help. (See the list of foods high in insoluble fiber that appear in "Fiber Facts at Your Fingertips," on page 152.) Another option for increasing your fiber intake is a bulking agent, such as Metamucil. You can find a selection of these in any drugstore. And if none of these do the job well enough, your doctor may add a painkiller or tranquilizer to your regimen to relieve severe pain and discomfort.

From Bad to Worse

Some people who have diverticulosis have all the luck—they don't even know that they have the condition. For others, though, diverticulosis not only causes troublesome symptoms but also progresses to diverticulitis. This happens to about one of every eight to ten patients.

You don't have to worry that diverticulitis will go unnoticed. It makes its presence known–with abdominal pain and tenderness, fever, and change in bowel habits. More worrisome are further complications–severe inflammation, excessive bleeding, or development of an obstruction in the digestive tract.

Obviously, these possibilities mean that prompt medical attention is essential. Hopefully, bed rest, antibiotics, and/or intravenous fluids will bring things under control. Occasionally, however, the doctor may decide that surgery offers the best hope for alleviating the condition.

FIBROCYSTIC BREAST DISEASE

The Food Connection

For some women, it's a monthly ritual. Each month, on cue, breast pain and tenderness make their presence felt. Suddenly a lump–sometimes several –can be felt in the breast. Or lumps already present get dramatically bigger. But shortly after the menstrual period begins, the symptoms subside. The troubles seem to vanish as quickly as they came.

Describe a pattern like this to your doctors, and they will tell you, "Sounds like fibrocystic breast disease (FBD)." Or, they might call it chronic cystic mastitis or mammary dysplasia. Some people just refer to the syndrome as breast lumps. Take your choice!

If you have breast lumps that cycle with your menstrual period, you've got plenty of company. A majority of women–as many as 80 percent–experience the condition at least occasionally. Can something that regularly happens to so many truly be considered a disease? Some experts say no, and insist that FBD is a normal condition during a woman's childbearing years. But others warn against taking too cavalier an attitude. They say that for some women, the pain of FBD or its potential for complications is too serious to ignore.

Facts about Fibrocystic Disease

Before looking at nutritional approches to FBD, a few basic facts are in order.

- Hormonal changes that occur during the menstrual cycle are the cause of FBD. More specifically, doctors suspect that an imbalance of estrogens over progesterone is responsible.
- Early signs of FBD may occur in women aged 20 to 25, but most patients are in the 30-plus age range. Symptoms are usually most severe during the years that precede menopause.
- Women who suffer from symptoms of premenstrual syndrome are predisposed to FBD also, no doubt because both conditions are influenced by similar hormonal factors.

182

- If you began menstruating at a young age, do not use birth control pills, have no children, or have a history of miscarriage, your chances of developing FBD are increased.
- Ten to 15 percent of those who have FBD experience no discomfort, while in others the pain may become constant and severe. Heavy menstrual bleeding, ovarian cysts, and irregular periods commonly accompany this pain in more severely affected women.
- Although FBD originates in the breasts, the pain and tenderness may spread to the underarm area, where the lymph glands may become enlarged at the same time that other symptoms occur.

The Cancer Question

Here's one more fact—the one we consider most important: Fibrocystic lumps are *noncancerous*. That is, they are classified as benign by tumor experts. Of course, it's essential to have firm evidence that a lump is fibrocystic before taking reassurance on this point.

For starters, here are some general guidelines: If the lumpy area causes pain, or the lumps fluctuate in size or occur in multiples, the condition is more likely to be FBD than cancer. Secretion of fluid from nipples also occurs in women who have FBD, but you should see a doctor right away if the fluid has a bloody appearance; this may be a warning of cancer.

To rule out cancer for sure, however, one or more tests will be needed. These can include the following.

Biopsy. Often a simple needle biopsy done in the doctor's office is sufficient, but sometimes surgical biopsy may be needed.

Ultrasound. This high-tech breakthrough spots FBD without requiring that the skin be broken or exposed to x-rays.

Mammogram. This familiar x-ray technique can reveal both FBD and breast cancer.

All of these have good track records for detecting FBD and will spot 80 percent or more of cases.

FBD and Future Health

For years conventional wisdom has held that although benign, FBD is an omen that a woman is at greater risk of developing breast cancer someday. But thanks to new research, the picture now looks rosier.

According to the College of American Pathologists, FBD is not one condition but many. Researchers have identified 13 different kinds of fibrocystic tissue. Most forms appear not to increase breast cancer risk, although an estimated 25 percent of affected women have a form that does. A biopsy of the breast tissue will determine whether the type of fibrocystic tissue present is the higher-risk variety.

Helmuth Vorherr, M.D., an authority on FBD at the University of New Mexico School of Medicine, recommends that women with lumps such as these have their breasts examined by a physician every four to six months. In addition, he recommends a mammogram every one to two years for women with signs of higher risk.

The Caffeine Question

Nutrition has become a hot issue in FBD for two reasons. First, some research has linked fibrocystic disease to consumption of coffee, tea, and chocolate. These foods contain caffeine or related compounds suspected of playing a role in the condition.

Wendy Levinson, M.D., and Patrick M. Dunn, M.D., of the Good Samaritan Hospital in Portland, Oregon, reviewed available reports of this link. According to Dr. Levinson and Dr. Dunn, the two best studies on caffeine and FBD reached conflicting conclusions: One supported the link and the other did not.

Nevertheless, some women have reported that restricting these foods in their diets helps control their condition. John Minton, M.D., a surgeon at Ohio State University, asked 47 FBD patients to stop all caffeine-containing foods and drugs. Of the 20 women who completely eliminated these items, about two-thirds recovered fully–that is, they were lump free within six months. It's not worth waiting until this controversy is resolved; if you have FBD, it certainly can't hurt to try this approach and see if it works for you.

Recently, still another nutritional approach has been proposed. In 1987, David P. Rose and his co-workers at the American Health Foundation reported that lower fat intakes by women suffering from FBD improved their hormone profile. Presumably, FBD symptoms would also improve with long-term use of the low-fat diet that they tested, but this remains to be tested. Very low-fat meal plans are given in "Diet for a Picky Gallbladder," beginning on page 210. As they contain even less fat than the diets tested by these researchers, you need not follow them too rigidly if you decide to see whether they can affect your FBD symptoms.

Counting Up Your Caffeine Intake

Are you having problems with fibrocystic breast lumps? Some women have reported that *eliminating* caffeine from their diets noticeably improved the conditions.

The following should give you an idea where the caffeine in your diet is coming from. Values are per 6-ounce serving.

Beverage	Caffeine (mg)
Filtered drip coffee	110
Percolated coffee	85
Dark chocolate	80
Instant coffee	65
Leaf tea	40
Milk chocolate	35
Cola (not decaffeinated)	25
Cocoa	15
Decaffeinated coffee	2

NOTE: Coffee made from South American beans usually contains about half as much caffeine as that made from the robusta beans from Africa or India.

Enter Vitamin E

It's no secret that vitamin E has its share of skeptics. Imagine their surprise when the September 1980 issue of the *Journal of the American Medical Association* carried a headline that proclaimed "Vitamin E Relieves Most Cystic Breast Disease."

The article that followed cited work by Robert London, M.D., and his associates at Johns Hopkins University School of Medicine. They treated FBD patients with 600 international units of vitamin E daily for eight weeks. Twenty-two of the 26 women experienced fair to good improvement in their symptoms.

According to Dr. Vorherr, vitamin E is most valuable in FBD patients who have abnormal blood fats—that is, low levels of "good" HDL cholesterol or excessive levels of "bad" LDL cholesterol. He treats these women with both hormones and 400 to 1,200 international units daily of vitamin E. "It has no side effects," he says of the vitamin E, "and it can only be beneficial."

The Sure Cure

Is there a sure cure for FBD? Well, sort of. It's menopause. After menopause, a woman's ovaries secrete small amounts of estrogen for three to five years. After that, estrogen production all but ceases, and problems with FBD fall off dramatically.

Of course, if you take estrogen replacement therapy after menopause, FBD may persist. In fact, it commonly does. Unless the FBD is more trouble-some than the condition that called for estrogen therapy, however, it's unlikely to be grounds for stopping treatment.

If waiting until menopause isn't acceptable and other approaches fail, hormone treatment is another very successful option. The success rate with these medications is impressive.

Says Dr. Vorherr, "With thorough diagnostic evaluation, appropriate medication, and close follow-up, treatment success can be achieved in almost every [FBD] patient." He found that with treatment, FBD usually clears up in three to six months.

FIGS

Figure on Fiber

37 calories per medium fig (raw)
143 calories per 3 figs (dried)

Figs may have a biblical background, but they are a superfood of modern times. Years ago, nutritionists rarely gave them a thought, because their vitamin and mineral levels were too low to be impressive. But now that the focus is on eating more fiber and less fat and sodium, figs fit perfectly into the scheme of things.

A recent study on fiber–something that figs have aplenty–confirmed the rumor that figs contribute a feeling of fullness. June Kelsay, Ph.D., of the U.S. Department of Agriculture, tested three diets containing progressively higher amounts of fiber from foods such as figs and pumpkins. Although the calorie count of each diet was the same, her subjects complained of being asked to eat too much food when on the diet that contained more figs and fiber-rich foods. Dieters–take note!

At the Market: Figs come in light and dark varieties. The tastiest light varieties are the Calmyrnas, which should be golden yellow, and the Kadotas, which should be yellow-green. The best-tasting dark figs are the Brown Turkey and the Black Mission, which should be purple-black in color. Regardless of variety, fresh figs should be firm to the touch and have a wonderful fragrance. Avoid fresh figs that are soft or splotched with brown.

Kitchen Tips: Store figs in the refrigerator, loosely covered. They will not keep long, however–perhaps a few days. (You'll probably eat them a lot sooner.)

Accent on Enjoyment: Make room for figs on your menu with some of these ideas.

- Poach in fruit juices and serve warm or chilled.
- Serve whole, halved, or sliced with other fruits and cheeses.
- Puree and use as a filling for cookies and bars.
- Slice and sauté with strips of chicken.
- Stuff them with mild white cheese.

187

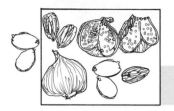

Almond-Fig Compote

12 ounces dried black
    figs
½ cup apricot nectar
1 tablespoon lemon
    juice
2 drops almond extract
2 tablespoons toasted
    slivered almonds

If the figs have stems, use a sharp paring knife to remove them. Then place figs in a nonmetal bowl and add nectar and juice. Cover and marinate in the refrigerator overnight.

In a small saucepan, simmer figs, marinade, and almond extract over medium heat until figs are heated through and plump, about 4 minutes. Place in individual serving bowls and sprinkle with almonds. Serve hot or warm for breakfast or dessert.

Makes 4 servings

FISH

Get Hooked on Health

(See also *Shellfish*)

Abalone: 90 calories per 4 ounces (canned)

Bass, striped: about 130 calories per 4 ounces (cooked)

Bluefish: 180 calories per 4 ounces (baked with butter)

Cod: 109 calories per 4 ounces (broiled without fat)

Croaker: 150 calories per 4 ounces (baked)

Flounder: 105 calories per 4 ounces (cooked without fat)

Haddock: 89 calories per 4 ounces (raw)

Halibut: 192 calories per 4 ounces (raw)

Herring: 236 calories per 4 ounces (canned)

Mackerel: 207 calories per 4 ounces (canned)

Perch: 113 calories per 4 ounces (raw)

Pollack: 107 calories per 4 ounces (raw)

Salmon: 233 calories per 4.5-ounce steak (cooked)

Sardines: 181 calories per 4 ounces (raw)

Shad: 226 calories per 4 ounces (baked with butter)

Swordfish: 200 calories per 4 ounces (cooked)

Trout, brook: 114 calories per 4 ounces (raw)

Tuna, fresh: 150 calories per 4 ounces (raw)

Tuna, water-packed: 126 calories per 3½ ounces

Whitefish: 175 calories per 4 ounces (raw)

Fish is in like never before, and its fan club just keeps growing. The latest additions to its list of followers are heart-health experts who have found, to their surprise, that the benefits of fish are even greater than previously realized.

The turning point came in 1985, when the *New England Journal of Medicine* published a series of papers linking fish to better heart health. So

189

impressive were the findings that a journal editorial advised that "the consumption of as little as one or two fish dishes per week may be of preventive importance in relation to coronary heart disease." Now that's the kind of "warning label" we like to see!

Here are just a few of the heart health benefits that fish has to offer.

Better bleeding time. Research at the University of Lund in Sweden shows that fish benefits the heart by making the blood less prone to the abnormal clotting process that can lead to heart attack. The omega-3 fats in fish are credited with this effect. (See "Fish Oil Facts," on page 138, for details on the best fish sources of this all-important nutrient.)

Better blood pressure. With generous amounts of potassium and only modest amounts of sodium, fresh fish rates high for keeping blood pressure in the healthy range. Use unsalted seasonings to keep the sodium content at the moderate level that Mother Nature put there. And stay tuned for new research that may confirm an effect of the omega-3 fish fats on blood pressure, too.

Better blood cholesterol. Yasuo Kagawa and co-workers at Jichi Medical School in Japan have shown that levels of the "good" HDL cholesterol are highest among Japanese who eat the most fish. Here in the United States, William E. Connor, M.D., and his research team at the University of Oregon have documented a dramatic effect of a diet rich in salmon oil. Ten days on the diet lowered blood cholesterol by as much as 20 percent–*and* cut blood triglycerides by as much as 40 to 67 percent.

At the Market: A good piece of fish has firm, springy flesh, tight scales, red gills, clear eyes, and a clean smell. To test a fillet for freshness, poke it with your finger; if the flesh is firm and springy, it's fresh. If a dimple remains where your finger was, pass it up for a fresher fillet. When choosing fish steaks such as swordfish or fresh tuna, accept only those that have few dark areas.

When shopping for canned fish, remember to watch for added salt and fat. More and more low-sodium and water-packed varieties have become available in recent years.

Kitchen Tips: To store fresh fish, wrap in waxed paper and keep in the coldest part of the refrigerator for up to two days. A few fish, such as mackerel and herring, really should be eaten the day that you purchase them. If the fish is absolutely fresh, you can blanch it for a few seconds before refrigerating to allow slightly longer storage–about four days.

If you need to keep the fish longer, wrap it in aluminum foil or freezer paper and freeze. Most fish will keep frozen for three to six months.

If you have leftovers from an opened can of fish, transfer them to a nonmetal container and store in the refrigerator. They should stay tasty for up to a week.

When preparing certain fresh fish, such as herring and salmon, you'll be confronted with bones–sometimes lots of them. Using tweezers makes removing them easier. In the case of whole shad, we suggest asking the seller to bone it for you; it's not an easy job.

Stuck with old-style, salty canned fish? Transfer the fish to a strainer and rinse under cool water for about 30 seconds. This will rinse much of the sodium away. Pat dry before using.

Accent on Enjoyment: What's the most important difference between various kinds of fish? Taste! Two fish may be similar nutritionally but worlds apart in flavor. Accordingly, we discuss how to enjoy each one best in the sections below.

Our policy, by the way, is to try each fish in at least three different ways before drawing conclusions about its culinary appeal. That's why we list a minimum of three ideas for preparing each one.

Here we go–from A to Z.

Abalone

To make abalone more tender, pound with a mallet as you would veal or marinate it several hours before cooking. We recommend these seasoning combinations for marinades and sauces:

• Garlic, ginger, and chives.
• Sweet onions, tomatoes, basil, and thyme.
• Saffron, leek, and tomatoes.

At cooking time, grill or bake it, or slice it against the grain and sauté it for several minutes on each side in a small amount of olive or peanut oil.

Striped Bass

This is a versatile fish. You can broil, bake, microwave, sauté, plank, poach, or grill it. It substitutes well for red snapper in recipes.

When you're in the mood for something unusual, stuff the fish's cavity with any of your favorite recipes; its large size makes it perfect for this. Or experiment with recipes that allow you to serve striped bass cold. It's surprisingly good chilled!

Bluefish

Bluefish is great to cook with. It will give excellent results – whether you poach, bake, smoke, grill, stir-fry, sauté, or marinate it for seviche. Some pointers for first-time users:

- Bluefish has a strong flavor that blends particularly well with strong sauces and marinades. We recommend garlic, tomato, and citrus as complementary seasonings.
- Poached bluefish is delicious served chilled, accompanied by mustard sauce.
- Microwaved bluefish is the perfect choice when company is coming and you're in a hurry. (See "Fish in a Flash" for details.)

Fish in a Flash

When it has to be elegant, delicious, and fast – make it bluefish. Microwaving a bluefish fillet is child's play. Just follow these easy steps:

- Arrange a 1-pound fillet in a 9-inch pie plate.
- Sprinkle with lemon juice.
- Cover with vented plastic wrap.
- Microwave about 2 minutes.
- Flip and rotate fish, then microwave until cooked through (about another 2 minutes).
- Let stand for 4 minutes.
- Season, serve, and enjoy!

Cod

Cod is at its best when baked, poached, microwaved, or used in chowders. Don't grill it, though; it will fall apart. Here are some more specific suggestions for dressing up this common fish.

- Bake cod at 425° F, allowing 10 minutes for each inch of thickness. Flavor the cod with chopped ripe tomatoes, chopped sweet onion, and oregano; minced fresh basil, minced fresh parsley, and toasted pine nuts; or lemon and lime slices and a splash of olive oil.
- Steam cod over aromatic liquids, such as water and a handful of lemongrass or water, bay leaves, and black peppercorns.
- Microwave or poach cod in aromatic liquids. Low-fat ones such as stock and juices work well and add few calories. Cooked, flaked cod can be added to fish cakes, pâtés, soups, and casseroles.

Croaker

Croaker may be baked, broiled, grilled, poached, or microwaved. When baking, set the oven at 425° F, allowing 10 minutes for each inch of thickness. Shallots and tarragon are good seasonings for baked croaker.

To broil, we prefer to marinate it first in tomato juice and fresh basil. Then we broil or grill it (about 3 to 4 inches from heat) until cooked through.

If poaching fish is your fancy, cover the croaker with an aromatic liquid. Stocks that contain chopped celery, carrot, and onion are good. Serve garnished with toasted sesame seeds or slivered almonds—nutty flavors complement this fish well.

Flounder

Flounder may be baked, sautéed, broiled, grilled, or poached. It blends well with:

- Fresh ginger, garlic, and scallions.
- Dill, basil, and lemon.
- Garlic and chilies.
- Crabmeat—of course!

Haddock

Haddock is great poached, broiled, or baked. It's just the thing to serve when the urge to experiment with herbs and spices strikes. We especially like to season it with dill, tarragon, garlic, ginger, basil, thyme, onion, or chilies, then serve with pasta or rice. Some other ideas:

- Smother haddock fillets with chopped tomatoes, onion, and sweet peppers and bake uncovered at 400° F until cooked through, about 30 minutes for 1 pound.
- Paint haddock with peanut oil, then broil for a quick and nutritious dish.
- Sprinkle just-cooked or chilled haddock with a vinaigrette made with orange juice and rosemary.

Halibut

Choose halibut steaks when you're in the mood to grill. They are a perfect choice for grilling or broiling because they won't fall apart. And although it's terrific when grilled, the delightful flavor of this fish also blends superbly with soups and stews.

For a new twist on this old favorite, you can:

- Paint halibut steaks with melted orange marmalade, then grill. Serve hot or cold.
- Poach halibut fillets, then cut into chunks and use in fish salad with scallions and tarragon.
- Set halibut fillets or steaks in a baking dish and drizzle with lemon juice. Then cover with thinly sliced potatoes and minced fresh mint and bake covered at 400° F until cooked through, about 30 minutes. Serve hot with yogurt and ripe tomatoes.

Herring

Herring is a Scandinavian favorite. It has a strong taste, and people tend to either love it or never eat it. Those who like it can tell you that it tastes great when:

- Baked with potatoes, onions, and milk–Norwegian-style.
- Marinated in herbed vinegar, then baked or broiled.
- Grilled and served cold with coarse mustard and crusty bread.

Mackerel

Save yourself the trouble of learning firsthand that skinning mackerel before cooking is almost impossible. Do remove dark areas of flesh as best you can, though; a chef's knife or kitchen scissors will make the job easier. From there you can poach, broil, bake, or braise it. Baking it whole helps preserve moisture and it's a snap to do. Just rub the fish with lemon juice and fresh snipped dill and set it in a casserole dish. Cover and bake at 425° F until cooked through, about 25 minutes.

Fresh mackerel is not easy to come by, so if you are lucky enough to get it, why not savor it? Here's what we would do to make it into a special treat.

- Sauté fillets in peanut oil, garlic, and gingerroot. Serve cold, sprinkled with scallions and toasted sesame seeds.
- Rub fillets with top-quality coarse mustard, then grill and serve garnished with lemon, parsley, and carrots.
- Poach fillets in a stock with sliced oranges, bay leaf, and peppercorns. Serve hot on cold days, or chilled in summer.

Perch

When you tire of the exotic, you can always count on perch as an old standby that is ultra-easy to prepare. Braise, poach, or bake perch and serve with baked potato and a salad. For a quick grilled dish, rub fillets with reduced-calorie mayonnaise, sprinkle with basil, and broil until cooked through –about 3 minutes on each side.

Of course, we can't forget the microwave option. Start with whole perch; marinate in garlic and lemon juice. Then wrap in plastic wrap and microwave on full power until cooked through. One pound of fish will only take about 4 to 4½ minutes–less than some frozen dinners!

Pollack

The key to great pollack is a good marinade. Before you bake, sauté, or broil, try something aromatic such as lemon and thyme. Of course, there are other great ways to prepare this fish:

- Bake pollack with chopped onion, minced jalapeños, chopped tomato, oregano, and a splash of olive oil.
- Stir-fry sliced pollack with scallions, water chestnuts, and broccoli. Toss with toasted sesame oil and serve with hot rice.
- Substitute pollack for cod or haddock in your favorite recipe–hot or cold.

Salmon

As any fan can tell you, salmon has a wonderful taste of its own that should be enhanced but never overpowered. Simple approaches are best – and make for easy preparation. Some possibilities:

• Brush salmon steaks with a lemon vinaigrette and grill. Drizzle with more vinaigrette before serving and garnish with orange sections.
• Poach salmon fillets, then break into chunks with your fingers. Toss gently with pasta, dill, and ricotta.
• Serve cold poached salmon with a variety of mustards, thinly sliced purple onions, and crusty bread.

Sardines

If you can get fresh sardines, do give them a try. You will find that quick cooking gives the most delicious results. That makes sautéing the ideal cooking method. Rather than varying the outcome with other cooking methods, stick with the sautéing but vary the seasonings. Why not try some of these ideas?

• Marinate sardines in lemon juice, garlic, and onion. Sauté in olive oil until cooked through. Sprinkle with minced fresh oregano or mint and serve hot.
• Sauté sardines with shallots in peanut oil. Then deglaze the pan with Dijon mustard and raspberry or other flavored vinegar. Pour the glaze over the sardines and serve hot.
• Marinate sardines in rice vinegar, garlic, and gingerroot. Dust with a bit of cornstarch, then sauté in peanut oil. Sprinkle with minced scallions and serve.

Shad

Shad stuffed with its own roe may be a classic, but not everyone wants to drown their fish in cream sauce. Substitute a low-fat, aromatic alternative such as herbed stock for that high-fat cream. Or forgo the classic approach entirely with these ideas.

• Sprinkle shad fillet with freshly grated Parmesan cheese and minced rosemary. Bake until cooked through and serve hot.

- Rub shad fillet with olive oil, dill, and caraway. Grill or broil until cooked through.
- Rub shad fillet with peanut oil, curry powder and minced fresh gingerroot. Bake until cooked through and serve hot with steamed vegetables.

If you have trouble finding recipes for shad, just use it to replace salmon or haddock in your favorite recipes. We doubt that you will be disappointed.

Swordfish

Although the wonderful meaty texture of swordfish keeps it from falling apart when grilled or broiled, it's not as hardy as it may seem. Swordfish needs a little TLC to prevent it from becoming too dry. To preserve its moisture, marinate it and use a quick-cooking method such as grilling or poaching. Alternatively, surround and cover steaks with chopped vegetables and bake until tender.

Here are some specific ideas for seasoning and preparing this delicious fish.

- Marinate swordfish chunks in an herbed vinaigrette. Then skewer the chunks and grill. Serve hot with rice.
- Marinate steaks in olive oil and lemon juice. Then top with purple onion slices and bake. Serve hot sprinkled with crumbled feta.
- Buy custom-sliced steaks that are no more than ½ inch thick. To cook, blacken them as you would redfish.

Brook Trout

When convenience counts—as it so often does these days—turn to whole brook trout. It's surprisingly simple to make because it needs no scaling and is a snap to bone. Whole small fish, 12 inches and under, are best sautéed or pan-fried, as quick cooking will keep them moist. For 12- to 16-inchers, though, baking and grilling are good options. For very large trout, stuff first, then bake; or fillet them and sauté.

Let the delicate flavor of trout come through by sticking with mild seasonings such as dill, lemon, basil, or fennel. (Hold the chilies for stronger-tasting food.)

Here are some suggestions to get you on your way to becoming a certified trout lover.

- Sauté tiny whole trout in peanut oil, minced shallots, orange peel ribbons, and thyme.
- Sprinkle trout fillets with chopped walnuts and julienne strips of carrot, celery, and onions. Bake and serve hot.
- Poach whole trout, then chill. Serve cold with chopped avocado, minced scallions, and a creamy mild mustard.

Here's a trout tip rumored to have come from Missouri fishermen. To help keep trout sweet and delicious during freezing, dip whole gutted fish in milk before wrapping and putting in the freezer.

Fresh Tuna

If you've never eaten fresh tuna, you don't know what you're missing. Here are some ideas that are sure to get you hooked on this flavorful and meaty fish.

- Paint tuna with a fruity olive oil, then grill. Serve hot with garlic bread.
- Cut tuna into meaty chunks and put on a skewer. Then rub the chunks with Dijon mustard and grill. Serve hot with a green salad.
- Poach tuna with bay and rosemary. Let it cool in the poaching liquid and serve chilled with a marinated vegetable salad.

Tuna, Water-Packed

Before you reach for that jar of mayonnaise, let us put in a word for some more interesting ways to prepare canned tuna. They take no more time but make all the difference when it comes to flavor.

- Prepare tuna salad as you normally do, but substitute a lemon vinaigrette for that dull mayonnaise.
- Toss canned tuna with marinated artichoke hearts and blanched button mushrooms. Serve chilled on crisp romaine petals.
- Make a plain omelet and fill with mild white cheese, scallions, and canned tuna.

Whitefish

Whitefish has a delicate troutlike flavor that calls for subtle seasonings such as lemon, parsley, almonds, asparagus, or mild white cheeses. Some other great ways to prepare it are:

• Stuff a whole gutted whitefish with sprigs of fresh dill. Rub the outside of the fish with olive oil, then grill until cooked through. Serve hot or cold.
• Poach whole gutted fish, then remove skin and bones. Serve with chopped avocado and lime juice for drizzling.
• Substitute flaked cooked whitefish for canned tuna or salmon in a fish salad recipe.

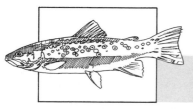

Flounder with Sweet Peppers and Toasted Pine Nuts

2 tablespoons pine nuts
1 pound flounder (or other small fillet)
2 tablespoons cornmeal
2 teaspoons sweet butter
1 shallot, minced
1 sweet red or yellow pepper, cut into julienne strips
1 teaspoon balsamic vinegar
¼ cup chicken stock

Toast pine nuts by placing them in a hot nonstick skillet and stirring frequently over medium-high heat until toasted, about 2 minutes. (Be careful not to let them burn.) Remove from heat and set aside.

Sprinkle fish with cornmeal.

In a large nonstick skillet, melt butter over medium heat. Add fish and sauté until cooked through, about 2 minutes on each side.

Remove fish from the pan and place on individual serving plates.

Add shallots and peppers strips to the hot pan and sauté until fragrant and slightly wilted, about 2 minutes. Then add vinegar and stock, increase the heat to high, and boil until liquid is reduced by half. Pour over fish, top with pine nuts, and serve hot.

Makes 4 servings

Steamed Whole Fish with Ginger and Chives

3 whole, dressed trout
    (about 8 ounces
    each) or 1½ pounds
    of other whole fish
2 tablespoons peeled,
    chopped gingerroot
2 tablespoons minced
    fresh chives

Rub the cavities of fish with oil, then stuff with ginger and chives.

Set fish in a steamer over boiling water and steam until cooked through, about 15 minutes. (Fish smaller than 8 ounces will take less time.)

To serve hot, remove ginger and chives, then fillet. To serve chilled, refrigerate before removing ginger and chives.

Makes 4 servings

Grilled Swordfish with Chili-Chive Butter

1 tablespoon sweet
    butter, softened
½ teaspoon chili powder
1 teaspoon minced fresh
    chives
1 pound swordfish steaks

Preheat the broiler or grill.

In a small bowl, combine butter, chili powder, and chives. Put a small amount of seasoned butter on the top side of each steak. Grill or broil for about 5 minutes, then turn steaks and put another small amount of seasoned butter on each steak. (Don't use all the butter.) Grill or broil 5 minutes more, then use remaining butter to top the grilled fish. Serve hot.

Makes 4 servings

FLATULENCE

Some Sensible Advice

For a symptom that rarely is a sign of serious health trouble, flatulence gets an awful lot of attention. Doctors hear plenty of complaints about it, yet they are convinced that the only thing most sufferers have to worry about is the embarrassment it might cause.

And they've got a point. Passing gas is a normal function of the body, just like sweating, sneezing, or going to the bathroom. But what, some plagued by the problem may ask, is considered normal?

That's a tough question, but there is at least one researcher who feels he knows the answer. According to David Altman, M.D., of the University of California, the average person passes gas about 14 times a day. So, lacking a better standard, this has become accepted as something of a norm.

So It's Normal, Now What?

Barring serious medical conditions (which we'll get to later), food is the major reason why your gassiness may be beyond normal.

Certain foods are natural gas producers. Fruits, vegetables, beans, and lactose-containing dairy products fall into this category. They contain carbohydrates that humans cannot digest completely. The synthetic sweetener sorbitol has the same characteristic. In fact, sorbitol's value as an artificial sweetener is due to the body's inability to digest it as completely as sugar. As a result, fewer calories are absorbed from sorbitol and the gas it produces is just proof positive that its carbohydrates are not being readily digested.

Foods that contain gas in their natural state also contribute to flatulence. Apples, for instance, are about 20 percent gas by weight. In addition, air whipped into foods during preparation can be a source of gas—soufflés, whipped toppings, and bread are but a few examples of gas-causing foods in this category.

"Foods That Fight Back" will get you started in your search for foods that may be responsible for excessive gas. Chances are you won't have to look further than these common gas-producing foods to control your symptoms. But you will have to eat less of them if you want to reduce gassiness.

201

Foods That Fight Back

The foods that cause flatulence in normal people vary from one person to the next. The best approach is to find those that cause you the most trouble. Doing so takes time, but it is not difficult.

A good starting point is a diet that contains as few of the following foods as possible. Try adding these suspects one at a time–just like the elimination diets used in diagnosing food allergy. Be alert for symptoms that develop within 1 to 4 hours of eating the foods. If they are unusually severe, you've probably found one of the foods you're most sensitive to. For the most reliable results, test each food more than once.

You'll note that the list includes dairy and wheat products. Those who are intolerant to these foods may experience severe gas from eating them. However, even those who can tolerate lactose well cannot digest all of it, so cutting down on lactose-containing foods can make a difference even if you don't have lactose intolerance.

Similarly, cutting back on wheat products makes a difference for some people free of celiac disease, although as a general rule, wheat products are normally not a major cause of flatulence. For those who have problems with wheat products, however, substitutes made from rice are good alternatives.

Apples
Beans*
Brussels sprouts
Broccoli
Cabbage
Carbonated beverages
Cauliflower
Dairy products high in lactose
Diet foods sweetened with sorbitol
Onions
Radishes
Wheat products

*See the entry on beans, beginning on page 55, for cooking methods that help reduce the flatulence factor.

This Fact's Not Hard to Swallow

Just for the sake of argument, suppose that you've eliminated all potentially troublesome foods from your diet, yet your problems with gas persist. What should you do? Refuse to give up!

Gas can be a problem even when the diet is virtually free of troublesome, gas-producing foods. A possible explanation is an indirect dietary factor—swallowed air.

You can't feel it, of course, but as you eat and drink, you swallow air along with your food. It can't be avoided completely, although gulping your food as if you haven't had a meal in days doesn't help any. Some people also swallow more air when they are tense or in pain.

Determining whether excessive gas comes from swallowed air or your choice of foods requires some detective work. If dietary changes clear up excess flatulence, chances are that abnormal air swallowing is not the problem. If they don't, try eating more slowly and using a straw for drinking. These approaches may bring some relief.

Some Other Solutions

Modifying your eating habits is a first step toward coping with gas. If more drastic measures become necessary, though, you have two options.

Activated charcoal is especially effective at absorbing gas. You can buy it in pill form. However, owing to concerns that it may absorb beneficial substances such as vitamins as well as excess gas, it's best to use it only occasionally—not as a daily fix.

Some over-the-counter antacids also help combat gas. Look for a product labeled "antiflatulent," or check the ingredient listing for the presence of simethicone—the anti-gas factor.

Signs of Trouble

Sometimes flatulence is not just a normal reaction to eating but a symptom of an underlying disorder. So if gas is particularly troublesome to you, you should not immediately dismiss it.

For those who truly suffer from abnormal gas production, the most common problem is lactose intolerance, a condition in which the body is unable to handle lactose, the sugar found in milk. Having drunk milk for decades without problem, those who develop lactose intolerance in later life don't suspect milk as a cause of their gas. If symptoms drop off dramatically after you remove lactose-rich foods from your diet for a few days, however, chances are that a growing intolerance to lactose is the cause. (For more on lactose intolerance, as well as a list of lactose-containing foods, see pages 276 to 285).

Less common than lactose intolerance as a cause of excessive gassiness are the malabsorption syndromes, such as celiac disease. In this condition, the body cannot handle gluten, a protein found in wheat products. (Turn to the entry on celiac disease, beginning on page 110, for the details on how conditions such as this one are diagnosed and treated.)

Making these diagnoses on your own is tough, if not impossible. If you believe your flatulence may be more than a personal inconvenience, it's best to see your doctor.

GALLBLADDER PROBLEMS

Food for Better Bile

The terms *cholecystitis* (ko-lee-sis-TI-tis) or *cholelithiasis* (ko-lee-li-THI-a-sis) may sound like Greek to you, but chances are you know both by other names. Cholecystitis refers simply to an inflamed gallbladder, and cholelithiasis is that all-too-familiar condition called gallstones.

Exactly what causes gallbladder disease remains the subject of some debate. Experts doubt that any one factor can be blamed; they believe that the sum total of several factors determines whether gallbladder trouble develops. So far, the finger has been pointed at the following factors.

Heredity. Gallbladder trouble clearly runs in families.

Infection. Infections no doubt account for some cases of gallbladder disorders.

Bile composition. The gallbladder's function is to store bile, a substance needed in the digestive process. Factors that increase the cholesterol content of the bile are now considered powerful influences on gallbladder health.

The last item is where nutrition comes in. As we'll be explaining shortly, the food you eat probably has major effects on bile composition.

The Sometimes-Silent Stone

Never had gallstones? That's great. There is one thing you should know, however; some people have gallstones but don't know it. Experience has shown that stones located in the gallbladder itself often cause no symptoms at all.

If the stones settle elsewhere—in the duct that leads out of the gallbladder, for example—the symptoms are likely to be anything but quiet. These stones may block the flow of bile out of the duct and as a result, cause severe pain, nausea, or vomiting. Unfortunately, the complaints don't end with these three symptoms; fever, jaundice, bloating, belching, and intolerance of fatty and spicy foods may accompany them.

It goes without saying that any of these symptoms is unpleasant. But doctors worry far more about the possible complications. Should the patient's condition go from bad to worse, the gallbladder may become infected or actually tear. And the trouble may spread to other organs, too; when gallstones block the bile duct, the liver sometimes becomes seriously diseased.

205

Who Gets Gallstones?

Gallstones are no stranger in the United States. Among middle-aged and older Americans, about 10 percent of men and 20 percent of women have gallstones. If that sounds high, consider that some population groups have it worse. As many as 70 percent of the Pima Indians aged 25 or older, for instance, have gallstones.

Obviously, growing older brings a higher risk of gallbladder disease. But the middle-aged and elderly are not the only ones affected. Other likely candidates include:

• Overweight women.
• American Indians from the southwestern United States.
• Diabetics.
• Patients with inflammation of the intestinal tract.

Geography, too, plays its part. Looking worldwide, you find that gallstones are common in Westernized societies but are usually rare among primitive peoples. For many years, these stones were uncommon in Japan, but now their incidence is on the rise.

The changing rate of gallstones in places such as Japan and the dramatic differences in patterns of the disease worldwide tell us that heredity alone can't account for the condition. Our lifestyle, too, obviously plays a role.

Is Prevention Possible?

If you have diabetes and a family history of gallstones, and you take drugs that make gallstone formation more likely, you may develop gallbladder trouble no matter how hard you try to prevent it. Nevertheless, experts are certain that many–although not all–cases of gallbladder disease can be prevented.

As we mentioned earlier, the composition of the digestive substance called bile strongly affects the odds of getting gallstones. Today experts are absolutely convinced that the food we eat has a major influence on bile composition. According to Scott Grundy, M.D., of the University of Texas, the intake of calories, fat, cholesterol, and fiber have been shown to affect bile composition.

In fact, studies that compare food habits between gallstone patients and those free of stones tie these and other factors to this condition. Here's the rundown, by suspect.

Calories. Australian scientist R. K. R. Scragg found that as a group, those who developed gallstones before age 50 ate more calories than those who did not develop stones.

Fat. In the same study, Dr. Scragg also linked increased chances of developing gallstones to higher intakes of fat. Although it remains possible that polyunsaturated fats in particular favor gallstone development, the research on this point has yielded conflicting results, and at present, all fats remain suspect.

Low fiber intake. British researcher K. W. Keaton, M.D., a well-known expert on dietary fiber, and his colleagues have shown that low fiber intakes affect the bile composition in a way that probably favors the development of gallstones.

Sugar. American Indians are extremely prone to gallstones, and the federal government's first health and nutrition survey (the HANES study) documented that they consume large amounts of sugar. Experts now wonder if their sweet tooth is affecting their risk of stones.

Of course, researchers are more sold on some of these relationships than others. Excessive calories—to the extent that obesity results—and dietary fat are widely accepted as likely troublemakers. On the matter of sugar and low fiber intake, though, it looks like many experts are reserving judgment.

The Trouble Can Be Treated

If you already have gallbladder trouble, good treatment is your top priority. Doctors use a variety of treatments, all with respectable rates of success. If your doctor suspects that obesity has contributed, for example, he'll probably recommend losing weight. Medication is another option, as is surgery.

Although surgery sounds like a rather drastic treatment, some doctors actually favor it as a preventive approach, too. Diabetics who have symptomless gallstones are considered particularly suitable candidates for this preventive surgery, which is performed to ensure that the now-silent gallstones don't make trouble in the future.

Then there are nutritional strategies. There is no one diet that is perfect for every patient with gallbladder disease, but you can bet that the diet will drastically restrict fat. This is because fat stimulates the gallbladder to contract— something that needs to be avoided when the organ is irritated.

Other irritants—such as spicy foods—can also be troublesome. While determining your particular sensitivities may involve some trial and error, you'll find some general guidelines in "Diet Dos and Don'ts." Also, in "Diet for a Picky Gallbladder," there's a week's worth of menus that show how to turn the list of allowed foods into a healthy diet.

Diet Dos and Don'ts

Diets for a problem gallbladder can be a little rough at first. This is because the "foods-to-avoid list" is longer than you'd like. But there's a bright side; some people can tolerate more of the banned foods than others.

Below you'll find a list of okay and not-okay foods designed for patients with gallbladder disease. Naturally, these are general guidelines; for some, they will turn out to be stricter than necessary.

Let's start with what you can eat before turning to the list of troublemakers.

Food Type	Allowed
Beverages	Whole milk, only 2 cups; skim milk as desired; coffee, coffee substitute, tea; fruit juices
Breads	All kinds except those with added fat
Cereals	All cooked or dry breakfast cereals, except possibly bran; macaroni, noodles, spaghetti, rice
Cheeses	Cottage only
Desserts	Angel food cake, fruit whip, fruit pudding, gelatin, ices and sherbets, milk and cereal puddings using part of milk allowance
Eggs	3 per week
Fats	Vegetable oil or margarine
Fish	All non-fatty varieties
Fruits	All kinds when tolerated
Meats	Broiled, baked, roasted, or stewed without fat: lean beef, chicken, lamb, pork, veal
Seasonings	In moderation: salt, pepper, spices, herbs, flavoring extracts
Soups	Clear
Sweets	All kinds: hard candy, jam, jelly, marmalade, sugars
Vegetables	All kinds when well tolerated; cooked without added butter or cream

Food Type	Avoid
Beverages	With cream; soda-fountain beverages with milk, cream, or ice cream
Breads	Griddle cakes, sweet rolls with fat, French toast
Cheeses	All whole-milk cheeses, both hard and soft
Desserts	Any containing chocolate, cream, nuts, or fats: cookies, cake, doughnuts, ice cream, pastries, pies, rich puddings
Eggs	Fried
Fats	Cooking fats, cream, salad dressings
Fish	All fatty varieties
Fruits	Avocado; raw apples, berries, melons may not be tolerated
Meats	Fatty meats or poultry, bacon, corned beef, duck, goose, ham, fish canned in oil, mackerel, pork, sausage, organ meats, smoked and spiced meats if they are poorly tolerated
Seasonings	Sometimes not tolerated: pepper, curries, meat sauces, excessive spices, vinegar
Soups	Creamed
Sweets	Candy with chocolate and nuts
Vegetables	Strongly flavored may be poorly tolerated: brussels sprouts, broccoli, cabbage, cauliflower, cucumbers, onions, peppers, radishes, turnips; dried cooked peas and beans
Miscellaneous	Fried foods, gravies, nuts, olives, peanut butter, pickles, popcorn, relishes

Diet for a Picky Gallbladder

Here is a menu plan tailor-made for Jack Sprat—that nursery-rhyme fellow who could eat no fat. Had he had the benefit of modern-day medical knowledge, we're sure that his trouble would have been diagnosed as a very picky gallbladder!

Because avoiding the fat in food is usually essential to calming a sensitive gallbladder, we've sharply restricted fat in these plans. Each of the menus provides less than 20 grams of fat per day. As fat intakes of 75 to 100 grams daily are common in the United States, you can see that this change is a dramatic one.

As you might expect, however, some people with gallbladder disease can handle more fat than others. It's a matter of determining personal tolerance. Should you be better able to digest fat than Jack Sprat, you will probably be able to add some butter, margarine, or oil, or other sources of fat to these plans. In testing the waters, though, be sure that you increase fat only in small, carefully controlled amounts.

Day 1

Breakfast
   1 cup oatmeal
   2 slices raisin bread
   1 tablespoon jelly
   1 orange
   1 cup skim milk
     coffee

Lunch
   3 ounces chicken breast (without skin)
   2 slices Italian bread
   ⅓ cup loose-leaf lettuce
   1 tomato
   1 apple
   1 cup skim milk

Snack
   1 banana
   1 cup skim milk

Dinner
   3 ounces steamed flounder
   1 baked potato
   ¾ cup green beans
   2 slices Italian bread
   1 tablespoon jelly
   1 cup skim milk
   1 cup fresh raspberries

Day 2

Breakfast
   1 scrambled egg
   1 apple
   2 slices Italian bread
   1 tablespoon jelly
1 ⅓ cups skim milk

Lunch
   1 cup oysters
1½ cups lettuce, tomato, and carrot salad
   2 slices Italian bread
   1 tablespoon jelly
   1 cup skim milk

Dinner
   3 ounces turkey breast (without skin)
   ⅓ cup cranberry sauce
   ¾ cup brussels sprouts
   1 baked sweet potato
   1 slice whole wheat bread
   1 cup skim milk
   1 cup cantaloupe

(continued)

Diet for a Picky Gallbladder–Continued

Day 3

Breakfast
   1 ounce 100% natural cereal, plain
   ½ white grapefruit
   2 slices raisin bread
   1⅓ cups skim milk
      coffee

Lunch
   2 slices whole wheat bread
   1 tablespoon jelly
   1 cup fresh spinach
   1 cup onions
   9 cucumber slices
   ½ cup grated carrots
   4 radishes
   ¾ cup green pepper
   1 cup skim milk

Snack
   1 papaya

Dinner
2½ ounces lean round steak (trimmed of fat)
   ½ cup brown rice
   ½ cup broccoli
   ½ cup lima beans
   1 slice Italian bread
   1 teaspoon jelly
   1 cup skim milk
   1 cup fresh fruit cocktail

Day 4

Breakfast
   1 ounce crisped rice cereal
   1 cup nectarine
   2 slices raisin bread
   1⅓ cups skim milk
      coffee

Lunch

 2 slices Italian bread
 1 tablespoon jelly
Salad medley (1 cup loose-leaf lettuce, ¾ cup green pepper, 1 tomato,
 ½ cup fresh bean sprouts, 6 cucumber slices, ½ cup raw bamboo
 shoots, ½ cup cooked chick-peas)
 1 cup skim milk

Snack

 1 banana

Dinner

 3 ounces chicken breast (without skin)
 ½ cup brown rice
 ½ cup pinto beans
 ½ cup cooked spinach
 ½ cup unsweetened applesauce
 2 slices Italian bread
 1 cup skim milk
 1 piece watermelon

Day 5

Breakfast

 1 cup cooked cream of wheat cereal
 1 tangerine
 2 slices Italian bread
 1 tablespoon jelly
1⅓ cups skim milk
 coffee

Lunch

 ¾ cup loose-leaf lettuce
 ¾ cup 2% low-fat cottage cheese
 ¾ cup juice-packed fruit cocktail
 1 cup raw broccoli
 1 cup raw cauliflower
 2 slices Italian bread
 1 tablespoon jelly
 1 cup skim milk

(continued)

Diet for a Picky Gallbladder–Continued

Dinner

2½ ounces lean round steak (trimmed of fat)
¾ cup baked winter squash
½ cup green beans
½ cup water chestnuts
1 slice Italian bread
½ tablespoon honey
1 cup skim milk
1 cup fresh raspberries

Day 6

Breakfast

1 cup cooked corn grits
2 slices raisin bread
1 tablespoon marmalade
1 cup orange sections
1 cup skim milk
  coffee

Lunch

3 ounces chicken or turkey breast (without skin)
2 slices whole wheat bread
1 cup honeydew melon
½ cup brown rice
1 cup skim milk

Snack

1 apple
1 cup skim milk

Dinner

3 ounces fillet of sole
¾ cup cooked eggplant
1 cup celery and lettuce mixture
1 cup green pepper

1 tomato
2 slices Italian bread
1 tablespoon honey
1 cup skim milk
1 cup fresh pineapple chunks

Day 7

Breakfast
¾ cup whole wheat flakes
½ pink or red grapefruit
1 slice Italian bread
½ tablespoon honey
1 cup skim milk
coffee

Lunch
Garden sandwich (1 pita bread, ¾ cup crisphead lettuce, ¼ cup grated
carrots, ½ cup alfalfa sprouts, ½ cup water-packed tuna)
1 cup skim milk
1 papaya

Snack
1 cup skim milk
½ cup seedless raisins

Dinner
3 ounces turkey breast (without skin)
1 baked potato
½ cup brussels sprouts
½ cup carrots
1 slice Italian bread
½ tablespoon jelly
1 cup skim milk
1 cup fresh strawberries

GARLIC

Hot Stuff for Your Heart

4 calories per clove

If you love garlic, you probably don't need any coaxing to eat it. Few seasonings go with as wide a range of food as garlic does, and nothing else can really compete with its distinctive flavor. But there's more to the garlic story than flavor alone.

For centuries it was said that garlic has special health properties, but the medical profession brushed off the idea as simple folklore. Today the tables have turned—and the latest results show that the "barefoot doctors" were truly on to something. Here are just a few highlights from recent research.

- In the laboratory, garlic juice inhibits the growth of many bacteria and fungi.
- Studies by Arun Bordia, M.D., of the Ravindra Nath Tagore Medical College in India, and others show that large amounts of garlic—on the order of 10 to 12 cloves a day—help reduce the "bad" cholesterol in the blood and increase levels of the "good" cholesterol.
- Dr. Bordia and others also have shown that the same large amounts of garlic enhance the process by which our bodies break up potentially dangerous blood clots.

Apparently, the active ingredient in garlic resides in the oil. It also seems to be unstable, so it remains to be established whether commercial garlic capsules have the same kind of effects seen in studies using fresh garlic or a just-prepared extract.

Unfortunately, large amounts of fresh garlic don't sit well with everyone. Volunteers who took large amounts of fresh garlic extracts—about 2 to 5 teaspoons—often experienced discomfort and burning sensations in the mouth, stomach, and esophagus. And although it is an impressive antibiotic in laboratory studies, it remains to be seen whether or not garlic works the same way when eaten.

For all that we don't know, the well-established facts about garlic have us sold. It's essentially sodium free, so it's just the thing for salt-deprived taste buds. Garlic also ranks among the best sources of the mineral selenium, which is one of the nutrients that cancer researchers have cited for its impressive antioxidant properties.

Good-bye to Garlic Breath

Love garlic but not what it does to your breath? Indulge anyway, then chew on a sprig of fresh parsley to relieve the effect on your breath.

To remove the aroma of garlic from your fingers, rub them with toothpaste, then rinse.

At the Market: California leads other states in garlic production, and most of its crop is known as the Italian type. It has large, white heads containing about 15 cloves with a mild flavor. Spanish garlic is smaller and has a purplish color and sharper flavor. Tahitian or "elephant garlic" has much larger heads than Italian garlic; its flavor is also somewhat mild and its texture a bit spongy.

The guidelines for choosing garlic are the same regardless of type. Heads should be firm, with a dry, papery sheath free of green sprouts. Avoid garlic that has green sprouts or a head that is soft or wet.

Kitchen Tips: Garlic keeps best in a cool, dry place with good circulation–in other words, not in the refrigerator. Very fresh heads may keep for months under good conditions, even if partially used. Bruised bulbs, however, will invite insects.

For easy peeling, just drop whole garlic cloves in boiling water for about 5 seconds. If adding garlic to uncooked dishes, strike the clove sharply with the flat part of a knife so that the skin splits.

Accent on Enjoyment: Here are some facts about garlic to keep in mind when cooking.

- Garlic adds a wonderful flavor to sautéed foods, but care should be taken to prevent it from burning, which makes the flavor bitter.
- Long, moist cooking, such as stewing, mellows garlic flavor.
- Roasting gives garlic a nutty flavor.
- Garlic goes well with countless foods, especially eggplant.
- Peeled cloves make a flavorful addition to herb vinegars and oils; you can also give your salad a touch of garlic flavor by rubbing the inside of the bowl with a clove before adding other ingredients.

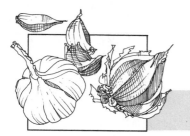

Garlic Soup with Summer Greens

1 tablespoon olive oil
1 bulb garlic, peeled
   and separated into
   cloves
2 onions, chopped
3 bay leaves
1 teaspoon dried thyme
2 allspice berries,
   crushed
3 cups chicken or beef
   stock
1 cup milk
1 cup shredded fresh
   spinach

In a large stockpot, warm oil over medium heat. Add garlic, onions, bay leaves, thyme, allspice, and stock and bring to a boil. Reduce heat to simmer and continue to simmer until garlic is tender, about 15 minutes.

Discard bay leaves, then use a slotted spoon to transfer garlic and onions to a food processor or blender. Add a splash of stock, then process until smooth.

Add garlic mixture to stock in the pot and heat over low heat while adding milk. Continue to heat gently and stir until the soup is hot. Add spinach, stir briefly, then serve. (The hot soup will blanch the spinach perfectly.)

Makes 4 servings

GOUT

Getting the Pain Out

Long ago, say the history books, a painful disease often struck those who participated in royal feasts rich in gourmet food and drink. They called it the "disease of kings"; today the condition is known as gout.

Gout is actually a form of arthritis that settles in the joints of the body–usually the big toe. For many years the pain was blamed on eating rich foods, but today we know that not all gout victims eat high on the hog. Just how much diet plays a part in the disease is a matter for debate.

What is well established, however, is what causes all the pain–a buildup of uric acid in the joint. Gout sufferers, for some reason, produce more uric acid than their body can handle. The result is the formation of needlelike crystals that get dropped around the affected joint.

Like other forms of arthritis, gout hurts–some say even more than other joint diseases. So when the pain strikes, the gout victim's only care is getting rid of it–not settling academic debates about its origin.

Know Thy Enemy

Fortunately, preventing and treating the pain of gout has become much easier during this century. Now that doctors understand the metabolic abnormality that accounts for the painful flare-ups, the prognosis is better than ever.

Obviously, keeping uric acid under control is the key to beating gout. That's where diet comes in. Experts established long ago that uric acid is a breakdown product of substances called purines that are found in certain foods. So it stands to reason that if you eliminate purine-rich foods, you'll eliminate gout.

But it turns out that that's only part of the story. According to British nutritionist Sir Stanley Davidson, diet contributes, at most, 50 percent of the uric acid present in the blood of normal people. Apparently much of the uric acid comes not from food but from the body overproducing it on its own.

Who Gets Gout?

For all that remains to be learned about gout, one thing is certain: This is not a disease that strikes indiscriminately. To the contrary, most patients share

Pruning Purines from Your Diet

Nowadays, strict diets are usually unnecessary for gout patients, thanks to the effectiveness of medicines now available. As a general rule, the following foods that are high in purines need to be avoided totally.

Anchovies
Brains
Gravies
Kidney
Liver
Meat extracts
Sweetbreads

If this approach doesn't work well enough, the next step is to also limit those foods with moderate purine content to three to five small servings a week. These foods are:

Dry beans
Dry peas
Lentils
Meats
Oatmeal
Poultry
Seafood
Spinach

If the strictest diet is necessary, totally eliminate the high- and moderate-purine foods and eat only the following foods.

Breads and cereals
Butter and other fats
Caviar
Cheese
Eggs
Fish roe
Fruits
Gelatin
Nuts
Sugar, sweets
Vegetables

certain characteristics that no doubt have much to do with the development of the disease.

Here are some typical characteristics of the gout patient.

Male. Most gout patients are male. In the United States, women account for less than 10 percent of all cases.

Over 30. Gout is more common among older age groups. Among males, few develop it before puberty; of those women who do succumb, the disease rarely strikes before menopause.

Family history. At least 25 percent of gout patients have a relative who also suffers from the disease.

Overweight. Many gout patients are overweight. J. T. Scott, M.D., a British authority on gout, reported that about half of patients are 15 percent or more above ideal weight.

Presence of certain diseases. Some patients develop gout as a result of other illnesses that compromise their ability to handle uric acid. Chronic kidney failure; high blood pressure; and the blood-related diseases of leukemia, polycythemia, and myelofibrosis are among the diseases that predispose their victims to gout. For these patients, gout is a complication of another disease, not a disease that exists on its own.

Defending Yourself

Fortunately, the painful attacks of gout are usually short-lived, lasting a few days or so. But the attacks often recur and at times become chronic. The joint damage that results from chronic gout forces some patients to have surgery.

If you have gout, you'll want to take action, not just to prevent it but also to minimize the chance of complications–especially kidney stones–which are all too common among gout sufferers.

Today, drugs are the first line of defense against gout. But they are not problem free; side effects can be such that alternative approaches may be needed. Even when drug treatment goes without a hitch, however, these other approaches can help increase their effectiveness.

Here's how to take a strong stand against gout.

Avoid both feast and famine. Meals rich in fat or high-purine foods raise the uric acid levels and can trigger gout attack. (See "Pruning Purines from Your Diet.") The other extreme–fasting–also causes a sharp increase in uric acid. That's why gout patients should avoid drastic approaches to weight reduction.

Minimize stress. Stress can precipitate an attack, so do what you can to avoid it. You can't avoid the stress of sudden illness or necessary surgery, but you can take steps to curtail stressful lifestyle.

Lose excess weight—slowly. Your weight affects the amount of uric acid in your blood. As Dr. Davidson and his co-workers point out, as weight creeps upward, so do uric acid levels.

Drink water, not alcohol. Alcohol is double trouble. It not only interferes with the body's efforts to excrete uric acid, it also encourages it to produce too much. Water, by contrast, offers benefits to gout sufferers because it helps discourage kidney stones from forming.

GRAPEFRUIT

Golden and Good for You

74 calories per medium grapefruit
96 calories per cup juice (unsweetened)

First came the Grapefruit Diet. The sequel will probably be the Grapefruit Fiber Diet–and James Cerda, M.D., of the University of Florida will know why.

Several years ago, Dr. Cerda tested the effect of grapefruit pectin–a kind of fiber–on blood cholesterol levels. His volunteers all had high cholesterol; rather than change their diets in any way, Dr. Cerda simply gave them supplements of grapefruit pectin that provided a whopping 15 grams of it daily. The results of the treatment were impressive: The total blood cholesterol level fell and the ratio of "bad" to "good" cholesterol improved.

Now, we don't expect that anyone could eat enough grapefruit to provide the same dose as the volunteers took. But grapefruit isn't the only pectin source in our diets; lots of fruits and vegetables have it. We estimate that you'll get enough pectin to make an impact on your cholesterol if you eat four to six servings of fruits and vegetables a day. (See "The Soluble Fiber Solution," on page 140, for more specific details.)

Grapefruit is perfect for heart-healthy diets on other counts too; its fat and sodium content is negligible, while its potassium content is good. (Hear that, blood pressure watchers?) And it's also among the foods that can meet the entire vitamin C allowance in one serving–a medium grapefruit provides 50 percent more than the Recommended Dietary Allowance for vitamin C; ditto for a cup of its juice. But when it comes to fiber, only the whole fruit is a good source.

Whole Grapefruits

At the Market: Grapefuits that are thin-skinned, round, and heavy for their size should be juicy and flavorful. Sniff before you buy, though; a sweet and fragrant scent is a sign of quality. Unfortunately, if the grapefruit is kept in a cold environment, you may not be able to detect its fragrance. If the shipping box is in sight, look for the name of the variety. Indian River, Orchid Island, Star Ruby, and Ruby Red are especially flavorful.

223

Kitchen Tips: To preserve juiciness, store grapefruits loosely covered at room temperature; they will keep for up to two weeks. For longer storage, refrigerate in the crisper drawer or inside a perforated plastic bag; they may last as long as a month this way.

At eating time, slice the fruit across its "equator," then use a grapefruit knife or other sharp, thin-bladed knife to loosen the sections enough to be scooped out. A grapefruit spoon is also helpful.

If you like peeled and sectioned grapefruit, use a grapefruit peeler such as The Snacker. Sold in cookware shops and many supermarkets, this plastic device has a point at one end that zips through the grapefruit skin and a flat blade at the other end to help coax the skin from the flesh.

Accent on Enjoyment: Before you reach for the sugar, remember that grapefruit is more flavorful at room temperature. To warm up a chilled grapefruit quickly, wrap half a grapefruit in waxed paper and microwave on full power until it's at room temperature, about 45 seconds.

Grapefruit is also tasty in fruit salads, hot or cold fruit compotes, chicken salads, marmalades, and preserves. You can substitute it for oranges in many recipes. The zest (finely grated skin with no white part) is excellent with sweet potatoes and in baking. Here are some specific approaches.

- Halve and sprinkle with cinnamon. Then broil until fragrant and serve as an appetizer, dessert, or breakfast.
- Toss grapefruit sections with sliced mango and tomato for a refreshing salad.
- Serve grapefruit sections as an accompaniment to spicy foods such as chili.

Grapefruit Juice

At the Market: Supermarkets sell grapefruit juice in canned and frozen forms, but specialty shops and juice bars are more likely to have freshly made juice. If you have a juicer, consider making your own–it takes a lot less time than you might think, and the fresher flavor is worth the effort.

Kitchen Tips: Store juice in a clean glass jar or bottle in the refrigerator. Reconstituted frozen and canned grapefruit juice will last for about a week in the refrigerator. Fresh juice is more perishable and should be used within two days.

Accent on Enjoyment: Grapefruit juice isn't just for breakfast. Explore its many culinary uses. For instance:

- Use in marinades for fish and poultry, or as a poaching liquid for chicken.
- Create a grapefruit ice or sorbet.
- Fill an ice cube tray half full of grapefruit juice, then freeze. Set a tiny mint sprig atop each cube, fill with more grapefruit juice, then freeze again. Use the cubes in punches, iced tea, or other refreshing beverages.
- Mix grapefruit juice half-and-half with club soda and garnish with a twist of lime.
- Use some grapefruit juice to vary the flavor of punches and dressings for fruit salads.

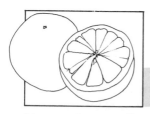

Scallop and Pink Grapefruit Salad

¾ pound sea scallops
2 pink grapefruits, sectioned
1 tablespoon minced fresh chives
2 tablespoons grapefruit juice
1 tablespoon hazelnut oil
½ teaspoon Dijon mustard
 red lettuce leaves

Cut larger scallops in half, then steam scallops in boiling water, covered, until cooked through, about 2 to 3 minutes.

In a large bowl, combine grapefruit sections and chives. Add scallops.

In a small bowl, whisk together grapefruit juice, oil, and mustard. Pour over scallop mixture and toss well to combine. Serve at room temperature or chilled on lettuce leaves.

Variation: Add a bit of chopped avocado to the salad before tossing with dressing.

Makes 4 servings

GREENS

Let's Hear It for Green Cuisine

Beet greens: 38 calories per cup (cooked)
Chicory greens (curly endive): 42 calories per cup (raw, chopped)
Collard greens: 26 calories per cup (cooked)
Kale: 42 calories per cup (cooked)
Mustard greens: 20 calories per cup (cooked)
Spinach: 12 calories per cup (raw)
       42 calories per cup (cooked)
Swiss chard: 36 calories per cup (cooked)
Turnip greens: 28 calories per cup (cooked)

Broccoli, take cover! Greens are out to give you some stiff competition, nutrition-wise. Their list of credits is getting longer, and already includes the following:

Vitamin A as carotene. Greens provide plenty—on the order of 50 to 100 percent of the Recommended Dietary Allowance (RDA) per cup.

Vitamin C. The carotene in greens comes with this cousin antioxidant—with levels varying from one-third to three-quarters of the RDA.

Fiber. Greens are great for fiber, too, with 2 to 5 grams per cup.

Low calorie count. How many foods give you so much nutrition for 50 or fewer calories per serving?

Low fat content. With so few calories, greens obviously can't pack in any fat to speak of.

And some greens—those of collards, mustard, turnips, and kale—boast still another distinction. They belong to the cabbage family of vegetables now in the cancer-prevention spotlight.

The bottom line, obviously, is that greens are winners. They are perfect for helping to lower cholesterol, prevent cancer, lose weight, and control diabetes.

At the Market: When shopping for greens, look for lively green, tender leaves. Avoid batches that look limp or yellowed. Those with the largest leaves are most likely to be bitter. As for chicory—sold by the head—look for a loose appearance, curly leaves, and ragged edges.

Can't find good fresh greens? Don't fret. Frozen will do.

Kitchen Tips: At home, wrap your greens in perforated plastic. Spinach and chard will keep for about five days; other greens for about a week.

Greens can be gritty, so rinse well (but don't soak) before cooking or adding to recipes. A salad spinner is ideal for the job. Then, if you like, simply chop the greens and cook in a covered saucepan or microwave-safe dish—you needn't pat dry or add water. (If your greens have tough stems, remove before cooking.)

Quick cooking also enhances the taste of greens—especially turnip greens. This makes them suitable for sautés and stir-fries.

Greens in a Flash

You may think of greens as old-fashioned, but they fit in well with our modern lifestyle. Now that the microwave has left its mark, plain greens can be turned into a great side dish in no time flat.

Here's the step-by-step procedure.

- Toss chopped collard greens into a 9-inch glass pie plate.
- Splash on a bit of stock and cover with vented plastic wrap.
- Microwave on full power until just tender, about 2 minutes for 2 cups of greens. Let stand for 2 minutes, then drain.
- Add to sautés, stir-fries, casseroles, and rice dishes for a simple presentation. For a more elegant touch, top with crumbled feta cheese and slivered almonds and serve with lamb.

Accent on Enjoyment: Greens are as versatile as they are nutritious. If you're short on ideas, you can:

- Liven up salads with tender greens of any kind, although chicory and spinach are probably the favorites for this purpose.
- Shred greens and add to soups, but be forewarned that beet greens will bleed and impart a red color to the broth.
- Make lasagna more healthful by using spinach or chard in place of some or all of the ground meat.
- Use greens of your choosing to replace spinach; most are more resistant to overcooking than spinach is, so novice cooks can feel more confident with them.

- Stuff greens the same as you would cabbage leaves.
- Serve poached chicken or main-dish salads on a bed of crisp raw greens.
- Season greens with fresh garlic, nutmeg, allspice, hot peppers, thyme, or oregano. Also worth a try are onions, chives, scallions, garlic, gingerroot, peanuts, or pine nuts. If you must add fat, favor olive oil for both flavor and health.
- Add shredded greens to Chinese-style fried rice a couple of minutes before cooking is finished, then crown with toasted almonds or sesame seeds.

Freeze-'Em-Yourself Greens

It's great to enjoy greens year-round, but supplies fluctuate with the seasons in many regions. Some people settle for frozen greens, but the truly

---

When Sodium Concerns You

Greens lack most of our modern-day gremlins, but sodium is an exception. The sodium content of greens varies—from a very low 22 milligrams per cup in cooked mustard greens to a high of 316 milligrams in a cup of Swiss chard. Needless to say, adding salt during preparation or at the table will send these values upward.

For most of us, the range of naturally occurring sodium in greens is not worrisome; many foods have far more sodium per serving and make more sense to cut back on. For those on strict low-sodium diets, though, every milligram counts, so take note of the numbers that follow and shop accordingly. Values are for 1 cup.

Type of Greens	Sodium (mg)
Mustard, cooked	22
Collard, cooked	36
Turnip, cooked	42
Kale, cooked	47
Chicory, raw	80
Beet, cooked	110
Spinach, cooked	126
Swiss chard, cooked	316

adventurous buy them fresh at peak season and freeze them at home. If they can do it, so can you. Here's how.

- Bring water to boil in a large kettle.
- Set a bunch of greens in a strainer with a handle; plunge the greens and strainer right into the boiling water.
- Allow to blanch for up to 2 minutes, keeping in mind that delicate young greens will take less time than older ones. (A bright green color is a good sign that the greens have been blanched long enough.)
- Plunge the blanched greens into ice water and let chill for about 30 seconds.
- Drain, then pack in freezer containers or divide into recipe-size portions and place in freezer bags. Pack the greens flat to allow for easy microwaving; they will also be easier to chop while frozen and added directly to soups, stews, gumbos, sauces, and casseroles.

Put them in the freezer until you are ready to use—just do it within six months or so.

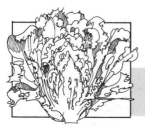

Oranges and Chicory with Poppy Seed Dressing

2 navel oranges, sectioned
2 cups chicory, ribs removed and torn into bite-size pieces
1 small red onion, thinly sliced
¼ cup sunflower seeds
1 tablespoon lemon juice
1 tablespoon orange juice
1 tablespoon olive oil
1 tablespoon poppy seeds

Slice each orange section into thirds and remove any seeds. Then combine them with chicory, onions, and sunflower seeds in a large salad bowl.

In a small bowl, whisk together juices and oil.

In a nonstick skillet, heat poppy seeds over medium-high heat until fragrant and toasted, about 3 minutes. Add poppy seeds to salad, then pour on dressing and toss well to combine. Serve at room temperature or chilled.

Makes 4 servings

Sautéed Collard Greens with Garlic and Scallions

2 teaspoons olive oil
3 cups shredded or
    chopped collard
    greens
1 clove garlic, minced
2 scallions, minced
1 tablespoon crumbled
    feta cheese

In a large nonstick skillet or a wok, heat oil over medium heat.

Add collards and garlic and sauté, stirring constantly, until collards are just wilted, about 4 minutes. Add scallions just before collards are finished cooking. Serve hot, sprinkled with feta.

Variation: Sauté a medium-size, chopped, ripe tomato with collards and garlic.

Makes 4 servings

Sautéed Greens with Potatoes and Rosemary

1 tablespoon olive oil
2 cloves garlic, minced
½ teaspoon rosemary,
    minced
2 medium potatoes
    (about ¾ pound)
    cubed and steamed
2 cups (about 6 ounces)
    chopped mustard
    greens
    freshly grated
    Parmesan cheese

In a well-seasoned cast-iron skillet, heat oil over medium heat. (If you don't have a cast-iron skillet, use a nonstick skillet.)

Add garlic, rosemary, potatoes, and greens and toss well to combine. Sauté until greens wilt, about 4 minutes. Then smash the mixture down to a pancake shape with a spatula. Continue to cook for another 3 to 4 minutes, then sprinkle with Parmesan and serve hot as an accompaniment to grilled meats. You can also serve the sauté with corn bread and a bowl of bean soup.

Makes 4 servings

HEADACHE

When Food Goes to Your Head

Even people in perfect health get headaches every now and then. Sometimes, however, headaches become an all-too-common occurrence. They may even become so frequent and painful as to make a normal life impossible.

Where do headaches come from? If only we could give you an easy answer! The reality is that no one factor can be singled out; the list of known causes is long. Among the best-known headhunters are allergies, medications, tension, hormonal factors, and lack of sleep. And another is food.

For years, doctors have listened to patients complaining that certain foods give them headaches, so much so that medical researchers have started to examine the food issue more seriously. The results are fascinating.

The Trigger's in the Gum

In searching for the obvious, you sometimes have to look at the obscure. Chewing gum, for instance, is a perfect example. Seymour Diamond, M.D., executive director of the Diamond Headache Clinic in Chicago, found that some of his gum-loving patients spent so much time chewing the stuff that they overworked the muscles of the jaw area, triggering a headache. The pain that goes with this kind of headache, says Dr. Diamond, is usually felt at the front and sides of the head.

Another unsuspected suspect is the all-American favorite–ice cream. For some, it quite literally is a food that packs a punch. Dr. Diamond explains that the cold temperature of ice cream activates nerves in the roof of the mouth, which send a message to the brain that trips the pain alarm.

A third suspect, he adds, is a substance that we all come across every day–salt. How it does its damage remains unclear, but Dr. Diamond finds that patients often develop headaches a few hours after eating salty food.

Sensitive Souls

The idea that chewing gum or cold food such as ice cream can trigger headaches by affecting the muscles and nerves in the head is not controversial. What is, however, is the notion that allergies, unusual sensitivities to certain

231

foods, or even food additives, might also be a cause of headaches. Some doctors dismiss the notion almost entirely. Others, however, do not.

Research by Dr. Norma Cornwell and co-workers at Royal North Shore Hospital in Sydney, Australia, however, suggests the problem is real–and not exactly rare. Dr. Cornwell's research team took a hard look at how chemicals in food affected symptoms among 26 patients who complained of recurrent headaches. Almost all of them (22 of the 26, to be precise) found marked relief when they followed a special diet designed to eliminate common food constituents such as monosodium glutamate (MSG), yellow food coloring, yeasts, and nitrites.

Those who improved on the special diet reported only half as many headaches while on this treatment. As if that weren't enough, they said that when they did get a headache, it was not as severe.

A basic "headache diet" that incorporates findings of reports such as this one is described in more detail in "The 'I-Have-a-Headache' Diet." It's not the most complicated diet to follow, but we know that some will say that too much effort is required. If you're really plagued by headaches and have found no metabolic cause, however, it might be worth giving it a try.

The "I-Have-a-Headache" Diet

Here's a list of foods that contain one or more potential headache triggers. Not everyone can expect to benefit from avoiding them, of course, but we're impressed with the success that some patients have had.

Beer
Coffee, tea, and other sources of caffeine
Other alcohol
Red wine
Beans (such as kidney beans, lima beans, baked beans; green beans or
    string beans are okay)
Cheese
Chocolate
Cured foods (cold cuts, hot dogs, smoked fish, salami, bacon)
MSG (monosodium glutamate)
Pork
Yogurt

Woe Is Wine

Doctors convinced of the food-headache connection expect, of course, that the list of troublemakers will vary from one patient to the next. And according to researcher Julia T. Littlewood of London's Queen Charlotte's Maternity Hospital, patients are far more likely to complain about some foods than others. Of these, she finds, "Alcoholic drinks, in particular red (but not white) wine, head the list."

Dr. Littlewood decided to conduct a research project on the red wine connection. She recruited 19 patients who reported that red wine brought on their headaches. Eleven were asked to drink a red wine-lemonade mixture. The others were offered vodka with their lemonade. Of the 11 who were given the red wine and lemonade, all but 2 experienced a migraine attack. Yet of the 8 who drank vodka and lemonade, none complained of headache symptoms. What's the link? The researchers believe it's tyramine, a substance found in red wine that causes blood vessels to contract.

The Desperation Diet

Hopefully, the Basic Headache Diet will make a major difference in your headaches. But we're great believers in having a contingency plan. If the basic diet doesn't work for you, there is one more diet that you may want to try.

We have to warn you that this is a very restrictive diet—at least at first. In fact, we probably wouldn't even mention it were it not for the benefits that have been reported to children who often suffered from severe migraine headaches.

Led by Dr. J. Egger of the London Hospital for Sick Children, the doctors involved put the children on a diet that consisted solely of one meat (lamb or chicken), one carbohydrate (rice or potato), one fruit (banana or apple), one cabbage-family vegetable, water, and vitamin supplements. Dr. Egger called it the "oligoantigenic diet," but we call it the Desperation Diet. Simple as it may be, we doubt that anyone would stick with it unless desperate.

The results, however, apparently provide plenty of motivation. Fully 93 percent of the children (there were 88) recovered on the diet. For some, headache symptoms disappeared once the diet was started; for others, a three-week period was needed before the troubles cleared up.

By reintroducing other foods after a trial on the Desperation Diet, Dr. Egger's research team was able to identify the trigger foods that were unique to 40 of the children. Milk was the most common trigger food; eggs, chocolate, orange, wheat, cheese, tomato, rye, and the food additives benzoic acid and tartrazine also provoked symptoms in at least 25 percent of the children tested. Although time-consuming to obtain, this information is worth having, for it allows patients to have a more varied diet as long as they avoid their own trigger foods.

Accounting for these findings is a matter for the experts. Because many of the children–as well as their immediate relatives–were known to have allergies, Dr. Egger and co-workers suspect that their headaches result from a true allergic reaction to the foods involved. (See the entry on allergy, beginning on page 5, for more details on the distinction between food allergy and food intolerance.)

But whether it's a true allergy or something else comes down to semantics. To the patients, it's the relief that counts.

HEARING PROBLEMS

Tune In to the Good News

Aging is a fact of life, but all the symptoms of getting older need not be. Hearing problems are a perfect example. Are you among those who consider loss of hearing an inevitable part of aging that no one can stop? If so, read on.

"Hearing problems," of course, is a general term. But one particular hearing disorder is Ménière's syndrome, a disease of the inner ear that affects not just the sense of sound but also of balance. In the process, it causes such symptoms as dizziness, progressive loss of hearing, and ringing in the ears–all of which make life pretty trying at times.

Listening for Clues

Fortunately for those who suffer from Ménière's, James T. Spencer, Jr., M.D., was not content to dismiss the problem simply as an inescapable part of aging. Dr. Spencer, a professor of medicine at West Virginia University, took a close look at the characteristics of more than 400 patients with symptoms of Ménière's disease. The vast majority proved to be obese and to have abnormal glucose (sugar) tolerance; half also had excessively high blood fats.

Convinced that these factors–notorious enemies of the healthy heart– might also be related to hearing woes, Dr. Spencer asked the patients to lose weight and follow a cholesterol-lowering diet.

For those who succeeded, the rewards were great. Some experienced "phenomenal" improvement in their hearing–it increased as much as 30 decibels, and that's a lot! What's more, improvement in some symptoms–headache and a feeling of pressure in the head or ears–came fairly quickly. Some patients reported relief in as little as a month or two.

Dr. Spencer noticed that successful patients also tend to "improve in appearance from weight loss, exhibit or admit to having more energy, and feel more youthful. They are very grateful patients." We can understand why!

Diet Does It Again

If your doctor is skeptical of these results, be sure to mention that others have reported similar success. Joel F. Lehrer, M.D., of the University of Medicine

235

and Dentistry of New Jersey, is one of them. He focused on patients who complained of dizziness–and proved to have Ménière's syndrome or a related problem termed "vestibular pathway disorder."

Dr. Lehrer checked the patients for abnormal blood fats or glucose tolerance; sure enough, there was no shortage of either. A diet appropriate to each one was recommended. Once again, the results were impressive, with dizziness occurring much less frequently–or not at all–in a vast majority of participants.

My Hearing, My Heart

Dr. Spencer has a hunch that his patients' troubles were an early sign of the process known as hardening of the arteries, which leads to heart attack and stroke. His beliefs are backed by findings by New York hearing expert Samuel Rosen, M.D. Dr. Rosen examined participants in a Finnish heart-health study that questioned if cholesterol-lowering diets help prevent heart disease. He found that in addition to better resistance to heart attack, participants had better hearing while on the cholesterol-lowering diet.

The way Dr. Spencer sees it, hearing troubles are not simply a nuisance in themselves but also a warning sign that more serious heart problems may be in the works. We're impressed with his reasoning and agree that those with Ménière's disease may have much to gain by giving his approach a chance.

HEART ATTACK

Closing the Case

(See also *Angina; Cholesterol; Triglycerides*)

Medicine is full of mysteries waiting to be solved. Fortunately, heart attack isn't one of them. Thanks to four decades of intensive research, our knowledge about America's number one health problem is enormous. In fact, we don't know of any heart scientists who doubt that nutrition is a major player in either prevention or treatment of this all-too-common condition.

You may think of heart attack as something that strikes suddenly, as if from out of the blue. But don't let the apparent drama fool you. Sudden though it may seem, a heart attack is merely the culmination of a process that has been going on behind the scenes for decades.

Here's how it works. The first (and longest) stage is as silent as can be. During this time, fat and cholesterol are deposited–ever so slowly–in the walls of blood vessels. Gradually, the fatty deposits grow larger; naturally the blood vessels become narrower and narrower as a result.

Sometimes, at some point along the way, this process, commonly known as hardening of the arteries, gives a warning–chest pains, or angina. But often it continues without the slightest sign until the bitter moment when a blood clot forms in one of the vessels supplying the heart with blood.

Only then are many heart attack victims put on notice that their blood vessels are in trouble. Fortunately, a majority survive the first attack. Then they want to know what caused it–and how to prevent it from happening again.

Just the Risk Factors, Ma'am

You have probably noticed that health professionals shy away from using the word "cause" when talking about common diseases. Although this may seem odd, it goes with the territory. In science and medicine, it seems that nothing is ever certain, and as a result terms such as "cause" seem out of place. Instead of causes, health professionals prefer to talk about risk factors.

A risk factor is exactly what its name implies: a habit, trait, or condition that increases the odds of developing a disease. It may relate to age, sex, family size, place of birth, or current residence. The possibilities are endless.

Of course, the chances of heart attack increase with age, and men are affected more often than women. But these risk factors are beyond our control.

Others, however, are just the opposite—they are determined in large part by our lifestyle. You can probably name these three major risk factors, but just in case, here they are again.

High blood cholesterol. For three decades now, heart experts have been tracking the health of thousands of residents of Framingham, Massachusetts. The results from this now-famous study and others like it show that people with cholesterol levels of 265 or more are four times more likely to have a heart attack than those with levels of 190 or less.

Smoking. Lung cancer is the best-known consequence of smoking. Yet, the 1964 landmark "Report on Smoking and Health," that warned about cigarettes and lung cancer, also cited smoking as a powerful risk factor for heart attack. Follow-up studies have confirmed the bad news but also added a bright spot. It seems that kicking the cigarette habit can allow the damage to heal. Ten years after quitting, an ex-smoker's risk of heart attack is about the same as that of a lifelong nonsmoker.

High blood pressure. This number one risk factor for strokes is also a culprit in heart attack. The Hypertension Detection and Follow-up Program, for instance, sponsored by the federal government, was probably the largest blood pressure study ever. Of the study's 10,000 participants, those who fared best at bringing their blood pressure under control were rewarded with less chance of having a heart attack.

These three risk factors have been in the news for decades. In recent years, you have probably heard also about HDL (high-density lipoprotein) cholesterol, often referred to as "good" cholesterol. New findings do show that the total blood cholesterol count isn't the best measure of risk; rather, it's the ratio of total cholesterol to HDL cholesterol that best determines risk.

Why, then, do heart-health experts still list total blood cholesterol as the risk factor to watch? One reason is to keep things simple; another is that when the total cholesterol is high, it's usually not because of a high HDL, as we'd all hope.

Of those who check in with a total cholesterol count that is too high, the vast majority have too much LDL (low-density lipoprotein) cholesterol—the "bad" kind. So unless you know for sure that a high total count is due to an unusually good HDL reading, consider it a serious warning. (Should your HDL be low, by the way, take a tip from those with higher levels. As a group, they exercise regularly, shun cigarettes, and keep their weight under control.)

The Verdict Is In

Research on heart attack continues, of course. But a few years ago, a final verdict, so to speak, came in on the issue of cholesterol and heart attack. It was

Cholesterol: Weighing the Risk

Where to draw the line between normal and unhealthy cholesterol levels has been a matter of debate for years. For a long time, many laboratories considered any level below 300 as "normal." But that level was normal only in the eyes of statisticians. To them, it's customary to call all but the highest (or lowest) 5 percent of readings normal.

Needless to say, what is "normal" to statisticians may be a far cry from healthy. The possibility was debated for years. Then along came the Multiple Risk Factor Intervention Trial, which showed a definite link between high cholesterol and the likelihood of heart attack. So, in 1984, the National Heart, Lung, and Blood Institute (NHLBI) took action and decided to define exactly what is a desirable cholesterol level.

Because cholesterol levels tend to rise as we get older, the NHLBI panel chose to set different standards for various age groups. Here they are.

Age	Moderate Risk (mg/dl)	High Risk (mg/dl)
2-19	Greater than 170	Greater than 185
20-29	Greater than 200	Greater than 220
30-39	Greater than 220	Greater than 240
40+	Greater than 240	Greater than 260

the result of a nationwide research project sponsored by the National Heart, Lung, and Blood Institute (NHLBI). NHLBI hoped that this unusually large study–called the Multiple Risk Factor Intervention Trial (MRFIT) would settle the cholesterol issue once and for all.

Many had been skeptical that the MRFIT study would show any positive effect from lowering cholesterol levels because the subjects were middle-aged men at high risk. There was an expectation that it was "too little, too late" for the men, who no doubt had been harboring high blood cholesterol for decades.

But the fears proved unfounded. Against the odds, the efforts to lower cholesterol yielded impressive results. In the words of the NHLBI, "The benefits of lowering cholesterol are real. Recently released results of a clinical trial showed beyond doubt that men with elevated blood cholesterol who took steps to reduce it experienced fewer heart attacks that did men whose cholesterol remained at a high level. . . . In looking at the trial results, the scientists found that each 1 percent reduction in blood cholesterol produced a 2 percent reduction in the number of heart attacks. Thus, men who reduced their cholesterol by 25 percent cut their risk of heart attack by half."

With the MRFIT results in, the NHLBI decided it was time to turn research into action. The institute launched the National High Blood Cholesterol Education Program to get the word out about the importance of blood cholesterol and how to lower it.

Your Action Plan

Charting a healthy course for your heart is a two-step process. The first order of business is to count up your risk factors so you can figure how good a chance you stand of beating premature heart disease.

For some risk factors, this is easy to do. You already know whether or not you smoke, and if you do, how heavily. As for blood pressure, finding out your reading isn't hard. If you have the equipment, you can do it at home; you've probably noticed high-tech machines that test blood pressure springing up in shopping areas, too. We are all for having these options available, but we recommend that you have a professional reading, too. (It goes without saying that you must seek out a professional reading if a machine or home test shows a level anywhere close to the danger zone.)

The third important piece of information, of course, is your blood fat profile. Obviously, you can't do this one on your own. It's well worth a trip to the doctor's office, clinic, or health fair to have the blood test taken, though. Besides, as medical tests go, this one is fairly easy on the budget.

Once you know where you stand, you'll want to take action against worrisome risk factors. We don't have a diet to help you stop smoking. But if you have high cholesterol, high blood pressure, or high triglycerides, we've outlined nutritional approaches for you in the sections that cover each of these topics. Just turn to the entries, beginning on pages 136, 247, and 395, to find out more.

Suppose you don't smoke and your blood pressure and blood fats are in the good range. If so, congratulations! We do hope, however, that you will still go easy on foods rich in fat, cholesterol, and sodium. This preventive strategy can pay off handsomely in the future, for although it's okay now, your blood pressure and blood cholesterol are likely to rise as you grow older. By watching your diet now you have a better chance of avoiding future problems. And you'll benefit not only your heart but your overall health as well.

HEARTS OF PALM

A Dieter's Balm

21 calories per cup

If you were naming a food that is silky in texture and blessed with a deliciously delicate flavor, would you call it "swamp cabbage" or "hearts of palm?" Actually, both terms are used to describe this favorite of gourmet cooks, but given its elegant taste, we think the latter term is more fitting.

Hearts of palm are famous in Brazilian and some African cuisines. They're even more famous, we suspect, among dieters, who delight that a food tasting so good has only 21 calories per cup. If that's not enough to sell you on them, rest assured that they do more for you. A 1-cup serving provides 100 percent of the Recommended Dietary Allowance for vitamin A!

At the Market: Because of their perishability, hearts of palm are almost always sold canned. At home, remove from the can, drain, wrap in plastic, and refrigerate–they will keep this way for a couple of weeks. Slim hearts have the best flavor and texture for eating raw and for cooking. (However, tough, fat hearts can be made better by peeling off the "skin" with a sharp paring knife, so don't worry too much about the size.)

Kitchen Tips: To prepare, use a sharp knife to slice hearts of palm into coins or julienne slivers. From there, add them raw to green salads, marinated vegetables, or pasta salads. They can also be baked in casseroles or sautéed.

Accent on Enjoyment: Thanks to their delicate flavor, hearts of palm can be added to countless foods without seeming out of place. Try some of our favorites.

* For a classic dish from Rio de Janeiro, combine hearts of palm chunks with shrimp, cooked rice, sweet peppers, and saffron and bake until cooked through.
* Slice hearts of palm into julienne strips. Then sauté in olive oil with julienne strips of leeks, sprinkle with chopped toasted walnuts and serve hot as a first course or side dish.
* Add hearts of palm coins to soups or stews. They're particularly delicious in seafood soups and gumbos.

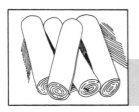

Hearts of Palm with Orange-Saffron Dressing

12 hearts of palm, rinsed
    and sliced into disks
½ teaspoon oregano
¼ teaspoon saffron
    threads, crumbled
2 tablespoons orange
    juice
2 tablespoons white
    wine vinegar
1 tablespoon peanut oil

Place hearts of palm in a serving bowl.

In a small custard cup, soak oregano and saffron in 1 tablespoon of orange juice. Let stand for 2 minutes.

In small bowl, whisk together remaining juice, vinegar, and oil. Add oregano, saffron, and orange juice to dressing and pour over the hearts of palm. Marinate for 1 hour before serving.

Makes 4 servings

HEMORRHOIDS

A Nuisance That Nutrition Can Fight

You know the old saying no one dies of a broken heart? Well, we doubt that anyone dies of hemorrhoids either, but somehow, there's not much consolation in that for someone who suffers from this age-old complaint. Although hardly what the doctor considers a serious threat to health, hemorrhoid attacks can be so intolerable that the only consolation is a treatment that works—preferably immediately.

If you've had hemorrhoids, you know the standard symptoms: lumps, pain, or itching in the rectal area. Bright red blood is also a sign of hemorrhoids, and it's also a sign that you should see your doctor. Bleeding could indicate a serious condition of the intestinal tract.

When a condition is as annoying as hemorrhoids are, it's only natural to wonder what brought it on in the first place. Not surprisingly, the possibilities are many. Some of the more common are:

- Frequent lifting of heavy objects.
- Pregnancy, especially the later months.
- Prolonged standing or sitting.
- Low fluid intake.
- Overuse of laxatives and/or enemas.

But still another factor is probably most important of all. It's the low fiber content of typical American diets. That, in turn, leads to constipation and straining. The increased pressure that accompanies these encourages the veins in the anal area to swell and become what we know as hemorrhoids.

Fortunately, you can do something about them!

What to Do

Treating a hemorrhoid attack and preventing one require different approaches. Bran, for instance, often works wonders for preventing attacks, but in the midst of one it is more likely to make things worse than better. During an attack, drink lots of water but go easy on coarse, whole grain foods, spicy items, or any foods such as raw fruits and vegetables that cause you to experience diarrhea.

When you're sure that the attack is over, you can start to think prevention. Fluids and insoluble fiber are the keys because of their ability to relieve constipation. You'll need to experiment with different levels of fiber in your diet and fine-tune your intake to give you best results. For all the how-tos, including meal plans, turn to the entry on constipation, beginning on page 151.

You may see results in no time at all. Melvin P. Bubrick, M.D., and Robert B. Benjamin, M.D., of the Park Nicollet Medical Center, Minneapolis, report that adding bulk to the diet in the form of psyllium (Metamucil and similar products) can help reduce anal pain and bleeding within six weeks. That's hardly a long time when you consider how long hemorrhoids have been in the works before causing trouble.

In addition to the dietary approach, consider these commonsense strategies for preventing future troubles.

- Exercise regularly, especially if you have a sedentary job.
- Take stretch breaks during periods of prolonged sitting.
- Don't linger on the toilet; a 5-minute maximum is recommended.
- Steer clear of laxatives or use them but rarely. In the long run, they are counterproductive.
- To the extent possible, avoid lifting heavy objects.

HIATAL HERNIA

How to Put Out Heartburn's Flames

Are you suddenly finding that there are foods you like that don't like you? Do large meals leave you with more than a feeling of fullness–like a burning pain under the breastbone? If so, you could have a hiatal hernia.

A hiatal hernia is actually a small part of the stomach that has slipped through an opening and managed to "ride up" into the chest, often taking stomach acid along with it. As you can imagine, the area above the stomach isn't designed to withstand the acids that the stomach produces. The result is heartburn. Pain, discomfort, and belching may also occur. But it needn't be a life sentence. With a little effort, you should be able to bring the fire of hiatal hernia under control.

Putting Pressure Where You Want It

Controlling the symptoms of hiatal hernia is a two-step process. The first part is increasing pressure on the esophageal sphincter muscle. You can think of it as a trapdoor between the food pipe and the stomach. Pressure there helps keep food and acid in the stomach, where it's supposed to be. For this reason, you'll want to avoid foods that lower the pressure in this area. These include:

- Alcoholic beverages.
- Coffee, tea, and other caffeine sources.
- Fatty foods.
- Peppermint or spearmint.

Now for the flip side. It's also important to reduce pressure inside the stomach, for pressure there gets things going the wrong way. Here are some no-no's that may increase pressure in the stomach and make matters worse.

- Wearing clothes that are too tight.
- Bending over when the stomach is full.
- Lying down shortly after eating, especially eating right before going to bed.

245

A Few More Tips

Don't pour fuel on heartburn's flames by eating foods that make conditions in the stomach more acidic. In this category are coffee and tea and acidic foods such as citrus juices or tomato-based products. (See "Putting Beverages to the Acid Test," on page 172, for a list of acidic beverages.) Needless to say, you should also avoid any other foods that trigger your symptoms. Your doctor is likely to suggest using antacids during a flare-up of heartburn symptoms.

In addition, be aware that overweight is no friend of hiatal hernia. If you can lose some weight, chances are that your symptoms will improve noticeably. Ditto for cigarettes. If you smoke, try to stop or at least cut down.

Friendly Fiber

With hiatal hernia often causing few if any symptoms, most doctors have not put energy into trying to prevent them. Nevertheless, Denis Burkitt, M.D., professor of medicine at St. Thomas's Hospital Medical School in London, thinks that hiatal hernia is preventable.

Dr. Burkitt, who ushered in the fiber revolution by proposing that this long-neglected nutrient helps prevent colon cancer, believes that high-fiber diets also make hiatal hernia less likely. Here are some of his reasons.

• Hiatal hernia is less common among vegetarians than among meat-eaters; vegetarian diets, of course, contain more fiber.
• American blacks are just as likely to develop hiatal hernia as the white population in the United States, yet the condition is extremely rare among blacks in Africa who are known for their high fiber intake.
• Hiatal hernia tends to occur in parts of the world where gallstones and diverticular disease are common, so there is some chance that all three share a common cause. Low fiber intake is a well-established factor in diverticular disease and is also considered a factor in gallstones. So there's reason to suspect that it influences hiatal hernia, too.

We'd like to have some more facts before we take a strong stand in this debate. But based on what we know today, it seems to us that once again, Dr. Burkitt is more likely than not to be right.

HIGH BLOOD PRESSURE

The Time Bomb Ticking Within

Whoever said ignorance is bliss didn't have high blood pressure. After all, who wants to be on a collision course with heart attack, stroke, or kidney failure?

Yet that's exactly where many of us are headed without even knowing it. Why? Simply because some of us don't check out our blood pressure—a harmless procedure that can prevent potential problems.

Fortunately, a growing awareness of the importance of normal blood pressure has encouraged millions to have theirs checked. A blood pressure reading, of course, includes two numbers. The top and larger number is called the systolic pressure; the bottom, smaller number is the diastolic pressure. High blood pressure is present when either one, or both, are elevated. Generally, a doctor will take action if the systolic tops 140 and/or the diastolic exceeds 90.

What's usually absent, however, is a clear set of symptoms. Nosebleeds and headaches are possible signs, but both have plenty of causes other than excessive blood pressure. Kidney changes and enlargement of one of the heart's chambers occur eventually, but not in the early stages. In short, high blood pressure needs to be looked for even when there are no signs that it exists.

Of course, we know enough to say that some people are more likely to develop the condition than others. Blacks, for instance, are at higher risk than whites. You should also count yourself in the "higher-risk" group if you:

• Have a family history of high blood pressure.
• Have a rapid heartbeat not readily explained by any other factor.
• Are overweight or drink heavily.

Having your blood pressure checked is simple, inexpensive and painless. So do it regularly.

Minerals in the Spotlight

If you are watching your blood pressure as a precaution or as treatment for a level already diagnosed as too high, you probably know all too well what

(continued on page 252)

247

Making Sodium Watching Simpler

Watching your sodium intake can seem complicated, we know. We, too, have longed for a simpler way, and think that this is it. Here, we focus on the best foods in each food category instead of all the foods that you should avoid. Those listed below provide less than 100 mg of sodium per standard serving. That means they qualify for the Food and Drug Administration's low-sodium label.

Needless to say, if you are on a strict sodium-restricted diet, you will want to follow advice tailored to your own personal needs.

Food	Sodium Range per Serving (mg)
Alcoholic beverages beer, distilled spirits, wine	0-25
Beans, cooked any unsalted beans and tofu (bean curd)	2-14
Beef, fresh most cuts	53-87
Cakes, prepared fruitcake	29
Cereals, cold 100% natural, Frosted Mini-Wheats, puffed rice, puffed wheat, shredded wheat	1-40
Cereals, hot, prepared, noninstant only farina, grits, oatmeal, cream of wheat	1-10
Cheeses dry curd cottage cheese, natural Swiss	17-74
Chicken and fowl most cuts of chicken, duck, or goose	56-86
Condiments apple butter, bitters, imitation ketchup, garlic clove; also horseradish, mayonnaise, Miracle Whip	0-9 50-80

Food	Sodium Range per Serving (mg)
Cookies (approx. 1 oz.) sugar wafers, macaroons	14-50
Crackers (approx. 1 oz.) melba toast, zweiback	1-80

Creams and creamers
  whipped toppings, half-and-half,
  imitation coffee whiteners
	4-29

Eggs egg white or whole egg	50-59
Fats and oils vegetable oil, any type	0
Fish and shellfish tuna, low-sodium, canned in water	46
Flour white, whole wheat, wheat-rye blend	3-4
Frozen desserts Creamsicle, Fudgsicle, Popsicle	9-37

Fruit, canned, plain
  applesauce, apricots, cherries, pears,
  peaches, pineapple, plums
	5-27

Fruit, dried apples, apricots, peaches, pears, prunes, raisins	2-18
Fruit, frozen mixed, raspberries, strawberries	3-8
Fruit, fresh most varieties	0-24
Grains barley	9-12

(continued)

Food	Sodium Range per Serving (mg)
Juices, canned or bottled apple, apricot, cranberry cocktail, grape, grapefruit, orange, pineapple, prune	5-9
Juices, fresh lemon, lime, orange	2
Juices, from frozen concentrate most varieties	1-20
Lamb leg, loin chop, rib chop, shoulder roast	56-77
Miscellaneous cocoa, jam, jelly, vinegar, yeast	0-2
Nuts (unsalted) and coconut almonds, brazil nuts, cashews, chestnuts, coconut, filberts, pecans, walnuts	0-7
Pasta egg noodles or macaroni, unsalted	1-2
Pork, fresh loin chop or roast	68-82
Rice and rice dishes instant, white long-grain, or converted	2-6
Seeds sunflower	11

Food	Sodium Range per Serving (mg)
Snacks	
unsalted popcorn or unsalted pretzels,	2-30
Nature Valley Granola Bars	65-80
Soups, prepared as directed	
many low-sodium varieties	35-75
Sugar	
granulated	0
Syrups	
corn syrup, chocolate syrup, honey	1-20
Turkey, fresh	
light meat or light and dark meat with skin	59-79
Veal	
cubes, cutlet, loin chop, rib chop, rump roast	56-83
Vegetables, fresh, cooked	
many if unseasoned	1-73
Vegetables, frozen, cooked, plain	
asparagus, broccoli, brussels sprouts,	
cauliflower, kale, yellow corn	1-82
Vegetables, raw	
cabbage, carrots, celery, cucumbers, lettuce,	
mushrooms, onions, spinach, tomatoes	2-52

to avoid–salty foods! Well, brighter days have arrived for you. While the time-honored advice to avoid the mineral sodium remains solid, it no longer stands alone. The new focus is on getting more–not less–of certain other minerals.

The two currently in the spotlight are calcium and potassium. And the findings are impressive. Here are some highlights from a few of the many studies that link these two minerals to better blood pressure.

- Mario R. Garcia-Palmieri, M.D., and his co-workers in the Puerto Rico Heart Health Program Study analyzed food habits and blood pressure among almost 8,000 men. Those who drank no milk–a leading source of calcium –were almost twice as likely to have high blood pressure as those who drank a quart or more per day.
- Putting calcium to a direct test, Marvin L. Bierenbaum, M.D., of the Jordan Research Group in Montclair, New Jersey, asked several hundred volunteers to drink milk fortified with extra calcium. They drank a quart a day, and as the study progressed, their blood pressures fell from an average of 126/82 to 119/76.
- At the University of California, Kay-Tee Khaw and Elizabeth Barrett-Connor, M.D., collected information on potassium intake for almost 900 men and women. They then followed their medical history for 12 years. Those who had the lowest potassium intakes at the beginning of the program had 2½ to 4 times the risk of stroke as those with more generous intakes.

Should you increase your intake of calcium and potassium based on findings such as these? Some say not yet; we see the issue differently. To us, the question is why shouldn't you increase your intake of these minerals when the signs are good that you can benefit? We haven't heard any reason not to, so we say "go for it." (See the entries on potassium and calcium, in the Appendix, for the best food sources of these minerals.)

Focus on Fat

Here's a puzzler for you from Australian researcher Ian L. Rouse, M.D. Impressed to learn that Seventh-Day Adventists–who follow a vegetarian diet–tend to have lower blood pressures, he decided to test a meat-free diet directly. He switched 60 volunteers from a typical diet to a meat-free diet, measuring their blood pressures at each step of the way. After six weeks without meat, blood pressures had fallen significantly, and analysis showed that changes in neither sodium nor potassium intakes could explain the difference. So what can?

Dr. Rouse concluded that the most likely explanation was a change in the type of fat that his subjects ate. Typically, vegetarian diets have a higher "P/S ratio"–that's nutritionist's jargon for a more favorable balance between polyunsaturated fat and saturated fat.

Research by James M. Iacono, Ph.D., and co-workers at the U.S. Department of Agriculture has supported the notion that this balance of fats positively affects blood pressure. In one of his own studies, for instance, Dr. Iacono tested the effects of just this kind of diet on blood pressure in 30 couples. While eating the diet with the higher P/S ratio, their systolic blood pressure fell by about 8 points and their diastolic by almost 3 points.

These diets, by the way, are similar to the standard cholesterol-lowering diet: Sources of polyunsaturated fat, such as oils and fish, are emphasized, and meat and dairy fats are minimized. We fully expect that someday soon, these diets will become as common for blood pressure control as they already are for controlling cholesterol.

Under the Influence of Alcohol (and Weight)

We hear so much about the negative effects of alcohol, and not surprisingly, the focus is on its obvious effects on judgment and behavior. But the effects of alcohol are far-reaching, and some, in fact, are completely hidden from our view–in particular, alcohol's effect on the risk of stroke. This effect may well be related to its impact on blood pressure.

Dr. H. Malhotra of Jaipur, India, looked at the effect of alcohol consumption on his patients with high blood pressure. He divided them into two groups: nondrinkers and regular drinkers. In both groups, he found that consuming alcohol did raise blood pressure in some way.

Remember, too, that alcohol packs in plenty of calories that can add up quickly. And we all know that excess calories can turn into excess weight.

So why should this be of concern to you if you're concerned with blood pressure? Because high body weight has been linked to high blood pressure. Swedish scientist Bjorn Fagerberg, M.D., for instance, found that modest weight loss–less than 20 pounds–was enough to make blood pressure fall significantly in overweight men afflicted with high blood pressure.

A New Slant on Sodium

If you are already watching sodium in hopes of controlling your blood pressure, you can get some extra mileage from your efforts by emphasizing low-sodium foods that also contain calcium—clearly a rising star in blood pressure research.

It's easier than you think. In fact, we've arranged for our computer to do it for you. All the foods in this list meet the Food and Drug Administration's (FDA) standards for low-sodium content. In addition, each provides a minimum of 100 milligrams of calcium.

We've divided the food list into three categories based on sodium content. They are:

Blue-ribbon foods. These contain less than 5 milligrams of sodium per serving, the FDA's standard for foods labeled sodium-free.

Red-ribbon foods. These contain 5 to 35 milligrams of sodium per serving, the FDA's standard for foods labeled "very low sodium."

Yellow-ribbon foods. These provide 36 to 140 milligrams of sodium per serving, the FDA's standard for foods labeled "low-sodium."

Here's the list of winners.

Blue-Ribbon Foods

Food	*Serving*
Almonds, chopped	⅓ cup
Dates, chopped	1 cup
Farina	1 cup
Navy beans, cooked	1 cup
Okra pods, cooked	10
Soybeans, cooked	1 cup

Red-Ribbon Foods

Food	*Serving*
Broccoli, fresh cooked or frozen	1 cup
Cocoa mix, Nestlé	1 cup
Cream of wheat, instant	⅔ cup
Fudgsicle	1

Food	Serving
Greens, collard, fresh, cooked	1 cup
Greens, mustard, fresh, cooked	1 cup
Greens, turnip, frozen	1 cup
Kale, frozen, cooked	1 cup
Masa harina, Quaker	1 cup
Molasses, blackstrap	1 tbsp.
Tofu (bean curd)	4 oz.

Yellow-Ribbon Foods

Food	Serving
Cheese, mozzarella, whole milk	1 oz.
Cheese, mozzarella, part-skim	1 oz.
Cheese, Swiss	1 oz.
Cream of wheat, quick	2/3 cup
Custard, baked with salt	1/2 cup
D-Zerta pudding, chocolate	1/2 cup
Eggnog	1 cup
Greens, collard, frozen, cooked	1 cup
Greens, dandelion, fresh, cooked	1 cup
Ice cream or ice milk	1 cup
Kale, fresh, cooked	1 cup
Milk, low-fat, skim, or whole	1 cup
Oysters, raw	4 oz.
Sherbet	1 cup
Yogurt, low-fat, fruit flavor	1 cup
Yogurt, whole milk, plain	1 cup

Going Down Slowly

These meal plans are part of our promise to make things as simple as can be. In this week's worth of meals, we've combined the latest strategies for controlling blood pressure—a minimum of sodium and saturated fat and good intakes of calcium, potassium, and polyunsaturated fat. And they taste good too!

Please remember, however, that as beneficial as diet can be in reducing blood pressure, you need to keep in mind that this, in turn, may affect the amount of medication you need. So be sure to give your doctor the opportunity to make any necessary adjustments.

Day 1

Breakfast
  1 ounce All-Bran cereal
  ½ cup 1% milk
  1 cup grapefruit
    coffee or tea

Lunch
  4 ounces water-packed white tuna
  1 tablespoon reduced-calorie mayonnaise or low-calorie salad dressing
  1 cup broccoli
  1 cup 1% milk

Snack
  1 cup low-fat fruit yogurt

Dinner
  4 ounces roasted veal rib
  1 baked potato
  1 cup cooked collard greens
  1 cup 1% milk
  ½ tablespoon unsalted high-polyunsaturated margarine

Day 2

Breakfast
  1 slice toasted mixed grain bread
  1 tablespoon unsalted diet margarine
  1 banana
  1 cup 1% milk

Lunch
Fruit 'n' cheese plate (1 cup part-skim ricotta cheese, 1 cup juice-packed
  peaches, 1 tomato, sliced, 2 teaspoons salad oil)
    iced tea

Snack
  ½ cup raisins

Dinner
  4 ounces roasted turkey
  1 cup broccoli
  1 pat unsalted high-polyunsaturated margarine
  1 cup cooked rhubarb, sweetened to taste
  1 cup 1% milk

Day 3

Breakfast
  1 cup sliced papaya
  2 slices toasted mixed grain bread
  1 pat margarine
  ¾ cup 1% milk
    coffee

(continued)

Going Down Slowly–Continued

Lunch
   1 cube (1 inch) natural cheddar cheese
   4 ounces flounder or sole, baked without fat
   1 cup brown rice
   1 tablespoon unsalted diet margarine or ½ tablespoon oil
   1 tablespoon lemon juice
   1 cup 1% milk

Dinner
   1 cup spaghetti with unsalted tomato sauce and cheese
   1 cup lima beans
   1 pat unsalted high-polyunsaturated margarine
   1 stalk celery
   1 cup fresh strawberries
   1 cup 1% milk

Day 4

Breakfast
   1 ounce All-Bran cereal
   ½ cup 1% milk
   ¾ cup pineapple-grapefruit juice drink
      coffee or tea

Lunch
   2 pieces roasted turkey breast
   1 ounce natural Swiss cheese
   1 tablespoon reduced-calorie mayonnaise
   1 slice rye bread
   1 cup low-fat fruit yogurt
   1 cup 1% milk

Snack
   1 cup sherbet

Dinner
 3 ounces baked salmon
 1 cup brussels sprouts
 1 tablespoon unsalted high-polyunsaturated margarine or ½ tablespoon oil
 1 apple, baked or raw
 1 cup 1% milk

Day 5

Breakfast
 1 cup unsalted cream of wheat cereal
 1 banana
 1 cup 1% milk
  coffee or tea

Lunch
Salad plate (¾ cup part-skim ricotta cheese, 2 lettuce leaves, 1 cup
  diced fresh pineapple)
 1 slice mixed grain bread
 1 pat unsalted high-polyunsaturated margarine
 1 cup 1% milk

Snack
 1 cup low-fat fruit yogurt
 ¼ cup unsalted almonds

Dinner
 ½ cup unsweetened canned applesauce
 2½ ounces lean broiled sirloin steak
 ½ cup cooked turnip greens
  1 pat unsalted high-polyunsaturated margarine
  1 cup 1% milk

(continued)

Going Down Slowly–Continued

Day 6

Breakfast
   1 ounce All-Bran cereal
  ½ cup 1% milk
    coffee

Lunch
  ¾ cup homemade macaroni and cheese, made with unsalted high-
      polyunsaturated margarine
  4 asparagus spears
  1 cup 1% milk
  1 orange

Dinner
Salad (1 carrot, 1 celery stalk, 1 tomato, 1 tablespoon salad oil,
   1 teaspoon white wine vinegar)
  3 ounces roasted chicken breast
  ½ cup lima beans
  1 cup 1% milk
  1 cup baked custard, homemade with low-fat milk

Day 7

Breakfast
  1 cup papaya
  1 ounce shredded wheat cereal
  ¾ cup 1% milk
    coffee or tea

Lunch
   3 ounces water-packed white tuna
   1 tablespoon reduced-calorie mayonnaise or salad dressing
   1 cup raw spinach
   1 pat unsalted high-polyunsaturated margarine
   1 fresh pear
   1 bagel
   2 tablespoons reduced-calorie cream cheese
   ¾ cup orange juice

Snack
   1 cup fresh blueberries
   2 tablespoons fresh whipped cream
   1 cup 1% milk

Dinner
   1 lean pork chop (trimmed of fat)
   ½ cup red kidney beans
   1 slice oatmeal bread
   2 pats unsalted high-polyunsaturated margarine
   1 cup 1% milk
      coffee or tea

INSOMNIA

Nutrition for a Good Night's Sleep

Most people credit good nutrition with helping them keep that "raring-to-go" feeling that we prize so much. Yet, odd as it may seem, nutrition also appears capable of doing the opposite. In fact, some nutrients are fast earning a reputation as the insomniac's best friend.

Is their reputation deserved? Well, the facts on hand are hardly conclusive, but they are far too compelling to be dismissed.

The Case of Tryptophan

These days, the amino acid tryptophan is getting its share of attention. Most notably, tryptophan *supplements* were implicated in 1989 in several deaths from a rare disorder called eosinophilla myalgia syndrome (EMS). Because of the potential seriousness of EMS, the federal Food and Drug Administration, as of this printing, has asked manufacturers to withdraw the supplements from the market and has strongly urged consumers not to take them. Even small doses of the supplement should not be taken. Tryptophan-containing *foods,* however, have not been implicated.

Tryptophan gained public interest in the first place because of its link to better sleep. For example, four or five tightly monitored studies showed that tryptophan has "high and reliable effects" against abnormal sleep patterns, according to sleep researcher Dietrich Schneider-Helmert of the University of Amsterdam. And at the Hospital of the University of Frankfurt, researchers tested tryptophan on patients with sleep problems. A dose of 2,000 milligrams of tryptophan proved beneficial against insomnia in about three-quarters of the patients. The treatment was very well tolerated, too–with the exception of one patient who developed nausea and diarrhea.

Naturally, even the most promising studies showed that tryptophan supplementation didn't work for everyone. As for getting enough tryptophan from food to induce sleepiness, it probably can't be done. Turkey, for example, contains a good amount of tryptophan, but it is also a high-protein food. And protein makes it harder for tryptophan to get into the brain, where the sleep center is located. Other amino acids in tryptophan-containing foods also end up as competitors. It seems tryptophan prefers to play sleep fairy on its own.

262

These facts notwithstanding, however, it appears you'd have to eat a huge amount of foods containing tryptophan to get the sleep-inducing effects.

Advice about Caffeine and Calcium

Though it may be the most controversial, tryptophan is hardly the only approach to insomnia. The time-honored advice to avoid caffeine-rich foods–especially in the evening hours–remains solid. For maximum effect, coffee, tea, and other sources of caffeine should be avoided throughout the day. Fortunately, the selection of caffeine-free alternatives has grown in the last few years, making this advice much easier to follow.

As for the sleep-inducing effects of calcium, we're on the fence. Some say that it works; others say it doesn't. As for warm milk, it has pluses and minuses. It provides calcium and tryptophan–but its high protein content reduces the ability of tryptophan to get into the brain.

Our advice? If a glass of warm milk helps you sleep, drink it.

IRRITABLE BOWEL SYNDROME

Friendly Foods to the Rescue

Gastroenterologists–the doctors who treat digestive disorders–are in great demand these days. The list of digestive disorders in the medical books is long–and growing longer. Yet, one condition accounts for almost half of the patients who see gastroenterologists. That condition is irritable bowel syndrome, or IBS for short. (It's also known as mucous colitis, spastic colon, and variations of these, but IBS is the preferred term these days.)

As any IBS patient can tell you, living with this condition is not easy. Naturally, symptoms vary from one affected patient to the next. As you can see from the following list, however, even one of the symptoms is likely to be at best annoying–and at worst, possibly disabling. The most typical are:

- Abdominal pain, bloating, or gas.
- Erratic bowel movements or diarrhea.
- Nausea or weight loss.
- Headache, fatigue, and/or impaired concentration.
- Anxiety and/or depression.

Usually, the IBS patient sees a pattern to the attacks. Although some bouts may seem to appear out of the blue, the symptoms are more commonly triggered by factors such as stress; overuse of laxatives, alcohol, tobacco, coffee, or tea; other troublesome foods; or lack of sleep.

IBS Basics

With so many patients to learn from, doctors have no shortage of experience from which to glean some basic facts about IBS. They've also intensified their research efforts. As a result, we now know far more about IBS than we did even a decade ago.

Here are some basic facts that should be understood by all who have IBS or suspect that they might.

264

- IBS symptoms result from abnormal muscle activity in the intestinal tract.
- IBS is a "functional" disorder. There is no damage to the digestive tract involved; only the bowel's function–not its structure–is disturbed.
- Women are three times as likely to develop IBS as men are. Female IBS patients also have a high rate of menstrual complaints, such as premenstrual syndrome.
- Some people are probably born with a predisposition to develop IBS. They have a built-in tendency to develop disorders of "smooth" muscle, of which IBS is but one example.

Obviously, facts such as these make clear that IBS is no condition for amateurs. Professional help is important–not only to identify possible causes and to design treatment–but also to keep an eye out for potential complications. IBS may lead to nutrient malabsorption or diverticulosis, for instance, so it's wise to find a knowledgeable physician and have regular follow-ups.

Because a variety of factors influence IBS, the doctors may favor a "whole person" approach to treament. Rather than rely on any one measure, this involves a broader plan that includes stress management, good sleep and exercise habits, control of alcohol and tobacco intake, and of course, nutritional strategies. This is not to say, however, one method by itself never works; for some patients, adding a single drug or food (or avoiding a certain food) makes all the difference in the world.

The Fiber Fix

We'll tell you right here that nutrition isn't the answer for every IBS patient. But one nutritional treatment has a record that we consider remarkable. It's bran–and it has been the saving grace for many IBS patients, especially those whose condition includes bouts with constipation.

A research study done by A. P. Manning, M.D., of the Bristol Royal Infirmary in England, sums up the benefits of bran as well as any we've seen. Dr. Manning divided IBS patients into two groups, and put one group on a diet high in insoluble wheat fiber, the other on a low-fiber diet. Here's how the two groups fared on key symptoms of IBS.

- Those on the high-fiber diet reported a reduction in pain, but those on the low-fiber diet did not.
- Bowel habits improved in about half of the patients on the high-fiber diet, but on the low-fiber diet, only one patient in seven had improvement.

• Many of the IBS patients originally reported that they passed mucus. The low-fiber diet made no difference on this count, but the high-fiber diet alleviated the problem for more than three-quarters of the patients who had it.

In a survey of gastroenterologists taken by mail, Dr. Manning and his colleague Dr. K. W. Heaton found that 93 percent were prescribing wheat bran, diets high in insoluble fiber, or both for IBS patients with constipation. About 84 percent of the doctors also prescribed similar treatment for IBS patients with diarrhea. With success rates such as those experienced by Dr. Manning's patients, it's easy to see why so many doctors are sold.

How do you turn talk of a high-fiber diet into action? You'll find meal plans rich in insoluble fiber in "Filling Up on Fiber," beginning on page 156. Some find, however, that no fiber source works as well as coarse bran. So as a general rule, it makes sense to first try adding unprocessed bran. We like this approach –it's nice and simple, not to mention remarkably effective for many.

The Allergy Angle

Nutritional approaches to IBS begin with fiber, but they don't end there. It's becoming clear that for some IBS patients, avoiding certain "trigger foods" helps enormously. In some cases, we're convinced, it's a true allergy to the food that provokes symptoms of IBS. For others, though, the problem is not a true allergy but rather a simple food intolerance. (See the entry on allergy, beginning on page 5, for more details on difference between allergies and intolerances.)

Suspecting that food sensitivities were causing symptoms in some of his IBS patients, Swiss researcher M. Petitpierre, M.D., put his hunch to the test. He asked 24 patients to follow a diet that eliminated foods that commonly cause allergy. The basic diet consisted of lake fish, apricots, rice, and bread made of corn and soy flour. Then, test foods were added–one at a time–to see if symptoms flared up. About half of the patients reacted to one or more foods. The most common offenders were milk, wheat, eggs, nuts, potatoes, and tomatoes. Of this list, the first four are well known to be common causes of food allergy.

Naturally, the food-sensitive patients were instructed to avoid offending foods. The result? After doing so for six months, about two-thirds of them were symptom-free.

We're impressed with these findings. We want to stress, however, as Dr. Petitpierre did, that only some of the food-sensitive patients were truly allergic to the problem foods. Others whose IBS was provoked by food were simply intolerant. Of course, whether allergy or intolerance, what's most important is that the treatment succeed.

In another study, J. F. Fielding, M.D., and dietitian Kathleen Melvin asked IBS patients about foods that provoked their symptoms. As you might guess, the list was long and varied. Rather than mention all the foods, we've included only the most commonly accused foods. They were:

- Fruits: apples, bananas, oranges, dried fruit.
- Vegetables: greens, onions, peas, potatoes.
- Smoked or fried foods: bacon, french fries, sausages.

No doubt, the IBS experts will be arguing the merit of these studies for a long time. Nonetheless, we don't think that the ongoing debate is grounds to dismiss these approaches as unproven. If avoiding one or more foods might lead to relief of your symptoms, why shouldn't you give it a try?

KIDNEY STONES

A Pain We Can Live Without

Although kidney stones and gallstones differ in many ways, there are similarities. Both tend to form in one place, then travel to another site where they cause trouble. For kidney stones, this new site is most frequently the ureter, where a lodged stone may block the flow of urine and lead to trouble that can't be ignored.

Of course, not all kidney stones lead to symptoms. Like gallstones that stay in the gallbladder, kidney stones that remain in the kidney and don't irritate or obstruct anything there may produce no symptoms. Like silent gallstones, these kidney stones go unnoticed until autopsy. We should all be so lucky as to have this kind, for kidney stones that do cause symptoms can bring excruciating pain. The severe pain is the best-known symptom, but others include:

- Nausea and vomiting.
- Fever and chills.
- Blood in the urine.
- Bladder irritability.
- Abdominal bloating.

Strangely enough, stones may be as small as a grain of sand, although some are many times larger. If you ever have the chance to see one, you will probably wonder how anything so small can cause so much pain.

Who Gets Them and Why

Anyone can have a kidney stone, but some of us are far more likely to get one than others. You're at higher risk if you can count yourself among any of the following:

- Men aged 40 and older.
- Patients who have gout or overabsorb calcium.
- People with a family history of stones.
- Heavy users of alcohol.
- Patients who have taken prolonged bed rest.

Probably the most important factor here is the composition of the urine. Conditions such as those listed above often affect the amount of calcium, oxalate, or other substances in the urine. These factors create a more favorable climate for stones to form.

Doctors also suspect that our water-drinking habits may influence the risk of kidney stones. They're confident that one simple habit–drinking plenty of water–can help prevent kidney stones from forming.

Treatment with a Future

The best treatment for troubling kidney stones is one that deals with the problem today but keeps an eye firmly focused on the future. Although most stones are passed eventually, an assist from modern medicine often is in order. Drugs, surgery, and ultrasonic therapy are available to do the job. Steps to prevent infection and damage to the kidney itself may be necessary, too.

Once the crisis passes, you may want to try to forget about it. But as your doctor can tell you, this is no time to close the book. Rather it's time to turn to the next chapter–which, naturally is about warding off a repeat experience.

Once retrieved, a kidney stone should be sent for chemical analysis. This information will help you plan for the future. The stone may contain large amounts of calcium or oxalate, for instance. Because both are found in food, a diet restricted in one or both may be in order. "Out with Oxalates!" gives details.

Some Supplemental Advice

The "stones and supplements" issue has been a controversial one in the nutrition field. We find that the likelihood of developing kidney stones as a result of nutrient supplementation has been exaggerated. That doesn't mean that we discount the possibility entirely, however.

In particular, we'd like to pass along some thoughts about three nutrients.

Vitamin C. Some vitamin C is converted to oxalic acid, which is a common substance in kidney stones. High doses of vitamin C (usually 4,000 milligrams or more) have been linked to recurrences of stones in a handful of cases. As a precaution, it makes sense for those at high risk to beware of high doses of C.

Calcium. Many kidney stones contain calcium. If yours do, you may be among those who overabsorb this mineral. Therefore, you should use supplements only with your doctor's consent.

Out with Oxalates!

If you are advised to restrict kidney-stone-forming oxalates from your diet, here is a list for you. We warn you, though, that on first reading, you may hardly believe your eyes. Many of the foods to avoid are the ones that nutritionists normally praise lavishly.

Even though these foods are all-stars when it comes to preventing heart disease, cancer, and other common health woes, if you have kidney stones, you have to put your kidney problems first. Regardless of their good properties, you'll want to avoid or cut back on these oxalate-rich items. Ask your doctor how strict you should be in keeping this diet.

If you are also advised to limit calcium intake, turn to the calcium entry, in the Appendix, for a list of calcium-rich foods.

Fruits

Blackberries
Cranberries
Currants
Figs
Gooseberries
Grapes, Concord
Lemon peel
Oranges
Plums
Raspberries, black
Rhubarb
Strawberries*

Vegetables

Asparagus
Beans, green and wax
Beets*

Vitamin D. This vitamin strongly influences calcium absorption—in some cases, even more than calcium intake does. Obviously, if you tend to overabsorb calcium, the last thing you need is a high intake of this vitamin.

*Beet greens**
*Chard**
Endive
*Lamb's-quarters**
Okra
*Parsley**
*Purslane**
*Spinach**
Sweet potato
Tomato

Nuts

*Almonds**
*Cashews**
*Pepper**
*Poppy seeds**

Beverages

*Chocolate**
*Cocoa**
Colas

*These foods contain the highest concentrations of oxalate.

Although we're not sold on the notion that supplements account for many kidney stones, we can certainly understand that those who have experienced one are likely to prefer a cautious approach.

KIWIFRUIT

Or Gooseberry, As They Say in China

46 calories per medium kiwifruit (skinned)

In China, kiwifruit is known as "Chinese gooseberry," and it originally was known in the United States by the same name. But New Zealand growers suspected that a more exotic name would fare better in the marketplace and changed the name to "kiwi" in honor of their national bird.

Some value kiwifruit for its striking appearance, others for its unique flavor. But in China, where it is still known as the gooseberry, the emphasis is on kiwifruit's healthfulness.

The appreciation for fruit emerged as part of a major research effort to conquer the astonishingly high rates of esophageal cancer that afflicted Chinese provinces such as Lin Xian. Suspecting that compounds called nitrites played a major role, scientists measured how much nitrite the residents carried in their bodies–and found very high levels.

Their next goal was to track down the cause of the abnormally high nitrite levels. Following leads from earlier research, attention focused on vitamin C. Sure enough, the high levels went hand in hand with the low levels of vitamin C. The scientists supplied vitamin C to a group of women, and within a week, their high nitrite readings had dropped dramatically.

Obviously, the virtual absence of fruits rich in vitamin C explained why the residents had so little vitamin C in their bodies. A campaign to explain the benefits of fruit was begun. Today, the barefoot doctors preach about the importance of fruit the same way that our doctors warn us about high blood pressure. (Kiwifruit is perfect on the high blood pressure front, too, because it's rich in potassium yet virtually free of sodium and fat.)

At the Market: If you're all thumbs when it comes to selecting good produce, kiwi is the fruit for you. Kiwifruit stores so well that finding a bad one takes effort. Unless the fruit is mushy, very hard, withered, or bruised, it's far more likely than not to be good. If a delightful strawberry/banana/lime fragrance is present in room-temperature fruit, this too, signals good quality.

Kitchen Tips: Wrap kiwifruit in perforated plastic. Stored in the refrigerator, it will last for about a month. Most people prefer kiwifruit peeled, which is easily done with a sharp paring knife. But the fuzzy skin is edible if you like it.

Raw kiwifruit contains an enzyme that inhibits gelling, so the fruit must be cooked before added to dishes that contain gelatin.

Accent on Enjoyment: No matter when you serve kiwifruit, you are unlikely to get complaints. Although great any time of the year, they make a great picnic food. Should you have any left:

- Slice and add to fruit salads or pies.
- Peel, puree, and create a sorbet or sherbet.
- Slice and use as an edible garnish for pies, cakes, fish, or chicken.

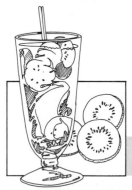

Kiwifruit Frappé

4 kiwifruit, peeled and coarsely chopped
½ cup ice cubes
⅔ cup milk
1 tablespoon maple syrup

Combine all ingredients in a food processor or blender and process until smooth. Pour into juice glasses and serve chilled for breakfast or a snack.

Makes 4 servings

KOHLRABI

A Cabbage by Any Other Name

48 calories per cup (cooked)

It looks and even sounds like it's from another planet, but actually, kohlrabi is quite earthy. Peculiar as its name is in the English-speaking world, it's as common as can be in other countries. The word *kohlrabi* means "cabbage turnip" in German. A rather mundane-sounding food after all!

Once you know the German translation, you can guess its first good point. Kohlrabi is a member of the now-famous cabbage family of foods. That alone makes it a healing food.

But wait—there's more. Kohlrabi is actually more nutritious than some of the better-known cabbage-family foods. Like the common turnip, it also earns kudos for its low sodium and fat content. When it comes to vitamin C and potassium, however, kohlrabi takes the lead. A cup of cooked kohlrabi supplies more than 100 percent of the Recommended Dietary Allowance for vitamin C.

At the Market: To ensure mellow flavor and texture, choose globes that are no larger than 3 inches in diameter. With the exception of the one variety that is vivid purple, the color should resemble clear pea green. Make sure that attached leaves are crisp and unblemished so you can add them to salads.

Kitchen Tips: To store kohlrabi, separate the bulbs from the leaves. Toss into separate perforated plastic bags and store in the refrigerator. The globes will last for about two weeks, but the leaves are more perishable and will only last for several days.

To prepare the globes, slice or chunk—but don't try to peel them—and simmer in water to cover until tender, about 25 minutes. Drain, and when cool enough to handle, remove the skin. As a result of cooking, it can be removed easily.

Kohlrabi is also a snap to microwave. To cook a pound, quarter and place in a 9-inch glass pie plate. Add 2 tablespoons of water and cover with vented plastic wrap. Microwave on full power for about 6 minutes, stirring after about 3 minutes. Let stand for 5 minutes, then zip off the skins and serve.

Accent on Enjoyment: Kohlrabi is versatile, as the suggestions below demonstrate.

- Substitute cooked kohlrabi chunks for potatoes in potato salad recipes.
- Kohlrabi is compatible with caraway, fennel seed, onion, dill, carrots, and parsnips.
- Mash cooked kohlrabi and serve half-and-half with mashed potatoes.

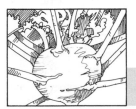

Creamy Kohlrabi Salad

1 pound kohlrabi globes, each about 2 inches across
3 scallions, minced
1 tablespoon minced red onion
¼ cup part-skim ricotta cheese
2 tablespoons reduced-calorie mayonnaise
1 teaspoon coarse mustard

Cut kohlrabi into quarters and steam, covered, over boiling water until tender, about 25 minutes.

When kohlrabi are cool enough to handle, remove the skins with your fingers. Place kohlrabi in a medium bowl with scallions and onion.

In a food processor or blender, combine ricotta, mayonnaise, and mustard and process just until creamy. (Don't overprocess or it will become too watery.)

Pour ricotta mixture over kohlrabi mixture and toss well to combine. Serve warm or at room temperature.

Makes 4 servings

LACTOSE INTOLERANCE

The Sugar Blues Revisited

There's probably no digestive disorder more appropriately named than lactose intolerance. The bloating, gassiness, cramps, discomfort, and diarrhea that it brings are enough to make anyone complain!

It may seem little consolation, but you're in good company if you have lactose intolerance. Most of the world's people–an estimated 75 percent–are lactose intolerant. The condition is common among those of oriental, black, or Mediterranean ancestry, and to a lesser extent, those of northwestern European descent.

The cause of lactose intolerance is simple. In order to digest lactose–the sugar in milk–your body needs to "split" it into two smaller sugars. The key to making the split is an enzyme called lactase, which, like other needed enzymes, is made by the body. If your body makes too little lactase, milk sugar will go undigested, causing the unpleasant symptoms of lactose intolerance.

Perhaps you were once able to drink all the milk you wanted, only to become intolerant to it in your middle or later years. Rest assured that your experience is common. As we grow older, our bodies produce less lactase. Consequently, lactose intolerance may develop at any time during the adult years.

A Multitude of Causes

If your lactose intolerance is genetic, you have what doctors call the "primary" form. Simply stated, this means that your troubles are *not* the result of some other condition of which lactose intolerance is but one feature.

There's plenty of primary lactose intolerance in this world. Yet other causes often account for more than a few cases, too.

Infections or inflammation of the digestive tract. Bacterial or viral infections in the gastrointestinal tract can interfere with normal lactase production, causing lactose intolerance for some time.

Stomach or intestinal surgery. Surgery can have temporary or permanent effects on the ability to make lactase.

Irritable bowel syndrome or celiac disease. These two chronic digestive diseases are accompanied by lactose intolerance in some patients. (For more information, see the entries on celiac disease, beginning on page 110, and irritable bowel syndrome, beginning on page 264.)

Say "Cheese, Please"!

Cheeses usually contain less lactose than an equivalent amount of milk. That means that lactose-intolerant individuals can often enjoy these foods—at least in controlled amounts.

Be aware, however, that all cheeses are not the same on this count. Of course, you should avoid any cheese that triggers your symptoms, regardless of its place on this list. If you are very sensitive to lactose, you should study this list carefully.

Low-Lactose Cheeses

American
Blue
Brick
Caraway
Cheddar
Colby
Fontina
Gouda
Gruyère
Limburger
Lite-Line
Monterey Jack
Mozzarella
Parmesan
Port du Salut
Provolone
Roquefort
Swiss (natural)
Tilsit

High-Lactose Cheeses

Cottage
Mysost
Primost
Ricotta
Sapsago

Alcoholism. We've learned from experience that alcoholics have an elevated risk of lactose intolerance.

Drugs. It's an unfortunate fact that drugs have side effects, of which lactose intolerance is but one. Certain antibiotics and antiarthritis drugs in particular are linked to lactose intolerance–fortunately, it's usually temporary.

Radiation. Here's another from the department of unfortunate effects. Radiation therapy in the area of the stomach or pelvis may cause lactose intolerance by damaging the tissues that produce lactase enzyme.

Prematurity. Although lactose intolerance is uncommon among newborn babies, it can occur, and premature infants are even more likely to have a temporary bout with it.

Testing for Tolerance

Naturally, the symptoms of lactose intolerance occur after drinking milk or foods made with it–and they can linger for as long as half a day. If this happens to you, or if your digestive complaints vanish if you avoid milk for a few days, you have what doctors call "presumptive evidence" of lactose intolerance.

Of course, doctors favor tests that yield hard evidence over presumptions. To confirm the suspicion of lactose intolerance, several tests are available.

Tolerance test. This approach measures the effect of lactose on your blood sugar level. If your blood sugar rises as expected after you are "challenged" with a standard dose of milk sugar, you are responding normally. The blood sugar of lactose-intolerant patients, by contrast, shows little increase–because the milk sugar hasn't been digested properly. (Moreover, the test sugar may bring on symptoms that the doctor can witness firsthand.)

Breath hydrogen analysis. This high-tech test is based on the simple principle that hydrogen in our breath comes from undigested carbohydrate in the digestive tract. Abnormally high levels after lactose is consumed is an obvious sign of lactose intolerance.

Mucosal assay. At one time, the favored test for lactose intolerance was an analysis based on a biopsy of the digestive tract lining. It's no longer in vogue, however, as other tests are credited with giving more reliable information with less difficulty.

Life without Lactase

Perhaps you have a firm diagnosis of lactose intolerance already. Or maybe you simply want to see what happens if you cut back on lactose-containing foods. Either way, you need information that many nutritional tables don't provide–the lactose content of foods.

Fortunately, the goal of a lactose-restricted diet usually is to cut down– not out. So most patients need not worry about eliminating every possible speck of it from their menu. According to Armand Littman, M.D., an expert on lactose intolerance at the University of Chicago, most patients do well as long as their daily lactose intake does not exceed 10 to 12 grams, which is the equivalent of about one glass of milk. Take a look at "Your Lactose Counter" to

Your Lactose Counter

The following table can be your guide to keeping your lactose intake within whatever limit works best for you.

Food	Portion	Lactose (g)
Butter	2 pats	0.1
Camembert cheese	1 oz.	0.1
Cheddar cheese	1 oz.	0.4-0.6
Swiss cheese, processed	1 oz.	0.4-0.6
American cheese, processed	1 oz.	0.5
Half-and-half	1 tbsp.	0.6
Blue cheese	1 oz.	0.7
Colby cheese	1 oz.	0.7
Cream cheese	1 oz.	0.8
Sherbet, orange	1 cup	4
Cottage cheese, regular	1 cup	5-6
Cottage cheese, low-fat	1 cup	7-8
Ice cream, vanilla	1 cup	9
Low-fat milk	1 cup	9-13
Chocolate milk	1 cup	10-12
Whole milk	1 cup	11
Skim milk	1 cup	12-14

NOTE: If you are extremely sensitive to lactose, you may also have to avoid foods that contain any of the following: casein, cream, lactose, margarine, milk chocolate, milk solids, and whey.

see which foods supply lactose and how much of them you'll be able to consume while still staying within recommended limits.

If you are supersensitive, you may react to as little as 3 grams of lactose a day. If you're among the most severely affected, says Dr. Littman, you can try limiting lactose even more; however, proportionately better results don't always happen.

Nutritionists worry that lactose-intolerant patients will have poor intakes of the so-called milk nutrients—calcium, riboflavin, and vitamin D. A simple solution is to take a daily multivitamin, which will ensure that riboflavin and vitamin D allowances are met. Consider adding a calcium supplement if, in addition to avoiding milk, you avoid other dairy foods such as cheese and yogurt.

New Breakthroughs

Thanks to some important new findings, diets for lactose intolerance are no longer based solely on avoiding lactose-containing foods. You'll want to take note of some advances that broaden—not limit—the food choices available to you.

The meal factor. Eating lactose-containing foods with meals enables some patients to tolerate milk better. Noel W. Solomons, M.D., of the Institute of Nutrition of Central America, found that only about half as much of the lactose in milk went undigested when patients consumed it at the same time as solid foods such as corn flakes, banana, and hard-cooked egg.

The lactase enzyme factor. Thanks to modern technology, you can now buy packets of lactase enzyme that break down the lactose in food before you eat it. Sold under the brand name LactAid, it's widely available in drugstores, or it can be ordered directly from the manufacturer. Write to the LactAid Company, P.O. Box 111, Pleasantville, New Jersey 08232.

Lactose-reduced dairy products. Encouraged by the success of LactAid enzyme, its manufacturer has also begun to market LactAid-treated milk, cottage cheese, cheese, and ice cream. These products have been pretreated with the LactAid enzyme and are ready to use. If you can't find them in your supermarket, contact the manufacturer for a source near you.

The yogurt factor. It's not just the amount of lactose that matters but also the form it's in. Joseph C. Kolars, M.D., of Minneapolis, found that 80 percent of his lactose-intolerant subjects complained of symptoms after drinking milk, but only 20 percent did after taking yogurt that contained the same amount of lactose! Dr. Kolars concluded that yogurt culture provides enzymes that can digest lactose.

As Dr. Kolars points out, it's no wonder that yogurt is so popular in countries where lactose intolerance is the rule!

Low-Lactose Meal Plans

We hope that we've convinced you that lactose intolerance is no cause for despair. As we see it, plenty of tasty options for meeting your nutritional needs are still available–and here are some meal plans to prove it.

These plans provide a good intake (1,000 milligrams daily) of calcium without requiring you to drink a lot of milk. Should your age or health needs call for more calcium, consider a supplement to make up the difference.

Once you've determined your personal tolerance to dairy foods, you can adjust these plans so that they are tailor-made for you.

Day 1

Breakfast
  1 cup oatmeal
  1 cup orange juice
  1 cup low-fat yogurt

Lunch
  3 ounces canned Maine or Norwegian sardines (with bones)
  2 pieces Italian bread
  ½ cup butterhead lettuce
  9 cucumber slices
  1 ounce natural Swiss cheese
  1 cup canned apple juice

Snack
  1 piece honeydew melon

Dinner
  3 ounces lean sirloin steak
  1 cup broccoli
  ¼ cup shredded cheddar cheese
  1 baked potato
  ½ tablespoon margarine

(continued)

Low-Lactose Meal Plans–Continued

Day 2

Breakfast
  1 cup canned pineapple juice
  2 pieces Italian bread
  ½ tablespoon margarine
  1 cup cooked cream of wheat cereal

Lunch
  1 ounce natural Swiss cheese
  4 radishes
  ¾ cup green pepper
  ½ cup canned water chestnuts
  1 cup low-fat fruit yogurt

Snack
  2 ounces cheddar cheese

Dinner
  3 ounces chicken breast (without skin)
  ½ cup cooked collard greens
  ½ cup brown rice
  1 tablespoon margarine
  1 cup iced tea

Day 3

Breakfast
  1 banana
  1 ounce cereal of your choice
  ½ cup lactose-reduced milk
  1 piece raisin bread
  1 tablespoon margarine

Lunch
  3 ounces water-packed tuna
  ¾ tablespoon reduced-calorie mayonnaise
  2 pieces Italian bread

1 ounce Swiss cheese
¼ cup alfalfa sprouts
1 cup orange juice

Snack
1 cup fresh strawberries with 1 cup vanilla low-fat yogurt

Dinner
1 cup oysters
¾ cup broccoli with cheese sauce
1 baked potato
1 tablespoon margarine
1 cup cantaloupe with ½ cup lactose-reduced ice cream

Day 4

Breakfast
1 cup cream of wheat cereal
1 slice Italian bread
½ tablespoon jelly

Lunch
3 ounces ground round
2 slices Italian bread
1 ounce Swiss cheese
¾ cup broccoli
1 cup orange juice
1 cup low-fat fruit yogurt

Dinner
3 ounces turkey breast (without skin)
¾ cup peas
½ cup cooked collard greens
¾ cup cauliflower
1 tablespoon margarine

Snack
12 ounces club soda
1 fresh pear   *(continued)*

Low-Lactose Meal Plans–Continued

Day 5

Breakfast
 1 cup instant oatmeal
 1 piece raisin bread
 1 pat margarine
 ½ cup apple juice

Lunch
 ¾ cup fresh spinach
 ⅓ cup onions
 12 cucumber slices
  6 radishes
  2 ounces blue cheese, crumbled
  1 piece Italian bread with yogurt cheese
  1 yogurt drink

Snack
 1 ounce Camembert cheese
 2 plums
   Tea with lactose-reduced milk

Dinner
 4 ounces steamed scallops
 1 cup bok choy
 1 baked potato with yogurt
 1 tablespoon margarine

Day 6

Breakfast
 1 cup low-fat fruit yogurt
 1 piece Italian bread with 1 ounce melted provolone cheese
 1 cup orange juice

Lunch
 3 ounces canned Maine or Norwegian sardines (with bones)
 1 English muffin
 1 slice low-fat cheese
   mustard to taste
 1 cup fruit cocktail with ½ cup vanilla yogurt

Snack
  coffee or tea with lactose-reduced milk
  1 baked apple

Dinner
  3 ounces chicken breast (without skin)
  1 cup broccoli
  1 cup baked beans
  1 cup club soda
  1 piece cantaloupe

Day 7

Breakfast
  1 piece whole wheat bread
  1 slice low-lactose cheese
  1 tomato slice
  1 cup cantaloupe
  ½ cup orange juice

Lunch
  4 ounces water-packed salmon
  1 tablespoon reduced-calorie mayonnaise
  2 pieces Italian bread
  1 cup low-fat yogurt
  1 cup fresh pineapple

Snack
  ⅔ cup almonds
  ½ cup low-fat fruit yogurt

Dinner
  3 ounces ground round
  ¾ cup okra
  ¾ cup broccoli
  1 baked potato
  1 tablespoon margarine
  1 cup iced tea
  1 cup fresh strawberries

LEEKS

To Know Them Is to Love Them

8 calories per ¼ cup (cooked)

Leeks may be a stranger to some Americans, but the way they liven up recipes makes them worth getting to know. We appreciate them for their culinary powers and also for what they lack. You don't have to give a thought to the calories, fat, or sodium that they add to a serving of food; the numbers are too close to zero to even bother counting. So if you've never tried them, please do.

At the Market: Leeks look like giant scallions, with white stalks and flat green leaves. Select those that appear moist, crisp, and unblemished. For best results in cooking, the stalks should all be similar in diameter, and those less than 1½ inches wide are usually best. Limp, dried-out leaves are a sign of leeks that may have been stored too long; bulb-shaped stalks can indicate woodiness.

Kitchen Tips: The leaves of leeks often harbor hidden sand, so rinse them carefully before cooking. It helps to mince them and put in a strainer, then rinse with cool water; the sand will flush right out. When using whole leeks, such as for braising or poaching, trim and spread the leaves, then rinse the sand away under cool water.

Accent on Enjoyment: You have to prepare leeks a few different ways to see how you like them best. Because chopped leeks can be substituted for onions in recipes, the possibilities are endless. Some other suggestions:

- Poach halved leeks for about 8 minutes, then marinate in an herbed vinaigrette. Serve chilled as a first course, salad, or side dish.
- Cook leeks, then season with cheeses, fine mustards, or herbs.
- Simmer leeks until tender, then puree in a food processor or blender. Serve warm with roasted meats or poultry.

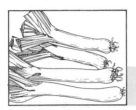

Leeks with Tangy Vinaigrette

1 cup chicken stock
1 bay leaf
1 pound leeks, trimmed,
    cleaned, and halved
1 yellow or red pepper,
    cut into julienne
    strips
  juice and pulp of
    1 lemon
2 teaspoons olive oil
½ teaspoon dried
    tarragon
½ teaspoon dried basil
1 clove garlic, minced
    freshly ground black
    pepper

Pour stock into a large skillet, add bay leaf, and bring to a simmer. Add leeks, cover, and simmer until tender, about 9 to 10 minutes.

Remove leeks from stock with a slotted spoon and arrange them on a serving platter, along with pepper strips.

In a small bowl, combine lemon juice and pulp, oil, tarragon, basil, garlic, and black pepper and whisk until combined. Sprinkle over leeks, then serve warm or chilled.

Makes 4 servings

LEG OF LAMB

Lean and Luscious

211 calories per 4 ounces (cooked)

Lamb is loved the world over and for many of us is a special treat. We're delighted to find that our favorite cut of lamb–the leg–is also the leanest and most nutritious.

Lamb is one of those foods so rich in protein that a single serving goes a long way toward meeting the day's allowance. More important, as a lean cut, leg of lamb does this without excessive calories and fat. In fact, a 4-ounce serving, trimmed of fat, has only 8 grams of fat–a moderate level compared to fatty meats.

Like other lean meats, lamb also supplies plenty of the "Big Three" B vitamins–thiamine, riboflavin, and niacin. But most of us get all we need of these easily, so we'd rather concentrate on something in lamb that too many of us run short on–the mineral iron.

A serving of lamb provides a healthy dose of iron, but the amount alone is not the only issue. Some of the iron in lamb is the heme type that is most easily absorbed by the body. In addition, lamb has some yet-unidentified factor that also helps us absorb more of the iron in other foods. Two of the world's foremost experts on iron absorption–James D. Cook, M.D., and Elaine R. Monsen, Ph.D., of the Kansas University Medical Center–have shown that two to four times as much iron was absorbed when lamb or other flesh food replaced egg protein in the diet. Naturally, nutritionists are impressed.

At the Market: Choose lamb that is pink- to red-fleshed and tightly grained. The fat should be cream colored and flaky, not greasy in appearance.

On the average, a whole leg of lamb weighs about 7 pounds. You can buy it several ways. For a big crowd, try it boned and butterflied; for a smaller group, buy half a leg that includes either the sirloin or shank portion. Get to know your butcher and he'll cut your lamb to order.

Kitchen Tips: Wrap lamb loosely in waxed paper and store in the coldest part of the refrigerator. It will last about five days. For longer storage, freeze it wrapped in freezer paper; frozen lamb will keep for up to a year. If you buy frozen lamb, however, don't refreeze it.

A whole leg of lamb (and often the sirloin and shanks section) has a covering of fat called "silver" or "fell" that should be removed before cooking–it simply can't be chewed. Again, call on a friendly butcher. Order in advance so the fell can be removed for you before you reach the store.

To cook lamb, roast, grill, broil, bake, or braise it. Robust barbecue-type marinades as well as lemon, garlic, rosemary, onion, citrus, or mustard complement it well. You'll get best results with short cooking at high heat; long, slow, dry methods will leave the meat tough and stringy. We recommend roasting at about 450° F until a thermometer shows an internal temperature of 170° F.

Accent on Enjoyment: Lamb is classic with eggplant or mint; our own favorite is curried lamb with apples and onions, served over pasta or rice. Some other ideas:

- Chunks of lamb can be used instead of beef in kabob recipes.
- Lime juice and hot pepper sauce will make a tasty low-calorie marinade.
- Ground lamb makes good burgers and is terrific in lasagna.
- Thinly sliced leftover roasted lamb can be added to a pasta or marinated vegetable salad.

One final note: Lamb is from a young animal; flavor and texture are best from those slaughtered young. Meat from an animal that was more than 18 months old is actually not lamb but mutton. It has a stronger flavor and can be substituted in most lamb recipes if the cooking time is increased by about 7 minutes per pound. Moist cooking methods, such as stewing, are best for mutton.

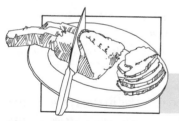

Marinated Sirloin of Lamb

3½ pounds sirloin of lamb, boned and butterflied
1½ teaspoons frozen orange juice concentrate
1 tablespoon soy sauce
2 teaspoons honey
2 teaspoons peanut oil
2 cloves garlic, mashed

Using a sharp knife, remove the visible fat, membrane, and fell from lamb. Then place it in a 13 × 9-inch ovenproof glass casserole.

In a small bowl, combine orange juice concentrate, soy sauce, honey, oil, and garlic. Pour over lamb and rub in until lamb is completely coated. Marinate for at least 4 hours or overnight.

Preheat the broiler.

Broil lamb until it is done the way you like it, about 7 to 10 minutes on each side for medium-rare. Let it stand for about 5 minutes before cutting it into thin slices, then serve warm or chilled.

Makes 4 servings

LENTILS

Beans without the Bother

212 calories per cup (cooked)

For those who'd like to eat less meat but worry about getting enough protein, consider the lentil.

For total protein, lentils can hold their own against meat and dairy foods. A cup of cooked lentils has 16 grams of protein, compared to 15 in a 3-ounce patty of lean ground beef. And while the protein in beef is said to be better in quality, the facts show that adults who have enough to eat rarely have to concern themselves with protein quality. We get enough even if we don't take advantage of the so-called best sources.

And even though lentils have more protein than the beef, they have less fat. In fact, lentils are virtually fat free, a claim that the hamburger—with 18 grams of fat per patty—can hardly make.

At the Market: Lentils look like tiny disks and are usually red-brown in color; occasionally you will find them in bright orange, khaki, olive green, or gray. They are sold dry, and in choosing them look for whole, unbroken ones that smell fresh and faintly nutty.

Kitchen Tips: Store lentils in a tightly covered glass jar in the refrigerator. These hardy legumes will last for up to a year. The longer you store them, however, the longer you will need to cook them.

Unlike beans—also members of the legume clan—lentils are a snap to prepare. Just combine 1 cup of dried lentils with 4 cups of water. Bring to a boil, reduce to a simmer, and continue cooking, loosely covered, until tender—about 30 minutes. You'll get about 2¾ cups of cooked lentils, which can be used in casseroles, soups, stews, salads, or rice dishes.

Hard water can toughen lentils during cooking. In hard-water areas, consider cooking lentils in bottled water.

Accent on Enjoyment: Lentils are excellent when seasoned with garlic, onions, leeks, coriander, cumin, curry, sweet peppers, chilies, yogurt, or cheese. We like to puree them and use in spreads and dips. We also make a "stuffing" of cooked lentils and cooked rice; it's perfect to use in stuffing eggplant or sweet peppers. Top with mild white cheese and bake until the cheese has melted; you'll convert even the most skeptical palate.

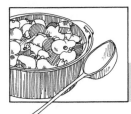

Lentil Stew with Curry Paste

1 tablespoon olive oil
1 medium onion,
   chopped
1 medium carrot,
   chopped
1 stalk celery with
   leaves, chopped
4 cups chicken or beef
   stock
   juice and pulp of
   1 lemon
½ cup lentils
1 cup sweet corn kernels
2 cloves garlic
1 teaspoon cumin seed
1 teaspoon coriander
   seed
½ teaspoon turmeric
½ teaspoon hot pepper
   sauce, or to taste

In a large stockpot, warm oil over medium heat. Add onion, carrot, and celery and sauté, stirring occasionally, until vegetables have wilted and are fragrant, about 7 minutes.

Add stock, lemon juice and pulp, lentils, and corn and bring to a boil. Reduce heat and simmer, covered, for 20 minutes.

In a spice grinder or a mortar and pestle, combine garlic, cumin, coriander, turmeric, and hot pepper sauce, then grind into a paste.

When stew is ready, add paste and stir well to combine. Simmer for an additional 15 minutes, or until lentils are tender. Serve hot. This mixture is good with warm pitas or topped with plain low-fat yogurt.

Makes 4 servings

LETTUCE

Go for the Green

(See also *Greens*)

10 calories per cup romaine (raw)

Are you a salad lover? If so, you probably know that salads offer a delicious way to get more fruits and vegetables onto the menu.

You'll get the most nutrition, of course, if you favor lettuce that is deep green in color. It packs the same nutritional attributes as greens that are traditionally cooked—lots of carotene, some vitamin C, and a fat, sodium, and calorie count to make any heart glad.

One especially interesting fact about lettuce is how often the word appears in reports on cancer prevention. In its review on the prevention of stomach cancer, the Committee on Diet, Nutrition, and Cancer of the National Academy of Sciences commented that "protective factors may include consumption of milk, raw green or yellow vegetables, especially lettuce, and other foods containing vitamin C." So, to fight cancer with your fork, enjoy salads often.

At the Market: Lively heads that are crisp and colorful are the only ones to buy. Once lettuce dries out, it cannot be revived, so stay away from heads that are wilted and discolored.

Of course, you have a garden of varieties to choose from year-round, and each has a distinct personality. The butterhead group, which includes Boston and bibb, are small, delicate heads that are perfect with light vinaigrettes. Cos is a tougher group with darker, longer leaves; it includes the popular, unwilting romaine. Leaf lettuces can be red or green and are good, all-purpose varieties.

Kitchen Tips: Put unwashed, uncut lettuce in a tightly closed plastic bag and refrigerate. Most varieties will last for up to a week. Rinse lettuce in cool water before using. Pat dry or run through a salad spinner and it will hold dressing better. If cut with a knife, lettuce discolors at the edges, so always tear the leaves instead.

Accent on Enjoyment: Salads are the obvious use for lettuce, but there are others.

- Use crisp leaves, instead of crackers, to scoop up dip.
- Simmer shredded lettuce with fresh baby peas.
- Make use of lettuce that has lost its crispness; mince and add it to soups.
- Sauté chopped lettuce with a bit of onion, then cook down until soft and wilted. Puree with a bit of fresh dill and serve hot with grilled chicken.

Most of us serve salads before the entrée without a thought. Take a tip from the Italians, however, who serve them after the entrée. This is a refreshing idea that can take your mind off dessert!

Beyond the Iceberg

If you still rely on the old standby, iceberg lettuce, now is the time to explore some different varieties of greens. Watercress, beet greens, arugula, radicchio, dandelion greens, purslane, and even parsley can liven up a salad.

Choose several different greens for your salad so you'll have a good contrast of tastes and textures. Watercress, baby spinach, and curly kale, for instance, are a tasty trio.

Still, you can ruin a good green salad quickly by drowning it in a fatty dressing. Be sure not to use too much dressing. One tablespoon is enough to dress greens for four. Here are some ideas to keep your salad low in calories.

- Use pureed fresh tomato or peeled seeded cucumbers as a low-fat base for dressings. Add a bit of grated lemon peel to the tomato and lemon juice and dill to the cucumber.
- Try plain low-fat yogurt with fresh minced herbs as a good dressing for crisp greens.
- Try cider vinegar with citrus zest, for a surprisingly flavorful sprinkle.
- Combine buttermilk with a bit of Dijon mustard and use to dress sharp greens such as arugula and watercress.
- Toss your salad well. Thirty times, using large salad paddles, will distribute the dressing perfectly.
- Resist the urge to chill your salad. Cold numbs taste buds, and if you taste less, you'll be apt to pour on more dressing.

MANGOES

Treat from the Tropics

135 calories per mango

Some people brag that the only vegetable they eat is pickles. The way we see it, why argue with vegetable haters. If they turn up their noses at vegetables, we offer them fruit that boasts the same nutrients as the vegetables that they won't even try.

Mangoes, needless to say, fall into this select group. Few fruits are empowered with more than a day's worth of vitamin A per serving, but mango makes the grade with 30 percent more than the Recommended Dietary Allowance. And this vitamin A (as carotene) comes with the full allowance of vitamin C, too.

And you needn't give a thought to its fat or sodium content, either; these two are barely detectable. There is, however, a moderate level of insoluble fiber nestled within the tender flesh of the mango—perfect for anyone who brags that the only residents of his house who eat bran are the termites.

At the Market: Ripe mangoes are deep or grass green with touches of yellow and blush. They are often freckled in appearance. When ripe, a mango will yield slightly to gentle pressure.

Kitchen Tips: Refrigerated, mangoes will keep for a couple of weeks. To peel, rinse well, then cut lengthwise all the way around the stone. Next cut slices and pull them away from the stone. Finally, zip the skin off, just as you would with a banana. For best flavor, eat raw mangoes chilled, but also try them baked in pies or custards, sautéed or stewed with other fruits.

Accent on Enjoyment: Mangoes add richness and sweetness to recipes, without adding lots of fat or calories. To take advantage of what mangoes have to offer:

- Puree and use in ice creams, beverages, or puddings.
- Add to fruit salads.
- Sprinkle with lime juice for an extra low-fat dessert.

294

• Try mangoes the Brazilian way—speared on holders like those used for corn —and served for dessert.

Should you find yourself with an unripe mango, peel and chop it, then use in chutneys.

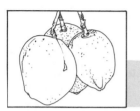

Mango with Tomatoes and Scallions

1 large mango or 2 small
  mangoes
2 medium tomatoes
2 scallions, minced
  juice and pulp of
  1 lemon
2 teaspoons safflower oil
pinch of dry mustard

To prepare mango, use a sharp paring knife to slice it in half lengthwise, around the large stone. Use the slice mark as a starting place to peel away the skin. Then slice off strips of mango flesh, working around the stone. Slice the strips into bite-size pieces and place them in a medium bowl. (The whole process is easiest if you do it over the sink.)

Cut tomatoes into chunks and add them to mango slices, then add scallions and toss well.

In a small bowl, whisk together lemon juice and pulp, oil, and mustard. Pour over mango mixture and toss well. Serve at room temperature or chilled on salad plates.

Makes 4 servings

MELONS

Sweetness Less the Calories

Cantaloupe: 93 calories per ½ melon

Casaba: 43 calories per ⅒ melon

Honeydew: 45 calories per ⅒ melon

Watermelon: 110 calories per ¹⁄₁₆ melon

Unless you live in a year-round warm climate, winters may leave you feeling that everything that tastes good is bad for you. But as soon as the warmer weather rolls in with a bumper crop of melons, you'll change your tune. There's no better example of great taste and great nutrition in the same package than a perfectly ripe melon.

Foods such as melon are attracting more attention in the scientific world, too. Research by Regina G. Ziegler, Ph.D., and her associates at National Cancer Institute has established a link between ample intakes of vitamin-rich fruits and protection from cancer of the esophagus. The best fruits, of course, are those that offer vitamin A or C. You can count on your choice of melons for the vitamin C and on cantaloupe for both in one package.

And that's just the beginning. Melons are also good for potassium–with a half of cantaloupe providing an incredible 825 milligrams. This potassium, along with low levels of sodium and fat, makes it the perfect treat for those concerned with blood pressure.

Cantaloupe

At the Market: Look for cantaloupe that is firm and unbruised, with an even gray netting. Hard green cantaloupes have been picked too soon and are best avoided. When ripe, cantaloupe has a characteristic sweet and delicate odor; if it's not fragrant, leave it at room temperature for a few days to ripen. Fully ripened fruit gives to gentle pressure on the base; overripe fruit feels sticky when you run your hand across it.

Kitchen Tips: Although cantaloupe must be ripened at room temperature, it should be refrigerated once ripe. Always cover cut cantaloupe with plastic wrap before storing.

296

Accent on Enjoyment: Cantaloupe is well loved, served plain or fancy. Some ideas on the latter count:

- Peel, slice, and toss with berries or other seasonal fruits.
- Halve and top with frozen yogurt.
- Make a main dish by filling cantaloupe halves with chicken or shrimp salad.
- Puree cantaloupe and make into a sorbet or sherbet for a real treat on a hot summer day.

Casaba

At the Market: Don't be surprised by the wrinkled skin that you see at the pointed stem end; it's normal. Casaba melons lack the sweet fragrance that cantaloupes have when ripe, but they signal ripeness with skin that is furrowed and pale yellow. The flesh will be creamy ivory and juicy.

Kitchen Tips: Like cantaloupe, casaba is stored at room temperature until ripe, then refrigerated.

Accent on Enjoyment: For a quick dessert:

- Drizzle chunks of casaba with lime juice and serve in chilled wine goblets.
- Puree casaba with some orange juice, then chill and enjoy later as a fruit-soup dessert.
- Fill rings of casaba with blueberries and serve on chilled plates garnished with mint sprigs.

One final word: Casaba and cassava are two very different foods. The latter, also known as manioc, is a root crop typically found in tropical climates.

Honeydew

At the Market: A honey of a honeydew smells pleasant and fragrant at the blossom end. The skin should be buttery in color and will feel velvety and probably somewhat sticky–the result of the sugars in the flesh. When you hold a good honeydew in your hand, it will feel heavy for its size.

If you suspect that a melon is overripe, shake it; seeds and juice sloshing around inside indicate overripeness. If the flesh is broken or looks frozen when you cut it open, the melon is overripe and should not be eaten.

Kitchen Tips: Honeydews should be refrigerated. If you cut them into chunks, wrap them as tightly as you can to avoid drying.

Accent on Enjoyment: We find that honeydew disappears before we can do anything special with it. But if you can keep it on hand, try some of these ideas.

- Puree honeydew to make a chilled soup. Serve in chilled melon halves garnished with mint sprigs.
- Serve sliced melon with smoked turkey as an appetizer or light entrée.
- Drizzle honeydew with its classic accompaniment–lime juice–and top with other fruits.

Watermelon

At the Market: When eyeing cut melon, look for flesh that appears moist and tight, not mealy. Judging whole melons is trickier, but start by checking the underbelly–that is, the part that rested on the ground when it was growing. A pale yellow color indicates a ripe, flavorful melon; a white or sprout green means the melon was picked too soon and will be short on flavor. A shriveled stem also signals ripeness.

Kitchen Tips: Store whole watermelon at room temperature. Cut sections should be wrapped and refrigerated.

Accent on Enjoyment: Watermelon is great eaten fresh in slices; the rind is often saved and pickled. For a more novel dish, seed a watermelon, then puree and make sherbet or sorbet. Or puree seeded watermelon with other soft fruits. Sprinkle in a bit of lemon juice and serve chilled as a dessert soup.

Melon Compote with Strawberry Dressing

2 cups melon chunks or
   balls (honeydew,
   cantaloupe, crenshaw,
   or your choice)
1 cup fresh strawberries
   honey (optional)
1 teaspoon lime juice
3 tablespoons orange
   juice
   mint sprigs for garnish

Arrange melon in wine goblets or pretty dessert dishes.

Place strawberries in a food processor or blender. If strawberries are very sweet, you won't need honey, but if not, add some honey, to taste. (1 teaspoon may be enough for the whole cup.) Add juices and process until smooth.

Pour dressing over melon and garnish with mint sprigs. Serve at room temperature or chilled.

Makes 4 servings

Icy Watermelon Soup

2 cups watermelon
2 cups orange juice
1 tablespoon frozen
   orange juice
   concentrate
   orange peel ribbons or
   mint sprigs for
   garnish

Combine watermelon, juice, and concentrate in a food processor or blender and process until smooth. Chill mixture (in the processor bowl or blender jar) for at least an hour. Reblend briefly before serving.

Pour into chilled bowls and garnish with orange peel or mint sprigs, then serve as an appetizer or dessert.

Makes 4 servings

MILK

Love It Low-Fat

Nonfat dry milk: 31 calories per 2 tablespoons
Fresh skim: 80 calories per cup
Fresh low-fat (1 percent): 102 calories per cup

As we see it, healthful milks are for those who like them. We're not ones to insist that you drink milk if you'd rather not; there are other sources of the good things found in milk. But if you're going to drink it, drink only the low-fat varieties–that is, preferably skim milk or 1 percent milk. Whole milk, though high in calcium, is just too high in fat to rate as a healing food.

So, if milk is your thing (and we do know adults who drink more of it than their children do), stay tuned for the latest in health news about this age-old beverage. We'd like to mention three health issues where milk is a hot topic.

Better blood pressure. Scott Ackley and his co-workers at the American Heart Association surveyed 5,000 California residents and found that men with normal blood pressure typically drank twice as much milk as those who suffered from high blood pressure.

Better bone health. At the University of Pittsburgh, Rivka Black Sandler, Ph.D., and her associates interviewed middle-aged women about their lifelong food habits. The women who recalled drinking milk with every meal during their childhood and adolescence had denser, healthier bones than women who had drunk milk less often. When Dr. Sandler compared women who said they drank milk with every meal up to the age of 35 to those who said they rarely drank it, the differences in bone health were even more dramatic.

Better resistance to cancer. Analyzing nutrition and health statistics collected during a 20-year study of heart health among manufacturing workers, Dr. Cedric Garland and his co-workers found that those who drank no milk were nearly three times as likely to develop colorectal cancer as those who drank several glasses a day.

In every one of these studies, of course, it appears that the protective factor is not milk itself but its calcium. So the point is to get your fair share of this important mineral. And to avoid taking in excess fat at the same time, make sure you drink low-fat milk. It has the same amount of calcium that whole milk does.

300

Nonfat Dry Milk

At the Market: Nonfat dry milk comes two ways: instant and regular. The regular is usually cheaper and is fine for baking, but instant is easier to dissolve in liquids and is favored for drinking.

Kitchen Tips: Keep nonfat dry milk fresh by storing in a tightly closed glass jar in the refrigerator. To mix a lump-free batch, process it in a food processor or blender. When heating, use a heavy-bottom pan over medium-low heat or a double boiler to keep the milk from scorching.

Accent on Enjoyment: You don't have to turn dry milk into liquid milk to reap its benefits to your health and food budget. As an alternative, add dry milk powder directly to pancake and waffle batter, bread dough, hot cereals, or soups. Many people who want more calcium in their diets keep a canister of dry milk handy and add a spoonful or two to a wide range of foods.

To cultivate a taste for milk made from dry powder, start out mixing the dry powder with skim milk. Then gradually reduce the amount of skim milk, replacing it with water.

Liquid Milk

At the Market: Milk processors sometimes label low-fat milks with names such as Lite or Jog. But any brand that indicates a milk fat content of 1 percent or 2 percent (preferably the former) or is labeled skim or nonfat will be fine.

With something that we buy so often, it's easy to forget simple but important guidelines. But try to get in the habit of checking the expiration date on the carton and be sure to run your hand across the bottom so you don't take home a carton that is leaking.

Kitchen Tips: It goes without saying that fresh milk must be stored in the refrigerator—and the sooner, the better.

Milk can be fussy when used in cooking. Heat it gently, and whisk occasionally to prevent a skin from forming on top. When combining low-fat milk with an acid ingredient such as tomatoes or lemon, slowly add the acidic food to the milk, not vice-versa. This will help prevent curdling.

Accent on Enjoyment: Just because you're counting calories doesn't mean you don't enjoy that creamy dairy texture. Try some of these ideas to keep your taste buds happy.

- Replace cream or whole milk with low-fat milk in soups, baked goods, casseroles, and puddings.
- Create creamy fruit shakes by combining chilled low-fat milk with pureed fruit or fruit juice. For example, combine 1 cup of low-fat milk with ½ cup of fresh strawberries in a food processor or blender and process until combined. Serve chilled.
- Whip up a healthy alternative to whipped cream with low-fat milk. Simply pour the milk into a bowl and freeze just until tiny crystals begin to form on top. Then whip as you would cream. Whipped low-fat milk won't hold its peaks as long as cream, but it's a great dessert topping for dieters.

Try a Health Shake

For two servings, combine each set of ingredients in a food processor or a blender and process until combined.

- 2 cups low-fat milk, 1 cup pitted canned apricots, 2 tablespoons maple syrup.
- 1 cup low-fat milk, 1 cup plain low-fat yogurt, 1 banana, ¼ cup creamy peanut butter, 2 tablespoons honey.
- 2 cups low-fat milk, 1 peeled and pitted avocado, ½ teaspoon grated lemon peel.
- 1 cup low-fat milk, 1 cup apple juice, ½ cup applesauce, 1 tablespoon maple syrup, dash of ground cinnamon.
- 1 cup low-fat milk, 1 cup orange juice, 1 peeled and pitted peach, dash of freshly ground nutmeg.

MILLET

A Grain That Grows on You

About 100 calories per cup (cooked)

Thirty years ago, researchers at the Harvard School of Public Health began a unique study that focused on the age-old debate about heredity versus environment. They enlisted about 500 men who had been born in Ireland but who had immigrated to Boston and an equal number of brothers of these men who had remained in Ireland. Several hundred Bostonians of Irish descent also participated.

For several decades now, the "Boston Brothers Study," as it has been nicknamed, has been yielding impressive clues about healthy lifestyles. In 1982, the researchers reported that about 150 of the participants had died so far of heart disease. Those who succumbed to its ill effects tended to have diets lower in carbohydrates, fiber, and vegetable protein than those who survived.

Which brings us to millet. Although less commonly eaten in the United States than grains such as wheat and rice, millet, too, is just the thing to boost your intake of the protective trio of carbohydrates, fiber, and vegetable protein. It's got all three, and in addition, it's richer in iron than grain foods such as pasta, rice, and barley. Add a little meat or a source of vitamin C to the meal and you'll get the most that you can out of the iron it contains.

At the Market: Millet looks more like a seed than a typical grain. For the best quality, choose tiny, round, red or yellow dots that are evenly colored and sized. Good millet smells faintly nutty with no mustiness.

Kitchen Tips: Keep millet in a tightly covered jar in the refrigerator. If you don't use it frequently, you can freeze it without needing to defrost it before cooking.

The simplest way to cook millet is to combine 1 cup of grain with 3 cups of water in a medium saucepan and simmer, loosely covered, until tender, about 45 minutes. One cup of raw millet will yield about 3½ cups cooked– enough to feed about four people. You can also sauté the millet first, to create a pilaf; as a result, the simmering time will be reduced by about half.

Accent on Enjoyment: Light textured with a gentle crunch, millet is a lot of fun to eat. It gives character to combination grain dishes, or you can use the following ideas.

- Use in place of rice in salads, side dishes, and entrées.
- Make a great breakfast by combining millet with grilled apple slices and your favorite spices.
- Add cooked millet to yeast bread dough.
- Sprout it yourself! Like lentils, alfalfa seeds, and mung beans, millet can be sprouted and added to salads and sandwich fillings. One word of advice: Fresh millet is easier to sprout than grains that have been frozen or refrigerated for a while.

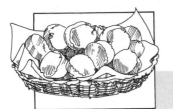

Millet Biscuits with Sage and Basil

1 cup whole wheat
    flour
1½ cups unbleached
    white flour
1 teaspoon baking soda
¼ teaspoon salt
1 teaspoon cream of
    tartar
1 teaspoon dried sage
1 teaspoon dried basil
1 cup cooked millet
3 tablespoons safflower
    oil
1 egg, beaten
½ cup plain low-fat
    yogurt

Preheat the oven to 425° F.

Into a large bowl, sift together flours, baking soda, salt, cream of tartar, sage, and basil. Then stir in millet.

In a medium bowl, whisk together oil, egg, and yogurt. Add wet ingredients to dry ingredients and use your hands to knead the dough until it is smooth.

Coat a baking sheet with vegetable cooking spray.

On a floured surface, use a floured rolling pin to roll the dough out to a ¼-inch thickness, then cut it into 2½-inch rounds. Set the rounds on the baking sheet and bake until puffed and slightly golden, about 15 minutes. Cool on a wire rack before serving for breakfast, appetizers, or snacks.

Makes about 2½ dozen

OATS AND OAT BRAN

Hearty–and Heart-Healthy–Food

Oat bran: 110 calories per ounce
Oatmeal: 110 calories per ounce

It's the same old story. A food becomes known as "old-fashioned" and is assumed to be out of place in contemporary diets. Then someone shows that this so-called old-fashioned food has health benefits that couldn't be more suited to modern times. Such is the case with oats.

Oats and oatmeal owe their new-found celebrity to James W. Anderson, M.D., a professor at the University of Kentucky College of Medicine. Dr. Anderson noticed that the high-fiber diets he had developed for his diabetic patients were bringing down not only their insulin requirements but also their blood cholesterol levels. So he decided to test the fiber in one food–oats–to see how it affected blood cholesterol.

Because oat bran is a more concentrated source of oat fiber than whole oats, Dr. Anderson chose a test diet containing 100 grams of oat bran a day (about a cup of dry oat bran). The oat bran was served as a hot cereal and as five oat bran muffins a day. The results couldn't have been better; blood cholesterol levels dropped about 20 percent–a very major improvement. As an unanticipated bonus, weight dropped an average of 3 pounds during the oat bran diet.

John Eisenberg, M.D., of the University of Pennsylvania, has looked at the practical side of Dr. Anderson's oat bran breakthrough. He reported in the *Journal of the American Medical Association* that oat bran is often a less expensive way to lower cholesterol than drugs.

As for its other pluses, oat bran is gremlin free–no fat or sodium worth worrying about. Regular or old-fashioned oats are also a source of the cholesterol-lowering fiber that oat bran contains, although they don't have as much. But regular oats are low in fat and sodium, too, and are just the kind of old-fashioned food that would do modern-day diets a world of good.

Oat Bran

At the Market: Oat bran is available in boxes and plastic bags or in bulk. The coarseness of the flakes differs slightly among different types but has little or no effect on flavor or cooking qualities. The signs of quality are an even, oatmeal color and a slightly nutty smell with no trace of mustiness.

Kitchen Tips: To preserve freshness, store oat bran covered and refrigerated. If you'll be using it strictly for breakfast and baking, tuck a vanilla bean into the container and the bran will take on its aroma.

For a fast breakfast for one, combine 1 cup of water with ⅓ cup of oat bran in a 9-inch glass pie plate. Cover with vented plastic wrap and microwave on full power until cooked, 1 to 2 minutes.

Accent on Enjoyment: Oat bran may be a wonder food, but you won't find yourself wondering what to do with it. It's versatile, so that you have lots of ways to enjoy it. Pick the one you like best—be it as a plain hot cereal, homemade muffins, yeast bread, or cooked and covered with fresh or dried fruit. (Peaches, apples, and berries are especially good with it.)

Whole Oats: Regular (Old-fashioned) or Quick Cooking

At the Market: The only difference between regular and quick oats is the size of the flake. Regular oats are whole flakes, while quick-cooking oats have been cut in a way that makes them cook faster. It's reassuring to know that wholesomeness, or lack of it, is not an issue between the two. (Instant oats, however, may contain added salt, so strict sodium-watchers should take note.)

In cooking, you will find that regular oats take slightly longer to cook and give a nuttier texture. Quick oats, however, can be used just as successfully in baking; the choice simply depends on your texture preference.

Kitchen Tips: Keep oats in tightly covered containers in the refrigerator. They will last for up to a year.

How to cook oats for cereal depends on the texture you want. If you are in the mood for a coarse texture, add the oats to boiling water or juice. If you're in a creamy frame of mind, add the oats to room-temperature water or juice, then cook. Either way, use a heavy-bottom pan and slow, steady heat to prevent scorching.

Accent on Enjoyment: From the three bears' porridge to this morning's breakfast, oats have been a favorite way to start the day. Here are some ways to incorporate them into lunch and dinner, too.

- Add to soups for a creamier texture without added fat.
- Substitute oats for some of the meat in meatball and meat loaf recipes.
- Add to pie crusts and quick bread and cookie batters.
- Toss some oats into a food processor or blender and process until they're powdered. Now you have oat flour; you can add it to baked goods or use to dredge chicken before sautéing.

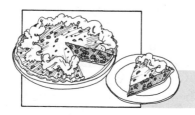

Oat Crust for Pies

1 cup quick-cooking oats
½ cup oat bran
2 egg whites
1 tablespoon sweet
    butter or margarine,
    melted

Preheat the oven to 350° F.

In a medium bowl, combine oats and oat bran.

In another medium bowl, use a hand mixer to beat egg whites until foamy and slightly thick, about 25 seconds.

Pour butter into oats and toss well to combine. Then add egg whites and continue to combine well.

Lightly oil a 9-inch pie plate. Pour the oat mixture into the pie plate and use a sheet of waxed paper to press it into a crust on the bottom and up the sides.

Bake until light brown, firm, and dry to the touch, about 15 minutes. Fill with fruit mousse or vanilla pudding and chill, or fill with pumpkin pie filling, then chill until set. You can also prebake for 7 minutes, then fill with a vegetable quiche batter and continue to bake until the quiche is set, about 20 minutes.

Makes one 9-inch crust

ONIONS

The Stuff of Serious Science

6 calories per 2 tablespoons (chopped)

History always spoke kindly of the onion. A U.S. Department of Agriculture report mentions that onions were treasured long ago by:

- Workers building the pyramids, for whom onions were a staple food.
- The Israelites, whose longing for onions while in the wilderness is mentioned in the Bible.
- General Ulysses Grant, who firmly believed that onions were a fine remedy for dysentery and other diseases typically found in hot climates. During the summer campaign of 1864, he reportedly wired the War Department, "I will not move my army without onions." The next day, three trainloads were started to the front.

Today, trainloads of onions are arriving in the scientists' laboratories. Among those who are taking their potential seriously are:

- Isabella Lipinska, Ph.D., a heart-health researcher at St. Elizabeth's Hospital in Brighton, Massachusetts. Dr. Lipinska's team has observed a significant improvement in levels of the "good," HDL, cholesterol after treating heart patients with a daily dose of onion extract equal to one to two whole onions. They have also seen beneficial effects against abnormal blood clots, similar to those reported for garlic.
- Dr. Michael Wargovich, Ph.D., of the M. D. Anderson Hospital and Tumor Institute in Houston. In the laboratory, says Dr. Wargovich, onion oils inhibit some of the activities considered part of the cancer process. Until we know more about the effect of onions on human cancer risk, we can only hope that humans benefit, too.
- Walter Dorsch, M.D., of the University of Munich. Looking for new treatments for the age-old problems of allergy and asthma, Dr. Dorsch tested the effects of onion extract on guinea pigs and documented an impressive antiasthma effect. Working with humans, he found that allergic patients reacted less severely to allergy-producing troublemakers when onion juice was rubbed on the skin where substances were injected. And in two of his patients, onion extract has inhibited bronchial asthma.

At the Market: A truly great onion is firm, dry, and well shaped, with a sweet aroma and no sprouts. Avoid those that are soft around the neck and smell acrid. White and yellow onions are most commonly cooked, but they can be eaten raw if they haven't been stored too long. If your taste generally runs toward sweet onions, favor the Vidalia, Maui, or Walla Walla varieties.

Scallions are actually immature onions. They should be firm and crisp.

Kitchen Tips: Store whole onions in a cool, dry place with good ventilation–not in the refrigerator. Scallions and cut onions, however, should be wrapped tightly in plastic wrap and refrigerated.

One medium onion equals about 1½ cups of chopped onions, which can be used raw, roasted, stewed, or sautéed. Long roasting leaves onions sweet and slow stewing makes them mellow.

Accent on Enjoyment: Tired of the same old onion routine? Here are three new ideas.

- Blanch whole onions, then peel, stuff, and bake.
- Sauté onions and use atop pizza or with pasta.
- Roast chopped onions and toss in vinaigrette. Serve chilled with curly lettuce.

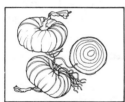

Grilled Onions en Brochette

1 pound small onions
1½ teaspoons frozen
   pineapple juice
   concentrate
1½ teaspoons frozen
   orange juice
   concentrate
½ teaspoon soy sauce

Preheat the broiler or prepare the grill.

Use a strainer to lower onions into boiling water and blanch for 5 to 6 minutes, then drain.

When onions are cool enough to handle, slip off the skins. (If the skins give you trouble, use a sharp paring knife to help remove them.) Place onions on skewers.

In a small bowl, combine juice concentrates and soy sauce. Use a pastry brush to paint the mixture onto onions. Broil or grill until onions are just burnished, about 6 minutes. Rotate and baste frequently so onions cook evenly. (This is easier to do on a grill than in a broiler.)

Serve hot as an appetizer or side dish.

Makes 4 servings

ORANGES

The Sweet Taste of Citrus

62 calories per medium orange
110 calories per cup juice (unsweetened)

Oranges and orange juice have long gotten good publicity, and there is every reason to believe that the trend will continue. Ultralow in sodium and fat, and a great way to get your vitamin C, both are loved by virtually everyone.

Occasionally we are asked whether the nutrients in oranges survive the transition from orange grove to frozen orange juice concentrate. The answer is yes. Analyses by the U.S. Department of Agriculture show that frozen orange juice concentrate has almost every milligram of vitamin C that was in the orange it came from.

Even more impressive is work by Barbara Rhode and her associates at Canada's McGill University. This research team temporarily fed diets low in folate–a B vitamin–to women so that their blood levels of the nutrient would drop. They then compared the ability of both folate supplements and orange juice made from frozen concentrate to restore normal folate levels. The juice and the vitamin pill did the job equally well–a testimony to the wholesomeness of juice from concentrate.

If you are wondering how orange juice stacks up against whole oranges, the answer is pretty well, with one exception. Apparently due to their fiber content, whole oranges have proved more filling than orange juice. If you are a dieter, you have probably noticed the difference yourself.

Whole Oranges

At the Market: The best way to find a tasty orange is simply to hold it in your hand. If it feels heavy for its size, it should have plenty of juice inside, so go for it! Smallish and medium fruit tend to be sweeter than large ones. If you have a good nose and the oranges aren't cold, sniff them to check for sweetness.

A note about the many different kinds of oranges. Navels are famous for seedless eating, Valencia and Temple are great for juicing, and Seville, which is tart to bitter in taste, is perfect for adding a salt-free zip to marinades, beverages, and desserts.

Kitchen Tips: If oranges will be used within a week, store at room temperature. A large orange will yield about ½ cup chopped.

Accent on Enjoyment: Of course, fresh oranges eaten out of hand make a refreshing and healthful snack. But don't forget how well oranges can brighten other foods. For example:

• Add the finely chopped pulp to marinades, sauces, punches, and cookie batter.
• Peel and section the fruit and add to pies, tarts, cakes, and salads.
• Use fresh oranges as an accompaniment to curries, chilies, and cheese plates.

Orange Juice

At the Market: Orange juice is as American as apple pie–with fewer calories and more vitamin C! Choose from frozen concentrate, fresh from a juice bar, fresh in containers, or canned. You can also choose from juices with pulp, without pulp, or even with extra pulp. But be sure to check expiration dates for freshness and ingredient lists for purity. For home juicing, try Valencia or Temple varieties.

Kitchen Tips: Store all orange juices in covered glass jars or bottles in the refrigerator; they will stay fresh for up to a week. When making your own juice, start by removing the peel, pith, and seeds to help prevent the juice from being bitter.

Accent on Enjoyment: The flavor of orange juices vary with type, and that gives you more ability to use juice in varying the flavor of other foods. Only an orange juice purist can resist trying mixtures of orange juice with other juices such as grapefruit, pineapple, or tangerine.

For a more novel approach, simmer orange juice with a bit of orange marmalade until the marmalade has melted. Then use as a glaze for fruit tarts or other confections. And on hot summer days, make "real orange soda." Mix ¼ cup of thawed frozen concentrate with ⅔ to 1 cup of club soda. The results will be far more nutritious and far more delicious than any orange soda that you buy in the store.

Orange and Red Onion Salad

3 navel oranges,
    sectioned
1 small red onion, sliced
    and separated into
    thin rings
1 tablespoon peanut oil
1 tablespoon lime juice
    pinch of freshly grated
    orange peel
    freshly ground black
    pepper
    watercress leaves
2 tablespoons toasted
    pumpkin seeds
    (pepitas)

In a medium bowl, combine oranges and onion.

In a small bowl, whisk together oil, lime juice, orange peel, and pepper. Pour over oranges and onion and toss well to combine.

Place watercress on serving plates and spoon salad on top. Sprinkle with pepitas before serving. This salad is great with spicy foods such as chili.

Makes 4 servings

OSTEOPOROSIS

Bone Up for Future Health

Like hardening of the arteries and other chronic diseases, osteoporosis is a long, slow process. The hallmark is thinning of the bones.

Naturally, bones that are too thin reach their "breaking point," and with osteoporosis present, even the slightest movement can cause enough stress to break a weak bone. Needless to say, countless American women are already well on their way to developing osteoporosis; in fact, experts estimate that, under present circumstances, up to 40 percent of them will eventually develop it.

Sadly, the effects of osteoporosis can be devastating. The pain and disability of a broken bone—be it in the wrist, hip, or spine—are but one part of the story; even more serious conditions can result from the lack of mobility that a fracture brings. These include infections, embolisms (lumpy blockages that interfere with blood flow to the lungs), and even death. No wonder osteoporosis is now considered a major killer disease.

What Are Your Odds?

Each and every one of us does lose bone with age. It is—to some extent—an inevitable part of growing older. However, losing some bone with age is *not* the same as developing osteoporosis. Osteopenia is the term for normal aging of bone. Osteoporosis is ostopenia that has advanced to a worrisome stage.

The issue obviously is not simply losing bone with age but losing large amounts of it. Today we know enough about osteoporosis to predict who the "big losers" will be. If one or more of the following descriptions apply to you, you're in the running for the big-loser label.

- A person with petite and/or thin body size.
- A person with a sedentary lifestyle.
- A woman who has never given birth.
- A smoker or heavy drinker.
- A descendant of someone who has lost height or fractured a hip in later life.

- A long-term user of drugs that interfere with calcium metabolism (such as anticonvulsants, cholestyramine, heparin, furosemide, high-dose thyroid preparations, cortisone, and isoniazid).
- A person with lactose-intolerance or lifelong low intake of calcium.

You may have noticed that a woman whose ovaries have been removed is not listed. Before the impact of this surgery on bone health became obvious, women who had it were frequent victims of osteoporosis. With drug therapy that replaces the ovary's naturally secreted hormones, however, this risk can be minimized.

Getting an Early Peek at Bones

If it were a perfect world, a warning would sound as soon as we start to lose bone. Even better would be a warning that would let us know during childhood and in our twenties that we weren't building strong enough bones to carry us through a long life. But it's not a perfect world—poor bone health usually goes undetected until it becomes obvious through stooped posture or a broken bone.

Bone health experts, of course, want things to be different. They've armed themselves with an arsenal of tests designed to discover the state of our bone health before trouble occurs. Their favorite techniques include:

X-rays. The familiar x-ray can detect bone loss, but only in its later stages. In general, osteoporosis is obvious on an x-ray only after about 30 percent of the bone has been lost. Nevertheless, this still offers a chance to detect the problem before a bone actually breaks.

Bone density test. This high-tech breakthrough is to bones what x-rays are to dentists. Using sophisticated new machinery, the strength of bones can now be measured and trouble detected in its earliest stages. For the patient, taking the test is similar to having an x-ray; the only drawback is its cost.

Appearance. Radiologists and bone experts insist that they can spot some osteoporotic women on sight. A woman who is petite, thin, and past menopause is bound to be suspected of harboring serious bone loss, and in some cases, a trained eye can spot it just by looking at her.

Thanks to a growing emphasis on bone health, more doctors are paying attention to the state of our bones, and osteoporosis centers are springing up throughout the country. Naturally, you can expect that these centers will be equipped with the machinery to test for bone density. If you don't have one nearby, contact the radiology department of your local hospital or medical school and ask for assistance in finding an expert in the diagnosis and treatment of osteoporosis.

It's Never Too Late to Try

The best way to have strong, healthy bones is to start young. A woman's bones, for instance, reach their maximum size and strength by about age 35. This best-they'll-ever-be state is known as "peak bone mass." It starts to fade shortly after it is reached, and from there on, the body fights to maintain bone.

If, like many who are concerned with their bone health, you are long past this peak period, there's no need for despair. There is still much that you can do for your bones. Here's how.

Exercise. Most exercise helps to strengthen bone. The one requirement is that the activity be "weight-bearing," that is, it must force your body to bear its weight. Walking is the perfect weight-bearing exercise; swimming is nonweight-bearing. Everett L. Smith, Ph.D., of the University of Wisconsin has documented that even women in their seventies and eighties can strengthen bone through a program of light weight-bearing exercise.

Estrogen replacement therapy. According to a Consensus Panel on Osteoporosis convened by the National Institutes of Health (NIH), one of the best ways to keep bones strong is to take estrogen therapy (you must start within a few years of menopause). Of course, there are risks, but they are not as great as once feared, and the panel believes that high-risk women should consider this option seriously. Talk to your doctor about it.

Increased calcium intake after menopause. If you don't take estrogen replacement, the sharp drop in this hormone at menopause will create a need for more calcium. Robert Heaney, M.D., authority on bone health at Creighton University, has long recommended increasing the recommended allowance for postmenopausal women to 1,500 milligrams a day. The NIH Consensus Panel endorsed this recommendation for postmenopausal women who do not take estrogen. All other women should aim for 1,000 milligrams a day.

Now let's look at how nutrition fits into the picture.

Bone Food for Every Palate

As with exercise, the nutritional approach is one that you can take into your own hands. And as we noted earlier, the sooner you do so, the better. It's especially important, by the way, for women to respect their bone health during pregnancy and breast feeding, so that bones will be strengthened rather than depleted during these periods.

The mainstays of a bone-healthy diet are:

• Calcium.
• Vitamin D, which allows you to absorb the calcium.

• Lactose, another factor that helps you absorb calcium, provided that you aren't intolerant to it.
• Phosphorus intake in balance with calcium; that is, equal amounts of both minerals.
• Alcohol in only moderate amounts, or not at all.

You'll find lists of the best sources of calcium and vitamin D in the Appendix. And if you aren't lactose intolerant, you can use the list in "Your Lactose Counter," on page 279, to find the richest sources. As for keeping

A Week of Bone-Building Meals

Although calcium has received the lion's share of attention, other nutrients also affect bone health. But managing all of the likely players can make things seem too complicated. So we've simplified things with a week's worth of bone-protecting meal plans.

Each day's plan provides at least 1,000 milligrams of calcium daily—but that's just the first step. These menus have also been designed to balance calcium with its fellow co-worker, phosphorus. There's some evidence that limiting fat and salt helps, too, so we've made our plans accordingly. And some studies also show that small amounts of coffee and tea may be best.

Don't forget, though, that if you're looking for more than 1,000 milligrams of calcium daily, the simplest step is to add a supplement that provides the extra amount desired.

Day 1

Breakfast
2 slices Italian bread
2 pats margarine
1 orange
1 cup 1% milk
   coffee or tea

Lunch
¾ cup homemade macaroni and cheese
¾ cup broccoli
1 pat margarine
1 cup 1% milk

phosphorus balanced with calcium, it's not as complicated as it sounds; eat meat only in moderation and don't overdose on colas.

Supplements are yet another alternative that deserve mention. You can simplify the bone-protecting process by using supplemental calcium. If you already take a multivitamin, you're taking care of the vitamin D. If you don't use a multiple or other source of D, however, reach for a calcium supplement that also contains this all-important vitamin. Remember, however, not to exceed a maximum D intake of 600 to 800 international units daily unless recommended by your doctor.

Snack
1 cup low-fat fruit yogurt

Dinner
3 ounces baked flounder or sole
¾ cup cooked spinach
½ cup brown rice
1 tablespoon margarine
1 cup 1% milk
1 baked apple

Day 2

Breakfast
1 hard roll
2 tablespoons low-calorie cream cheese
½ cup melon
1 cup 1% milk
   coffee or tea

Lunch
Garden salad (⅓ cup sprouted alfalfa seeds, ⅓ cup mung bean sprouts,
   2 spears broccoli, ⅓ cup cauliflower, ⅓ cup grated carrots, ⅓ cup
   celery, 6 cucumber slices with peel, ½ cup loose-leaf lettuce, ¼ cup
   low-calorie salad dressing)
1 cup 1% milk
1 cup low-fat cottage cheese
1 cup fresh strawberries

(continued)

A Week of Bone-Building Meals–Continued

Snack
  1 ounce Swiss cheese

Dinner
  1 broiled lamb chop
  ½ cup summer squash
  ¾ cup collard greens
  2 pats margarine
  1 cup 1% milk
  ¾ cup vanilla ice milk or frozen yogurt

Day 3

Breakfast
  1 ounce shredded wheat cereal
  ¾ cup skim milk
  1 cup diced pineapple
    coffee or tea

Lunch
  1 slice rye bread
  2 teaspoons mustard
  2 ounces Swiss cheese
  2 lettuce leaves
  1 cup skim milk
  1 tomato
  ¾ cup chopped dates

Snack
  1 ounce feta cheese

Dinner
  3 ounces roasted chicken breast
  1 cup red kidney beans
  1 slice cracked-wheat bread
  1 cup brussels sprouts
  3 pats margarine
  1 cup skim milk

Day 4

Breakfast
 1 hard roll
 1 ounce low-calorie cream cheese
 1 fresh pear
 1 cup 1% milk
  coffee or tea

Lunch
 3 ounces water-packed tuna
 ½ tablespoon reduced-calorie mayonnaise
 1 banana
 ½ cup loose-leaf lettuce
 1 cup 1% milk
 2 oatmeal cookies

Snack
 1 cup homemade banana smoothie (skim milk, banana, honey, ice
  cubes)

Dinner
 1 cup cranberry juice cocktail
 3 ounces broiled halibut
 ½ cup cooked eggplant
 ¾ cup spinach, cooked or raw
 1 tablespoon freshly grated Parmesan cheese
 1 cup 1% milk
 ¾ cup fresh raspberries
 2 pats margarine

Day 5

Breakfast
 1 cup cooked cream of wheat
 1 orange
 1 cup 1% milk
  coffee

(continued)

A Week of Bone-Building Meals–Continued

Lunch
¾ cup cooked pasta
 2 tablespoons freshly grated Parmesan cheese
½ teaspoon margarine
½ teaspoon parsley
 1 cup 1% milk
 1 cup juice-packed peaches
 4 rye crackers

Snack
 1 ounce Swiss cheese
 1 apple

Dinner
½ cup oysters
 1 baked potato
 2 tablespoons yogurt topping
¾ cup cooked kale
 2 raw carrots
 1 cup 1% milk
 6 cucumber slices, with peel
 2 pats margarine
 1 slice angel food cake with strawberry garnish

Day 6

Breakfast
¾ cup oatmeal
 1 cup fresh strawberries
 1 cup 1% milk
   coffee

Snack
½ cup chopped dates

Lunch
Cheesy garden pita (1 pita bread, ¼ cup bean sprouts, ½ cup crisphead
   lettuce, ¼ cup grated carrots, ¼ cup alfalfa sprouts, ½ cup shredded
   cheddar cheese, 2 tablespoons low-calorie Russian dressing)
 1 cup 1% milk

Dinner

 4 ounces turkey breast with fat-skimmed gravy
½ cup asparagus
½ cup unsweetened applesauce
 1 pat margarine
 2 tablespoons low-calorie salad dressing
½ cup raw sliced mushrooms
½ cup raw broccoli florets
 1 cup 1% milk

Day 7

Breakfast

 1 slice Italian bread
 1 pat margarine
 1 cup cooked plantain slices
 1 cup 1% milk
    coffee or tea

Snack

¾ cup fresh nectarine slices
 1 cup 1% milk

Lunch

Summer salad (½ cup escarole, ½ cup fresh spinach, 4 radishes,
    1 tomato, sliced, ½ cup grated carrots, ¼ cup onions, 6 cucumber
    slices with peel, ½ cup cauliflower, ¼ cup low-calorie salad dressing)
Cheese melt (1 slice whole wheat bread, with mustard to taste,
    1 teaspoon margarine, 2 ounces Swiss cheese)

Dinner

 3 ounces lean sirloin steak
 1 baked potato
 2 pats margarine
½ cup green beans
 1 baked apple with raisins
 1 cup 1% milk

OVERWEIGHT

Spotlight on Successful Strategies

How many times have you tried to lose weight? And how many times have you given up? If your answer to both questions is the same, you're like most people who try to lose weight.

But you know the old saying about try and try again. No one has taken it to heart more than weight-loss specialists—when one method has failed, they have gone back to the drawing board and come up with another. And some of them actually work! In this section, we'll share some findings on three strategies that have yielded impressive results.

But first, a few facts about "overweight." Although hardly a day goes by without someone mentioning the word, a firm definition is hard to come by. We're content to use one of the most common definitions—a body weight that is at least 20 percent above normal for one's height. Nevertheless, we are careful not to use this definition too strictly, for not everyone who meets this standard needs to take off pounds.

Defining overweight, however, is easier than explaining what causes it. In our view, its causes are many, and the old line that overweight occurs when you consume more calories than you expend just doesn't cut it. The plain truth is that some people can increase their caloric intake, keep their activity level the same, and not gain weight.

And here's another simple fact: Weight gain with age is all but universal in Western societies—so much so that we wonder whether putting on some pounds as we age isn't normal—and maybe even healthy.

Whose Fault Is It, Anyhow?

When weight-control efforts fail, everyone looks for someone or something to blame. And for too long, the dieters themselves have taken the rap—as if inability to control one's weight can only be for lack of trying. In some cases, dieters do in fact need to try harder—or be more patient—but the evidence just doesn't support the notion that weight is completely within our control.

Some conditions, for instance, do predispose us to weight gain. Prominent among them are diseases of the endocrine glands such as thyroid disorders or diabetes. Disorders affecting the area of the brain that controls the

322

desire to eat are also recognized for their role in weight gain—which may be unusually rapid.

Although weight loss is a classic sign of depression, some depressed patients actually gain weight. Recently, researchers at the Psychobiology Branch of the National Institutes of Mental Health have shown that some people experience overeating, oversleeping, and lack of energy in response to seasonal changes in the amount of sunlight. Researchers there, led by chief Thomas Wehr, M.D., have named the condition Seasonal Affective Disorder (SAD). But the weight gain doesn't seem to be the result of unusual hunger for just anything; rather, SAD sufferers report an intense craving for carbohydrates that no doubt accounts for their overeating.

Now for the converse. Although some people visit doctors as a result of conditions causing weight gain, others put on weight as a result of medications that doctors have prescribed for them. It's a painful fact of life that the following drugs, as essential as they may be in a wide range of conditions, have a tendency to promote weight gain:

- Tricyclic antidepressants, such as Elavil, Tofranil, Norpramin, and Sinequan.
- Antipsychotic drugs, such as Thorazine or Mellaril.
- Mood-stabilizing drugs, such as lithium.
- Some antimigraine drugs or antihistamines used in cases of severe migraine allergic conditions.
- Cortisone tablets.
- Birth control pills.

So, as you see, weight control isn't always just a matter of will power.

Proven Programs to Try

When overweight results from an underlying condition, you can bet that nothing is likely to matter unless the problem is brought under control. Similarly, if drug treatment is contributing to the problem, you'll be in that classic risk/benefit dilemma: Is the benefit of the medicine more compelling than the discomfort of the side effect?

The fact is, however, that for most people, no underlying cause for weight woes can be found. But that doesn't mean that you're without options. A diet and exercise program can make a big difference.

We'll leave the physical activity part to the exercise experts. Here are our thoughts, however, as to some nutritional strategies that have proven valuable.

Feeling Full: Take the Fiber Challenge

If you're convinced that nothing will curb your appetite, we have a challenge for you.

Time and time again, nutritionists have found that patients given high-fiber diets as a treatment for digestive problems or diabetes report feeling much less hungry. In some cases, patients have complained that high-fiber menus had "too much food" even though their calorie count was identical to that of a low-fiber diet that didn't make them feel stuffed at all.

Don't take their word for it. Try it yourself. Below you'll find two diets designed by James W. Anderson, M.D., of the University of Kentucky, who runs the High Carbohydrate and Fiber Research Foundation there. The calorie count of both is similar, but the fiber content varies. Try them both. If, as we expect, you feel less hungry on the high-fiber plan, you'll have firsthand evidence that your appetite can, in fact, be curbed.

800-calorie, fiber-rich diet

Breakfast
 4 ounces skim milk
 ⅓ cup All-Bran
 1 slice whole wheat toast
 ½ banana

Lunch
 ½ cup white beans seasoned with 1 ounce lean ham
 ½ cup beets
 ½ cup kale
 1 slice whole wheat bread
 1 teaspoon margarine

Dinner
 4 ounces broiled flounder with lemon
 ½ medium baked potato

½ cup broccoli
 1 slice whole wheat bread
 1 teaspoon margarine

Snack
 3 rye wafers

800-calorie fiber-poor diet

Breakfast
 4 ounces skim milk
⅔ cup Rice Krispies
 1 slice white bread, toasted
 4 ounces grapefruit juice

Lunch
Turkey sandwich (2 slices white bread, 1½ ounces turkey, 1 teaspoon
   mayonnaise)
 6 ounces V-8 juice

Dinner
 2 ounces roast beef
½ cup summer squash
⅓ cup white rice
 1 slice white bread
 1 teaspoon margarine

Snack
 5 saltine crackers

The Soup Scoop

Don't you love to hear examples of the plain, old-fashioned approach besting the latest technological breakthrough? If so, here's a weight-loss strategy for you.

We've long regarded a cup of hot soup as the simple way to warm up on cold days, but new research suggests that it is also a good way to make dieting easier. The story began when John P. Foreyt, Ph.D., a professor at Baylor College of Medicine, wondered whether eating soup might affect appetite or food intake. He and his co-workers recruited overweight subjects to compare a diet that included regular soup consumption to one that did not.

When all was said and done, here's what Dr. Foreyt found.

- Members of the soup group lost slightly more weight during the study than the other dieters.
- Weight loss among the soup group corresponded to the amount of soup consumed; the more soup consumed, the greater the weight loss.
- A year after the study, the researchers followed up on how well the weight was kept off. Members of the standard diet group had gained about 2½ pounds, but average weight gain among members of the soup group was only 1 pound.

Needless to say, not every soup can be recommended for use as part of a weight-loss plan. As a general rule, favor clear soups, vegetable soups, and the like. Whatever benefits soup provides to the dieter may be easily erased if the one you choose is rich in cream or meat fats.

Don't Dread Bread

Of course, dieters do not live by soup alone. If they are smart, they have some bread with their meal.

Hard as it may seem to believe, bread is "in" for weight loss. New research tells us that it's the high-fat stuff that we put on it or between it that makes for more of our weight troubles. Consider, for instance, the findings of Norwegian scientist Bjarne K. Jacobsen. While analyzing the results from a major study of heart health, Dr. Jacobsen found that people who ate less than two slices of bread daily weighed about 11 pounds more than those who ate large amounts of bread.

Needless to say, the bread lovers might have had other characteristics that accounted for their lower weight—such as more active lifestyles. Yet, researchers at Michigan State University have reported that some breads help reduce appetite. Working with college students there, Olaf Mickelson, Ph.D., and his co-workers compared the effects of two different breads—one white and one high in fiber. The students reported feeling less hungry when they ate the high-fiber bread (12 slices daily!), and not surprisingly, those on the high-fiber bread lost about 5 pounds more during the two-month experiment than those who ate equal amounts of the white bread.

Although weight loss was greater in the high-fiber group, even students who dined on the low-fiber bread managed to lose an average of 14 pounds in two months. Now how does that sit with the conventional belief that bread is the bane of the dieter?

Eat Less Fat, Make Less Fat

Score another defeat for conventional wisdom. It held that whether from protein, carbohydrate, alcohol, or fat in food, all calories were the same in terms of their effect on weight. In other words, 3,500 excess calories would make a pound of body fat whether the calories came from bread or butter.

But Lauren Lissner and her colleagues at Cornell University in Ithaca, New York, have collected some facts that turn this conventional wisdom upside down. They compared the effects of three diets of varying fat content on food intake and body weight. They found:

- On a diet that derived half its calories from fat, the women chose to eat about 2,700 calories a day and put on ⅔ of a pound in a two-week period.
- A moderate-fat diet (in which fat provided about one-third of the total calories) led to an average intake of 2,300 calories daily and body weight did not change.
- On a low-fat diet in which fat supplied only one-fifth of the calories, the women chose to eat only 2,100 calories a day. Over a two-week period, they lost almost a pound.

Is there a simple message here? You bet! It's that the fat we eat is more likely than anything else to become the fat we store. So you have another reason to enjoy your bread—just be careful what you spread on it.

Supplements Make Sense

Should you supplement during dieting? We think it's a good idea. Dieting is hard work, enough to make you feel that paying attention to the nutritional adequacy of your diet at the same time is unrealistic. Supplementation can seem like a much simpler solution, and often, it is.

As a general guide, we recommend a multivitamin and multimineral supplement while dieting (if you aren't already taking them, that is). And if you are cutting back on calories so that your diet contains few dairy products or calcium-rich foods, consider adding a calcium supplement, too.

Bonus Benefits

Feeling and looking better are the immediate rewards of successful weight loss. But keep your thoughts on the long-term benefits, too. Keeping

---

Diet for a Calorie-Conscious Planet

All set to go on a weight-loss program based on eating less fat and calories while eating more fiber and complex carbohydrates? This week's worth of menus will get you started. And for a head start, begin your lunch and/or dinner with a low-calorie soup. Good luck!

Day 1

Breakfast
  1 slice toast
  1 scrambled egg
  1 orange
  1 cup skim milk
    coffee

Lunch
Turkey pita (1 pita bread, 1 tablespoon low-calorie mayonnaise,
    2 tablespoons plain low-fat yogurt, 3 ounces white turkey meat,
    ¼ cup loose-leaf lettuce, 1 fresh tomato, ¾ cup celery)
  1 cup vegetable juice

Snack
  1 apple

Dinner
  1 cup cooked crab
  1 tablespoon low-calorie mayonnaise

weight under control has enormous benefits that you can't see. If your weight is normal, you are less likely to succumb to such conditions as high blood pressure and high cholesterol, diabetes, cancer of the endometrium in women, and arthritis.

When diabetes, high blood pressure, or high cholesterol are already present, losing weight also can go a long way toward correcting them. And tolerance for physical activity improves too, so that once the weight is off, exercising to keep it off doesn't feel so difficult.

Are these benefits worth it? Ask anyone who has succeeded!

¾ cup broccoli
1 teaspoon margarine
½ baked potato with 2 tablespoons low-fat yogurt
1 tablespoon chives
1 raw carrot
1 cup skim milk

Day 2

Breakfast
1 cup oatmeal
1 papaya
1 cup skim milk
coffee

Lunch
Salad (1 cup crisphead lettuce, 1 cup fresh spinach, ½ fresh tomato, 8 cucumber slices, ½ cup celery, ½ cup pink salmon)
1 piece Italian bread
1 cup iced tea

Snack
1 sliced banana with ½ cup fresh strawberries

(continued)

Diet for a Calorie-Conscious Planet–Continued

Dinner
  3 ounces chicken breast (without skin)
  ½ cup brown rice
  3 tomato slices
  ¾ cup Italian beans
  1½ teaspoons diet margarine

Day 3

Breakfast
  ½ pink or red grapefruit
  ½ cup plain low-fat yogurt
  2 slices whole wheat toast
  2 teaspoons diet margarine
  1 cup skim milk
    coffee

Lunch
  3 ounces water-packed tuna
  ½ tablespoon low-calorie mayonnaise
  ½ cup loose-leaf lettuce
  2 graham crackers
  1 cup cantaloupe

Snack
  1 cup juice-packed peaches
  1 cup iced tea

Dinner
  3 ounces lean sirloin steak (trimmed of fat)
  ¾ cup green beans
  ½ cup unsweetened applesauce
  ½ cup cooked summer squash
  1 teaspoon diet margarine
  1 cup skim milk

Day 4

Breakfast
  1 ounce wheat flakes
  ½ cup grapes
  1 cup skim milk
    coffee

Lunch
Chicken-cucumber sandwich (2 ounces chicken breast, without skin,
    2 slices whole wheat toast, 1 teaspoon low-calorie mayonnaise,
    10 thin cucumber slices)
  1 cup skim milk

Snack
  1 cup low-fat fruit yogurt or low-fat yogurt drink

Dinner
    3-ounce extra-lean hamburger patty
  1 baked potato
  ¼ cup low-fat yogurt
  1 fresh tomato
Spinach salad (¾ cup fresh spinach, ¼ cup mushrooms, 1 tablespoon
    low-calorie dressing)

Day 5

Breakfast
  ¾ cup multigrain cereal (such as Just Right)
  1 banana
  1 cup skim milk
    coffee

(continued)

Diet for a Calorie-Conscious Planet–Continued

Lunch
Salad (1½ cups crisphead lettuce, 1 fresh tomato, ¾ cup celery,
   10 cucumber slices, 5 radishes, 1 tablespoon low-calorie Italian
   dressing)
  1 cup skim milk

Snack
  1 cup broccoli, carrot, and cauliflower mixture
  ½ cup plain low-fat yogurt spiced with onion and garlic powder

Dinner
  ¾ cup oysters
  1 piece French bread
  1 teaspoon diet margarine
  ¾ cup asparagus
  1 baked apple

Day 6

Breakfast
  2 rice cakes
  1 cup plain low-fat yogurt
  ½ cup juice-packed peaches
  ½ cup skim milk
    coffee

Lunch
Turkey melt (2 slices whole wheat toast, 2 ounces turkey breast,
   without skin, ½ tablespoon low-calorie mayonnaise, ¼ cup loose-leaf
   lettuce, 1 ounce low-fat Swiss cheese)
  ¾ cup celery and carrot sticks
  1 cup vegetable juice

Snack
  1 cup fresh strawberries

Dinner
  3 ounces lean sirloin steak (trimmed of fat)
  ½ cup brown rice

¾ cup broccoli
½ fresh tomato
1 teaspoon diet margarine

Day 7

Breakfast
1 poached egg
1 slice toast with low-calorie jam
1 fresh pear
1 cup skim milk
   coffee

Lunch
Grilled cheese sandwich (2 slices whole wheat toast, 1 ounce Swiss
   cheese, 1 teaspoon diet margarine)

Snack
1 banana

Dinner
3 ounces broiled flounder
1 baked potato
¼ cup plain low-fat yogurt
½ cup broccoli
½ cup cauliflower
1 teaspoon diet margarine

PAPAYA

Temptation, Tropical-Style

119 calories per papaya

We're not alone in our view that nutrition has become far too complicated. Nor are we the only ones who have attempted to simplify it.

One of the approaches that has intrigued us is the concept of "nutrient density." It's a way of measuring bang for the buck: How much nutrition does a food deliver for each calorie that it provides?

When a food's content of essential nutrients is weighed alongside its calorie count, the results are often unexpected. For fruits, the most nutrient-dense proved to be not the orange or the legendary apple, but rather the cantaloupe and the papaya! Specifically, papaya stands out with a vitamin A level that exceeds the Recommended Dietary Allowance by 30 percent, plus enough vitamin C to meet a full day's allowance three times—all in one piece of this luscious fruit.

Not impressed yet? Consider the extremely high potassium content as well as the ample fiber that the papaya provides. Now we're sure you agree that even though expensive, papayas give you your money's worth.

At the Market: Ripe papayas are green with overtones of yellow and creamy orange. They will yield to gentle pressure and should be well shaped, reminding you of a large pear. The stem end should smell softly sweet, not acrid or harsh.

Kitchen Tips: Store ripe papayas in the refrigerator, where they will last for about a week. To prepare, use a sharp paring knife to peel, then scoop out the seeds with a spoon. Add raw to green or fruit salads—or puree and use in frozen desserts. Always use cooked papaya in dishes that rely on gelatin—raw papaya contains an enzyme that will prevent gelling. Unripe papaya is cooked and eaten like squash.

Accent on Enjoyment: If you are hesitant to try tropical fruits such as this one, don't be. You'll quickly become comfortable with the ease of using papaya and in no time will be hooked on its gentle sweetness and silky texture.

• Use half shells of ripe papaya to hold crab or shrimp salad.

334

- Sprinkle chilled papaya with lime juice and serve with smoked salmon or smoked shrimp.
- Add pureed ripe papaya to meat marinades for extra tenderness.
- Use papaya to replace pumpkin in a pie recipe. Unripe fruit is well suited to this use.
- Give papaya seeds a try–they are crisp and peppery. To prepare, rinse the seeds well, pat dry, and place in a jar. Cover with mild vinegar and refrigerate, then use as you would capers–in salads and sandwich fillings and as garnishes.

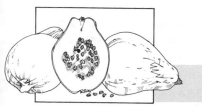

Fresh Papaya Parfaits

2 ripe papayas
2 tablespoons lime
   juice and pulp
1½ cups vanilla yogurt
   whole fresh berries

Using a sharp paring knife, halve and peel papayas. (It's best to do this over the sink.) Scoop out the remaining seeds with a spoon, then slice papaya flesh into a food processor or blender. Add lime juice and pulp, and process until smooth.

Spoon some papaya into the bottoms of four parfait glasses or wine goblets. Then add a layer of yogurt. Continue layering, using all of the papaya and yogurt. Sprinkle with whole fresh berries and serve for dessert or a fancy breakfast.

Makes 4 servings

PARSNIPS

Fiber-Rich and Flavorful, Too

126 calories per cup (cooked)

What do parsnips have that more common vegetables don't? The answer is an insoluble fiber content high enough to give bran cereals some serious competition.

We're fans of bran, of course, but we recognize that some people suspect that only termites truly like the stuff. Little do they realize that parsnips offer the perfect opportunity to get the digestive-tract benefits of insoluble fiber in the form of a vegetable whose flavor and texture don't resemble bran's at all.

And there is another side to the story. Parsnips provide nutritional benefits –including plenty of potassium–without fat or sodium to worry about.

At the Market: Pick parsnips that are small to medium in size, with a smooth, firm feel and creamy white color. Larger parsnips can be tough and woody.

Kitchen Tips: Store parsnips in the refrigerator in perforated plastic bags. They will last for about a month.

To cook parsnips, scrub them under cool water, chop, then simmer in stock to cover until tender–about 15 to 20 minutes. They can also be steamed, microwaved, baked, or pressure-cooked, then sauced the same way as chunks of cooked potato.

Accent on Enjoyment: Now don't turn up your nose. Parsnips are sweet, delicious, and very underrated. To prove it:

• Shred raw parsnips and add to green salads, slaws, or marinated vegetables.
• Puree cooked parsnips with a bit of rosemary and thyme. Serve hot with roasted meats.
• Team parsnips with carrots, onions, leeks, scallions, dill, tarragon, caraway, nutmeg, or citrus for a great combination of complementary flavors.

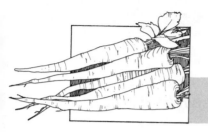

Parsnip Salad
with Carrots and Orange Vinaigrette

¾ pound parsnips, cut into ½-inch coins
¼ pound carrots, cut into ½-inch coins
2 tablespoons minced fresh chives
1 teaspoon celery seeds
2 tablespoons orange juice
1 teaspoon lemon juice
½ teaspoon Dijon mustard
2 teaspoons peanut oil

Peel parsnips and carrots, then cut into ½-inch cubes. Steam over boiling water until tender, about 15 minutes. Drain.

Place parsnips and carrots into a serving bowl and add chives and celery seeds.

In a small bowl, whisk together juices, mustard, and oil. Pour over parsnips and carrots and toss well to coat. Serve warm as an appetizer, side dish, or salad. Delicious with duck.

Makes 4 servings

PASTA

Ready for Prime Time

155 calories per cup elbow macaroni or spaghetti (cooked)

At last, pasta's undeserved reputation as fattening has faded. Its image is now one of a heart-healthy food low in fat and sodium (as long as you refrain from smothering it with salt or fat.)

And contrary to the long-held accusation that pasta is "just starch," the new emphasis is on a more accurate portrayal of its substantial nutritive value. Anaylses at the American Institute of Baking show that a plateful of pasta (about 2 cups) makes a significant contribution to the Recommended Dietary Allowance for six minerals, providing 31 percent of the manganese, 24 percent of the iron, 16 percent of the phosphorus and copper, 12 percent of the magnesium and 9 percent of the zinc that nutritionists recommend. Pasta retains its minerals well during cooking, tests show.

What more does a pasta lover need to hear?

At the Market: If the bounty of pasta shapes has left you confused, follow this simple rule: Thick, fat pastas work well with thick sauces; finer pastas are best with light sauces. For instance, rigatoni, a fairly thick cylinder, is great with a hearty tomato sauce.

When shopping, consider choosing one of the many flavored pastas available. Herbs, spices, and vegetable purees have made their way into pasta dough and add color and flavor without excess fat or calories.

Both plain and flavored pastas are available dry, fresh, or frozen. Regardless of form, the pasta should be unbroken and free of dark patches.

Kitchen Tips: Store dry pasta in tightly closed containers in a cool, dry place and it will keep for about a year. A pantry shelf is perfect. Fresh pasta should be tightly wrapped and refrigerated and used within a week. Toss a handful of cornmeal in with the fresh pasta to keep it from sticking to itself.

Pasta should be cooked in enough boiling water to prevent crowding. This is especially important with whole wheat pasta. Ideally, 1 pound of pasta will need about 7 to 8 quarts of boiling water to cook comfortably. Adding a splash of olive oil to the boiling water will prevent sticking. If you follow these procedures, you can drain and sauce your pasta without rinsing. Of course, dry pasta will take longer to cook than fresh.

338

Accent on Enjoyment: Like pizza, pasta is an all-American favorite that got its start elsewhere. In fact, pasta has such a great texture and is so versatile, it may be headed for an award as an all-time favorite food. Here are four easy, healthful ways to prepare it.

- Sauté garlic in olive oil, then toss with hot linguini or spaghetti. Sprinkle with toasted pine nuts and serve hot.
- Stuff cooked pasta shells with part-skim ricotta and minced fresh spinach. Serve with fresh tomato sauce.
- Toss cooked pasta with stir-fried vegetables.
- For dessert, toss hot pasta with chopped dates and raisins, then sprinkle with toasted coconut.

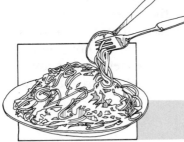

Spaghetti with Onions and Kale

2 teaspoons olive oil
1 onion, sliced and
    separated into rings
1 shallot, sliced
1 clove garlic, crushed
3 cups shredded curly
    kale
1 cup chicken stock
2 cups cooked spaghetti
    freshly grated Parmesan
    cheese

Heat a large skillet over medium-high heat. Then add oil, onion, shallot, and garlic. Reduce heat to medium and sauté until onion is just wilted, about 5 minutes. (Be careful not to burn garlic.)

Add kale and continue to sauté until it's moist and has brightened a bit in color, about 1 minute. Then add stock and cover loosely with crumpled foil. Reduce heat to simmer and simmer until most of the stock has evaporated and kale is soft but still a lively green, about 7 to 10 minutes. Stir in pasta and continue to simmer until heated through, about 1 minute. Serve hot, sprinkled with Parmesan.

Makes 4 servings

PEACHES

Smart Snacking

54 calories per 3 halves (canned)
37 calories per medium peach (fresh)

Peaches need no fancy ads or celebrity endorsements. Their juiciness and flavor say it all.

Of course, peaches are the perfect snack whether your priority is taste or nutrition. With modest levels of vitamins A and C, a low fat and sodium content, and potassium, too, they can be enjoyed without worry.

When you can, though, favor fresh peaches. Research by Jane K. Ross, Ph.D., of the University of Vermont, shows peaches lose more fiber during processing than other common fruits and vegetables. Nonetheless, canned peaches are a healthful addition to any menu—unless, of course, they are packed in sugary syrup.

Canned, Juice-Packed Peaches

At the Market: Be sure to check the label for purity of ingredients. Apart from that, buy the cut of peaches best suited to what you're preparing. Slices are best for salads and compotes; by contrast, halves are more dramatic for topping cakes.

Kitchen Tips: Once the can is open, peaches and their liquid should be placed in covered containers and stored in the refrigerator.

Accent on Enjoyment: Canned peaches offer convenience, nutrition, and good taste that few canned goods can match. Keep a can or two on hand, then:

- Chop and add to hot breakfast cereals.
- Fill halves with mild white cheese, then sprinkle with chopped almonds and broil until burnished. Serve for brunch or dessert.

- Chop and add to poultry stuffing.
- Don't forget to put the peach liquid to good use. Its fine aroma and flavor make it suitable for cooking oatmeal or as a liquid in a quick bread or muffin recipe.

Fresh Peaches

At the Market: Peaches are ripe when the last remainder of green has turned a creamy yellow. Gently press the flesh at the stem end with your finger; if it gives a bit, it's "firm-ripe." If it gives a lot, it's "tree-ripe," or slightly softer. Next smell the stem end of the peach. It should be sweet, aromatic, and fruity.

Kitchen Tips: To ripen peaches, keep them at room temperature and out of the sun. Refrigerated, firm-ripe peaches will keep for a couple of weeks, but to minimize bruising, it's best to spread them out in one layer. Tree-ripe peaches will keep refrigerated for up to five days.

For easiest peeling, blanch peaches in boiling water for about 30 seconds, then plunge immediately into ice water. Remove from the water; the skins should slip right off. (Use a sharp paring knife to get them started if they don't.)

To keep slices from turning brown, toss them with a bit of lemon juice. Note that two medium peaches are equal to about 1 cup of sliced peaches. When you're baking with peaches, taste them before you add the sweetener to the recipe. If the peaches taste sweet, you can reduce the amount of added sweetener.

Accent on Enjoyment: Peaches are perfect raw and can be baked, pureed, or microwaved. To prove their versatility:

- Flavor with different combinations of nutmeg, mace, cinnamon, almonds, currants, citrus, or gingerroot.
- Chop and add to chicken or smoked turkey salads.
- Chop and add to pancake or waffle batter.

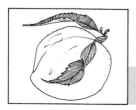

Ginger Chicken and Peach Sauté

⅔ pound chicken cutlets
2 teaspoons lemon juice
½ teaspoon fennel seeds, ground
½ teaspoon cumin seeds, ground
½ teaspoon curry powder
1 tablespoon minced fresh parsley or coriander
1 shallot, minced
2 teaspoons peanut oil
1 slice gingerroot
3 peaches, peeled and sliced
  unsalted shelled pistachio nuts

Slice chicken into finger-size ribbons and place in a nonmetal bowl. Add lemon juice, fennel, cumin, curry powder, parsley, and shallot and combine well. Marinate for an hour.

In a large wok or nonstick skillet, heat oil and ginger over medium-high heat until fragrant.

Discard ginger and add chicken mixture and marinade. Sauté over high heat until chicken is almost cooked through, about 4 minutes. Then add peaches and continue to sauté until peaches are heated through and chicken is cooked, about 1 minute more. Serve hot over rice or skinny noodles, sprinkled with pistachios.

Makes 4 servings

PEARS

A Spoonful of Sweetness
Helps the Fiber Go Down

100 calories per pear

If our mention of parsnips as a fiber-rich alternative to bran didn't send you to the vegetable aisle of the supermarket, we have another alternative to offer that we think will interest you: pears. Like parsnips, pears are low in fat and sodium yet rich in insoluble fiber. And *no one* would argue that pears taste like bran.

A single pear has a total fiber content of 5 grams–quite a bit–of which 4 grams is the insoluble kind with special benefits to digestive health. While superbran cereals contain higher levels per serving, the amount in pears compares favorably with part-bran and other whole grain cereals. (See "Fiber Facts at Your Fingertips," on page 152, for more details.)

At the Market: To avoid gritty texture, pears are picked from the tree before they ripen. They're shipped unripe and usually appear for sale in the same condition, so choosing pears can be chancy. Look for a light green to gold color with a bit of a blush in green Bartletts, Seckels, and some Boscs. Scars and surface blemishes make a less attractive pear but do not affect the quality.

Kitchen Tips: To store most pears, keep them at room temperature until ripe. A fruit ripener or simply a loosely closed brown paper bag are good ways to ripen pears. And try grouping together several at a time, because they release gases that help each other ripen. Anjou pears, unlike others, will ripen in the refrigerator.

Because pears ripen from the inside out, don't let them become soft on the outside, or you'll be faced with some mushy eating. They're ready when aromatic and the necks give a bit to the touch. At this point, eat them immediately or refrigerate for up to four days.

For canning and baking, use firm, unripe pears. To peel, dip each pear in boiling water for about 5 seconds. When cool enough to handle, peel with a sharp paring knife.

Accent on Enjoyment: The perfume of pears is perfect in desserts containing orange and vanilla. But they're equally alluring in other courses of the meal, including entrées containing meats and poultry. Here are some new ideas for an old favorite.

- Halve and core pears, then fill with a mixture of soft cheese, chives, and dill. Serve at room temperature as an appetizer or part of a light lunch or dinner.
- Puree peeled ripe pears in a food processor or blender. Then add to the batter for muffins, pancakes, or waffles. The puree adds a natural sweetness, so you can cut down on the sweetener in the recipe. You can also add the puree to marinades for pork or poultry.
- You may have noticed Asian pears in your market, and if you haven't tried them, you should. They're applelike, crisp, and keep well. Eat them raw, poached, sliced in fruit salads, or as you would an apple.

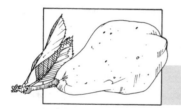

Baked Pears with Brie

⅓ cup raisins
¼ cup hazelnuts
2 teaspoons honey
2 ounces peeled Brie cheese
4 pears, peeled, halved, and cored
1 cup apple juice or sweet cider

Preheat the oven to 350° F.

Combine raisins and hazelnuts in a food processor or blender and process until finely chopped. Then, with the motor running, add honey and cheese and continue to process until a soft ball forms.

Spoon cheese mixture into cavities of pears and set them in an ovenproof casserole. Pour juice around them and bake until pears are tender, about 35 minutes. Serve hot as a dessert, breakfast, or snack.

Makes 4 servings

PEAS

Incredible and Edible as Ever

134 calories per cup (cooked)

Remember all that talk of milk as the most perfect food? As far as we're concerned, peas deserve at least equal billing. When it comes to the modern-day concerns in nutrition, it's hard to find any food that can outdo peas. They are perfect for:

- Keeping hearts healthy, because they have little or no fat, cholesterol, and sodium, yet are a good source of cholesterol-lowering soluble fiber.
- Helping to control diabetes, again because of their low fat and high fiber content.
- Preventing cancer, thanks to generous levels of fiber accompanied by carotene and vitamin C, but not fat.

At the Market: The small round peas that are often paired with carrots are called "garden" or "English" peas. They come fresh in pods that should be plump, firm, and lively green. Flat pods contain undeveloped peas; wilted, tired-looking pods contain old, starchy peas. Snow peas and sugar snaps are "edible-podded" peas. They should be crisp and without gray blotches.

If you can't find fresh garden peas, buy frozen. Canned peas are gray and tasteless and hardly resemble the original. Edible-podded peas are available frozen, but the texture is not alluring.

Kitchen Tips: To store, leave the peas in their pods and refrigerate in perforated plastic bags. Both garden and edible-podded peas will last for up to ten days but are sweetest when eaten right away.

To shell garden peas, grab the end of the pod and zip down the string, nudging the pod open at the same time. Then use your thumb to coax the peas out. One pound of peas only takes about 7 minutes to shell and yields about 1 cup of peas.

Accent on Enjoyment: Add peas to a stir-fry, sauté, soup, casserole, or omelet, and you'll add color, taste, texture, and nutrition all at once! Also consider:

- Varying the flavor of peas with thyme, marjoram, dill, mint, tarragon, ginger, garlic, toasted nuts, onion, scallions, or chives.
- Adding a handful of fresh peas to yeast bread dough before baking.
- Tossing steamed new potatoes with fresh peas, dill, and a splash of olive oil. This dish is best served hot.

The Incredible, Edible Pea

When you really consider how nutritious peas are, you wonder whether the "incredible edible egg" realizes that it has some serious competition. Check out these numbers:

	1 Large Egg, Hard-Cooked	Green Peas, Cooked, ¾ Cup
Calories	82	86
Cholesterol (mg)	252	0
Fat (g)	6	less than 1
Protein (g)	6	6
Vitamin A (I.U.)	590	645
Thiamine (mg)	0.04	0.34
Riboflavin (mg)	0.14	0.14
Niacin (mg)	trace	2.8
Vitamin C (mg)	0	24
Calcium (mg)	27	28
Iron (mg)	1.2	2.2
Phosphorus (mg)	103	118
Potassium (mg)	65	236

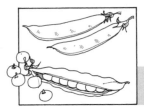

Five-Spice Beef with Peas

½ teaspoon cornstarch
1 teaspoon *mirin*
2 teaspoons soy sauce
1 teaspoon Chinese
   five-spice powder
¼ pound lean sirloin,
   thinly sliced against
   the grain
1½ cups fresh snow peas
1½ cups shelled garden
   peas (frozen peas
   may be used)
1 onion, chopped
2 teaspoons peanut oil

In a medium bowl, whisk together cornstarch, *mirin,* soy sauce, and five-spice powder. Add beef and combine well. Marinate for about 30 minutes.

Place a strainer in the sink and add peas and onion. Pour boiling water over them for about 10 seconds, then set aside. (If using frozen peas, do not blanch them.)

In a wok or large nonstick skillet, heat oil over medium-high heat. Then add beef, reserving the marinade, and stir-fry for about 2 minutes. Add peas, onions, and marinade and continue to stir-fry until beef is cooked, about 2 minutes more. (Be careful not to overcook the vegetables.) Serve hot with steamed rice or Chinese crepe-type pancakes.

Makes 4 servings

PEPPERS

A Bell of a Vegetable

18 calories per pepper (raw)

Chances are that everyone in your house likes sweet peppers, so you need not bother telling them about all their nutritional virtues.

Hardly anyone (including us, of course) would guess that peppers rate among our most nutrient-dense foods. (For more details about the meaning of "nutrient density," see the discussion in the entry on papaya, beginning on page 334.) Our most nutrient-dense fruits–papaya and cantaloupe–share honors with a long list of vegetables, and although these two fruits have very high ratings, some vegetables rank higher still. The highest honors, according to calculations by the Basic and Traditional Foods Association, go to various kinds of greens and, of course, to the popular bell pepper.

The most impressive characteristic of sweet peppers? We'd vote for their astonishing vitamin C content–a single pepper bests a cup of orange juice on this count.

At the Market: Select sweet peppers that have firm walls and are heavy and full size. Many peppers start green and turn red when mature, but some will turn yellow or purple instead. For visual appeal, choose two or three different colors and use them in the same recipe.

Kitchen Tips: Store peppers in tightly closed plastic bags in the crisper drawer of the refrigerator. They will last for up to two weeks. To freeze peppers that have tough skins, blanch them for about 3 minutes before freezing to prevent the skins from becoming even tougher in the freezer.

For a rich flavor without lots of calories and fat, roast peppers. The easiest way is to core and seed the peppers, then set them on a baking sheet. Broil about 5 inches from the heat source until charred and blistered on all sides. (Cooking time will average about 5 minutes on each side.) Then place the peppers in a large paper bag and let them cool. Finally, use your fingers and a sharp paring knife to remove the skins. Roasted peppers can be pureed and added to soups and sauces. Or chop and toss with rice or pasta.

Accent on Enjoyment: Sweet peppers let you enliven the flavor of surrounding foods without needing to add salt or fat. Or, try these ideas for preparing peppers.

- Sauté with garlic, rosemary, and olive oil until just wilted. Then serve as a snack on crusty bread.
- Add to stir-fries featuring pork or shrimp.
- Use thin strips of colorful sweet peppers to garnish clear soups.

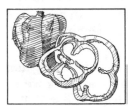

Roasted Sweet Pepper Soup

10 medium sweet red
   peppers, cored and
   seeded
1 tablespoon olive oil
1 cup thinly sliced fresh
   mushrooms
2 shallots, minced
1 teaspoon dried basil
½ teaspoon dried thyme
½ cup chicken stock
   minced chives

Preheat the broiler.

Arrange peppers on one or two large baking sheets. Broil until charred, 4 to 5 minutes on each side. Then set peppers in a large brown paper bag, fold the bag closed and let cool for 30 to 40 minutes.

In a large saucepan, heat oil over medium heat. Add mushrooms and shallots and sauté until tender and wilted. Then add basil and thyme and reduce heat to low.

Use your fingers and a sharp paring knife to remove the charred skins from peppers. Discard the skins and put peppers in a food processor or blender. Process until smooth.

Add peppers and stock to the saucepan and heat through, stirring frequently. Serve hot, sprinkled with chives.

Makes 4 servings

PINEAPPLE

Hawaii's Gift to the World

41 calories per slice
80 calories per cup

Pineapple may have more fans among gourmets than among nutritionists, and we can understand why. It has few of the nutrients that fruit is known for–such as vitamins A and C. But pineapple is surprisingly rich in a nutrient that most fruits–and most food, for that matter–have in far lesser amounts. It's manganese–one of the little-known trace minerals.

Nutritionists know that manganese is an essential part of certain enzymes needed to metabolize protein and carbohydrate. Not enough is known, however, to establish a firm recommended allowance. So nutritionists use the so-called Safe and Adequate Range of 2½ to 5 milligrams daily. One slice of fresh pineapple puts you more than halfway there–and that, to us, is no small accomplishment. And sodium and fat watchers need not worry about pineapple.

At the Market: Forget about plucking leaves out of the middle; your nose is the key to judging a good pineapple. A good one smells sweet at the base and feels firm when squeezed. The leaves should be green, and the body should be unbruised. At many supermarkets pineapple can be peeled and cored while you wait, so be sure to ask if this service is available.

Canned pineapple, of course, tastes different from fresh, but now that it's available packed in juice, it can be a great compromise when fresh isn't available. Always check the ingredient list for purity.

Kitchen Tips: Pineapple won't ripen after picking, but you can make it sweeter throughout by turning it upside down and leaving it overnight. This allows the sugars in the bottom half of the pineapple to circulate. In any case, always store uncut pineapples at room temperature to maximize flavor.

Always use cooked or canned pineapple in gelatin dishes. Fresh pineapple will prevent gelling.

Accent on Enjoyment: No matter where you are, eating a sweet, juicy pineapple can give you a delicious tropical feeling. Here are some ideas to encourage you to use pineapple more often.

- Add chopped pineapple to chicken salad, fruit salad, or stuffing for poultry or pork.
- For an easy breakfast, add chopped pineapple to vanilla yogurt and serve over cereal.
- Marinate chopped pineapple in orange juice and rum extract for about 30 minutes. Then serve with frozen vanilla yogurt in pretty glasses.

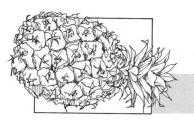

Pineapple-Mint Sorbet

2 cups pureed ripe
    pineapple
½ cup unsweetened
    pineapple juice
5 drops mint extract
    fresh mint for garnish

Combine pineapple, juice, and mint extract in an ice cream maker and process according to manufacturer's directions. Garnish with fresh mint and serve.

If you don't have an ice cream maker, combine the ingredients in a medium bowl, freeze for about 4 hours, then place in a food processor or blender and process before serving. If the sorbet is frozen solid, run it through a juicer before serving to improve the texture.

Makes 4 servings

PLANTAIN

Yes, We Look Like Bananas

178 calories per cup (cooked)

When confronted with a plantain for the first time, most people say, with some surprise, "Is that a banana?" Well, all that looks like a banana is not a banana. In both the culinary and the nutritional sense, the two have plenty of differences.

Plantains score higher than bananas for vitamin A and potassium, although both are similarly low in fat and sodium. We'd like to focus on another aspect of plantains, though–their fiber content. For despite their image as "off-limits" to dieters, if prepared without added fat, plantains have much going for them.

British scientist D. A. T. Southgate is one of the world's best-known authorities on fiber's effects on absorption of calories from food. Dr. Southgate has proposed that the fiber content of foods be measured in terms of how much must be eaten to supply a basic amount of fiber. The idea is to emphasize food sources that give you the most fiber for the fewest calories. And as "Buying Fiber for the Fewest Calories" shows, plantains are one of the foods that manage to deliver a gram of fiber with the fewest calories.

At the Market: Shaped like long bananas, plantains are green to black in color. They can usually be found in the exotic produce section at the supermarket, along with other tropical fruits and vegetables. Unlike the common banana, plantains are never sweet. Choose green plantains for frying and riper black plantains for steaming and mashing.

Kitchen Tips: Plantains are too starchy to eat raw amd must always be cooked. Store them at room temperature, then when you're ready, peel and remove the long, stringy fibers. If they give you trouble, use a sharp paring knife. Then simmer, bake, steam, or fry.

Accent on Enjoyment: With a little experimenting, you will be able to incorporate plantains into your diet easily. Here are some suggestions to get you started.

- Steam peeled, sliced plantains until tender–about 10 minutes. Then sauté with garlic and olive oil and serve as a side dish with roast pork or poultry.
- Mash steamed plantain by hand and stir in a bit of sweet butter and freshly grated Parmesan cheese. Serve hot as a side dish with grilled fish.
- Substitute plantains for potatoes in your favorite potato recipe. They have a similar texture and are delicious with similar seasonings.

Buying Fiber for the Fewest Calories

This table, compiled by fiber expert and researcher Dr. D. A. T. Southgate, shows how many calories of a food must be eaten in order to obtain 1 gram of fiber.

Food	Calories per Gram of Fiber	Amount Needed to Provide 1 Gram of Fiber
Cabbage, boiled	3	¹⁄₁₀ cup
Orange	18	¼ small fruit
Plantain, boiled	19	¹⁄₁₀ cup
Apple	23	⅓ small fruit
Whole meal bread	25	⅗ slice
Potato, boiled	79	½ potato
White bread	87	1¼ slices

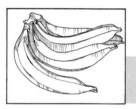

Baked Mashed Plantain, Caribbean Style

4 firm plantains
¾ cup milk
1 egg
2 tablespoons minced fresh chives
1 jalapeño pepper, cored, seeded, and minced
2 tomatoes, chopped

Preheat the oven to 400° F.

Use a sharp paring knife to peel and slice plantains, then steam over boiling water until tender, about 10 minutes.

Place plantains in a food processor or blender and add milk, egg, chives, and jalapeño. Use on/off pulses to process mixture until it's well combined and has the texture of cooked oatmeal. (If you overprocess, the mixture will be gummy.)

Lightly oil a 9-inch pie plate. Spoon mixture into the pie plate and pat it flat with your hand. Bake until heated through, about 10 minutes. Slice into wedges, top with tomatoes and serve warm.

Makes 8 servings as a side dish, 4 servings as an entrée

PORK

Shedding the Porky Image

275 calories per 4 ounces (lean shoulder)

You're known for the company you keep, and lean pork has had a rough time of it as a result. Because fatty pork products such as many luncheon meats and bacon are better known, their reputation as high-fat troublemakers has tarnished that of fresh lean pork. Yet, some cuts of lean pork actually contain no more fat than other foods that we consider healthful.

The latest figures from the U.S. Department of Agriculture show that a 4-ounce serving of roasted pork shoulder–picnic type–provides about 11 grams of fat when trimmed. That's not so bad–4 ounces of bacon and luncheon meats can provide several times this amount.

And the pork producers themselves can take a lot of credit for giving us this leaner alternative. The fresh pork you get now is often different from what you found in the market a few years ago. Many cuts are now leaner, accounting for the change in the amount of marbling you see. The change is especially obvious in the shoulder cuts.

And when you opt for less fat, you also opt for more nutritional value–the good stuff in meat is in the muscle, not the fat. Accordingly, lean pork supplies more of the nutrients pork is known for–like zinc and thiamine–than fatty cuts do.

At the Market: When choosing lean pork, make sure that the flesh is a pinkish color. Any visible fat should be clear white.

Kitchen Tips: Wrap lean fresh pork fairly loosely in waxed paper or foil and store in the coldest part of your refrigerator for up to five days. Fattier cuts should be wrapped the same way but stored for only about two days. Pork freezes well for three to four months.

One good way to cook the leaner pork is to slice it into thin ribbons against the grain and stir-fry until cooked through. Roasting in a clay cooker or an oven cooking bag is another great way to help keep it moist and juicy. Remember, of course, that pork should be cooked to an internal temperature of 175° F before eating.

Normally, a pork roast will need about 35 minutes of cooking for each pound of meat. If the roast is stuffed or rolled, however, it will need an extra 5 minutes of cooking time per pound.

Accent on Enjoyment: Pork's sweet taste and meaty texture are wonderful with marinades. Try an oriental one using soy sauce, garlic, and ginger, or:

* Marinate thin strips of pork in lime juice, ground cumin, and garlic. Sauté and serve with hot bread.
* Stew chunks of pork with onion, tomato, zucchini, and roasted chilies. Serve with soft flour tortillas.
* Rub pork chops with spicy mustard, then press on sprigs of thyme and grill.

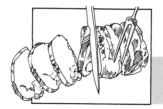

Pork with Broccoli and Hoisin Sauce

1 pound lean pork, thinly
    sliced against the
    grain
1 teaspoon soy sauce
1 teaspoon honey
2 teaspoons orange juice
2 teaspoons cornstarch
2 teaspoons peanut oil
1 cup chopped fresh or
    frozen broccoli
3 scallions, chopped
2 tablespoons hoisin
    sauce

In a medium bowl, mix pork, soy sauce, honey, juice, and cornstarch. Marinate for about an hour.

In a wok or large nonstick skillet, heat oil over medium heat. Add pork and stir-fry over high heat for about 3 minutes. Add broccoli and scallions and stir-fry for about 2 minutes more. Then stir in hoisin sauce and toss until meat and vegetables are coated with sauce and cooked through. Serve hot with rice or barley.

Makes 4 servings

Pork in Red Chili Sauce

¾ pound lean pork, cut into 1-inch chunks
3 to 4 tablespoons roasted chili powder
3 cloves garlic, coarsely chopped
1 teaspoon dried oregano
¼ teaspoon ground cinnamon
¼ teaspoon ground cloves
¼ teaspoon ground cumin
3 cups beef stock
4 large flour tortillas

Heat a well-seasoned cast-iron skillet, then add pork. (If you don't have a cast-iron skillet, use a nonstick one.) Sauté pork until brown, about 10 minutes.

Combine chili powder, garlic, oregano, cinnamon, cloves, cumin, and 1 cup stock in a food processor or blender and process until ingredients form a smooth paste.

Drain fat from the skillet if necessary, then add the puree. Sauté over medium heat, stirring with a spatula, until it darkens a bit, about 4 minutes.

Pour in the remaining 2 cups of stock and bring to a boil. Reduce heat, cover loosely with crumpled foil, and simmer, stirring occasionally, until pork is very tender, about 50 minutes. (If the sauce becomes too thick, pour in a bit more stock or water.) Serve hot with tortillas.

Makes 4 servings

POTATOES

Hot and Healthy

145 calories per potato (baked)
114 calories per cup (cooked and sliced)

Potatoes have been redeemed!

For a long time most folks had the notion that the potato was an unhealthful and fattening food loaded only with calories and starch. How far they were from the truth! Not only were potatoes falsely accused, but their good points went virtually unnoticed.

The tables have turned, of course, and none too soon. Concerns about fat and sodium (something potatoes have very little of unless you add it yourself) aren't the only reason. Fiber research is in its heyday, and potatoes have proved one of the best sources. What's more, potatoes have the kind of fiber that helps lower cholesterol. Add in the incredible potassium content of potatoes (enough to make oranges look mediocre) and you can understand why every heart expert in town wants potatoes on the menu.

Blood pressure experts have long suspected that a healthy potassium intake is beneficial. Recently, though, evidence linking potassium intake directly to protection from stroke has also come along. Kay-Tee Khaw and Elizabeth Barrett-Connor, M.D., of the University of California, compared food habits to the chances of having a stroke among residents of that state. They linked an extra 400 milligrams of potassium per day to a 40 percent reduction in the risk of having a stroke. Half a baked potato is all you need to pick up that additional amount.

To keep the potassium in the potato, it's best not to boil it. Nels Christian Henningsen and co-workers at the University of Lund in Sweden have found that 10 to 50 percent of the potassium in a potato may be lost during boiling, while only 3 to 6 percent is lost if it is steamed.

At the Market: Baking potatoes should be firm, well shaped, and without discolorations. Avoid any with green patches or sprouts. It's best to pick them out one by one rather than purchasing them by the bag, so you can carefully inspect them.

The green color sometimes seen in potatoes often causes concern. It signals the presence of solanine, a substance which in high amounts can cause drowsiness, itching, diarrhea, and vomiting. The chances of a single potato having levels even close to those needed to cause symptoms, however, are very, very, small. Nevertheless, potatoes riddled with green spots should be rejected because of solanine's adverse effect on flavor.

Kitchen Tips: Keep potatoes in a cool, dark place, but not in the refrigerator. Also, don't store potatoes near apples, as doing so may alter their taste.

When you're ready to cook, check for sprouts and green spots again; cut out any that are present. Scrub them well. To bake, use a sharp paring knife to puncture them in several places. Three medium baking potatoes weigh about a pound and will take about 50 minutes to bake in a preheated oven set at 400° F. By the way, some varieties of potato may turn blue if cooked in cast iron, so favor other kinds of utensils if possible.

Accent on Enjoyment: Sweet and nutty, potatoes are a fine foil for curries, members of the onion family, and most cheeses. For a quick lunch or dinner, top baked potatoes with one of the following combinations:

- Shredded cooked chicken, minced red onion, minced sweet red pepper, mashed avocado, and garlic.
- Chopped ripe tomato, rosemary, toasted walnuts, and freshly grated Parmesan cheese.
- Minced leeks, smoked salmon, fresh snipped dill, and plain yogurt.

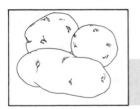

Potato Frittata with Sage and Onions

2 medium potatoes
  (about ¾ pound),
  cubed and steamed
1 medium onion,
  chopped
1 teaspoon dried sage
4 eggs, beaten
  freshly grated Parmesan
  cheese

Preheat the oven to 350° F.

Arrange potatoes in a 9-inch pie plate, along with onion and sage.

Pour in eggs and bake in the middle of the oven until set, about 20 minutes. Immediately sprinkle on Parmesan. Cut into wedges and serve warm for breakfast, brunch, lunch, or with soup and salad for a light dinner.

Makes 4 servings

PRUNES

Better Than Bran, Some Say

20 calories per prune

We know that lots of people wouldn't think of eating prunes. Perhaps we should be glad, because this lets us keep all the prunes in the house to ourselves. Knowing that prunes have so much to offer, though, we'd rather share them.

Maybe the new focus on fiber will help spruce up the image of prunes. After all, a serving of prunes at breakfast will give you almost as much fiber as a serving of an all-bran cereal. The prune's fiber is mostly the insoluble form found in bran—the kind that's best for digestive health. But unlike bran, prunes do contain substantial amounts of the other fiber—the soluble form that lowers blood cholesterol, too. We like to mix them with other fruits rich in soluble fiber, such as dried apples, in making healthful snack mixes. Prunes, though, contribute more in the way of vitamins and minerals—notably vitamin A, iron, and potassium.

At the Market: Choose prunes by matching them to the use planned. For instance, pitted prunes are a good selection for compotes; unpitted are fine for snacking. Some brands—especially in the newer vacuum-packed cans—are moister than others and can be eaten right out of the package, while others are drier and must be simmered to soften. If you want to see what you're getting, buy prunes in bulk or in see-through bags.

Kitchen Tips: Prunes will keep for months, tightly wrapped in a cool, dry place. If your pantry is on the warm side, refrigerate your prunes.

If prunes are very dry, simmer in a bit of apple or orange juice until tender. One cup of average-dry prunes will need about ½ cup of juice and 5 minutes of simmering. Tough prunes can be microwaved until tender. A half cup sprinkled with 1 tablespoon of juice and covered will take about 2 minutes on full power. For extra zip, add a drop or two of vanilla extract or a ribbon of lemon peel.

Accent on Enjoyment: If you think prunes are frumpy food, these ideas may be just the thing to change your mind.

• Stuff prunes with pureed cottage cheese and serve as a snack.

• Chop prunes and add to fruit salads, especially ones with fresh orange.
• Sauté prunes with chicken and walnuts. Serve with pasta and a green salad.

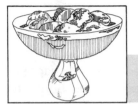

Sautéed Chicken with Prunes and Shallot

1 pound chicken cutlets
2 tablespoons flour
2 teaspoons peanut oil
⅓ cup chopped pitted
    prunes
1 shallot, minced
2 teaspoons Dijon
    mustard
¼ cup apple juice
¼ cup chicken stock
½ teaspoon dried basil

Dredge chicken lightly in flour.

In a large nonstick skillet, heat oil over medium heat. Add chicken and sauté over medium heat until cooked through, about 4 minutes on each side. Then transfer chicken to a heated plate.

Combine prunes, shallot, mustard, juice, stock, and basil in the skillet and stir to combine well. Increase the heat to high and boil the sauce, stirring and scraping up pieces from the bottom of the pan, until it is reduced by half, about 3 minutes. Spoon sauce over chicken and serve hot.

Makes 4 servings

PUMPKIN

More Than a Pie Filling

48 calories per cup (mashed)

Pumpkins are fun to decorate, fun to cook, and fun to eat–and even vegetable-snubbing children agree. Even adults who eat plenty of vegetables should consider eating more pumpkin; it couldn't be more nutritious, and it may even help curb your appetite.

That possibility was raised when June L. Kelsay, Ph.D., of the U.S. Department of Agriculture, set out to study how diets rich in fiber from fruit and vegetables affected mineral nutrition. The diets relied heavily on figs and pumpkin as fiber sources, and when the diet was richest in these two foods, the subjects complained that Dr. Kelsay was making them overeat! Yet, Dr. Kelsay had made sure that the calorie content of the diets stayed the same no matter how much or how little fiber was present. So the fiber itself–not more calories–obviously made the subjects feel full.

While on the high-fiber diet, Dr. Kelsay's subjects absorbed less fat and calories from their food. Yet they showed no signs of becoming deficient in calcium, magnesium, copper, or zinc.

Vitamin A was not an issue in this study, but as any nutritionist can tell you, the pumpkin pudding that the subjects ate provided plenty of it. And its orange color is the clue that it also contains plenty of beta-carotene (provitamin A), the nutrient getting credit for having cancer-preventing qualities.

At the Market: Most prized for eating are "neck pumpkins," which look like butternut squash with long necks. Jack-o'-lantern pumpkins can also be used for cooking and make great vessels in which to bake stews. Regardless of the type, choose one with clear, unbroken skin and no soft spots.

Kitchen Tips: Neck pumpkins, famous for pumpkin pies and puddings, should be stored in a cool place. Start preparing them for pie by cutting into chunks and simmering until tender–20 to 40 minutes, depending on size and age. Drain, and when cool enough to handle, remove the skin and puree. Use the puree immediately or freeze it for up to a year.

Jack-o'-lantern types may be stored and prepared the same way. As you'll find, however, their flavor is not as exciting.

Accent on Enjoyment: Pumpkin is also not just for pies. It can easily become the focal point of savory and hearty main-dish meals. For example:

• Add chunked and peeled pumpkin to beef stew.
• Toss diced pumpkin into a vegetable soup or side-dish sauté.
• Combine equal parts of pureed pumpkin and part-skim ricotta and use to fill ravioli, manicotti, or crepes.
• Try different combinations of the following friendly flavors: nutmeg, mace, cinnamon, allspice, ginger, rosemary, mustard, or mild white cheeses.

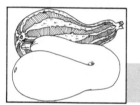

Savory Chunked Pumpkin

1 pound neck-type
    pumpkin, cut into
    chunks
¼ teaspoon ground mace
1 teaspoon dried thyme
2 teaspoons sweet butter
    or margarine

Steam pumpkin until tender, about 8 minutes.

Drain and peel pumpkin, then place in a medium bowl along with mace, thyme, and butter. Toss well to combine but take care not to crush the chunks. Serve hot over rice. It's fantastic with smoked turkey.

Makes 4 servings

RABBIT

Game Is Gaining Ground

246 calories per 4 ounces (cooked)

It used to be that the only place you'd be likely to find rabbit is on a hunter's dinner table. Today, however, retail meat markets are a good place to look, and with the growing preference for lean meat, the supermarket may well be next.

Do give rabbit a try, especially if you're concerned with blood pressure. It has more potassium and less sodium than more common meats, and as you may already know, getting more of the former and less of the latter looks like an important factor for healthier blood pressure. Rabbit is also rich in niacin, a B vitamin; a 4-ounce serving provides more than half the day's recommended allowance.

Although leaner than fatty meats, rabbit may still contain more fat than alternatives such as flounder or skinned chicken breast. This is especially true of rabbit that has been raised expressly to be sold as food. So as always, be on the lookout for the lean and trim away any separable fat that you can.

At the Market: These days, most poultry purveyors carry rabbit, but try to order ahead, especially around Christmas and Easter. Choose a rabbit that weighs 2 pounds or less to ensure tenderness. The flesh should be smooth and pale. To make handling and cooking easier, ask the butcher to cut your selection into seven pieces for you—four legs and three back pieces.

Kitchen Tips: Keep the rabbit in the coldest part of the refrigerator in a tightly closed plastic bag. Use it within two days. The back pieces have lots of meat on them, while the center piece will have side flaps reminiscent of veal scallops. During long cooking, tuck these under the center to prevent overcooking.

Accent on Enjoyment: To adopt rabbit into your culinary repertoire, use it in place of chicken in a favorite recipe. Rabbit flesh is slightly denser than chicken, however, so you'll need to increase cooking times slightly.

Here are some additional suggestions to get you started with rabbit.

• Simmer rabbit with chopped tomatoes, onions, sweet peppers, and bay leaf.

- Sauté rabbit with mushrooms and shallots, then simmer in stock with a pinch of mustard.
- Poach rabbit, then shred and add to fried rice or pasta.

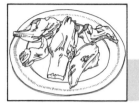

Spicy Rabbit Sauté

¼ teaspoon freshly
    ground black
    pepper
¼ teaspoon freshly
    ground white
    pepper
¼ teaspoon ground red
    pepper, or to taste
½ teaspoon dried thyme
½ teaspoon dried
    oregano
2 tablespoons flour
1 rabbit (about 2
    pounds), cut into
    7 pieces
1 tablespoon olive oil
2 cloves garlic, minced
3 bay leaves
1½ cups chicken stock

In a small bowl, combine black pepper, white pepper, red pepper, thyme, oregano, and flour. Then dredge rabbit in the mixture.

In a large nonstick skillet, heat oil over medium heat. Add rabbit and sauté over medium heat until fragrant and just brown, about 7 minutes.

Add garlic, bay leaves, and stock and bring to a boil. Immediately reduce heat to medium-low, cover loosely with crumpled foil, and simmer until rabbit has cooked through, about 25 minutes. Remove bay leaves. Serve hot with rice or corn bread and sautéed greens.

Makes 4 servings

RICE, BROWN

The Whole Grain and Nothing but the Grain

116 calories per ½ cup (cooked)

People have been eating rice for centuries, but it wasn't until the Kempner Rice Diet was developed in the 1940s that its nutritional value became widely appreciated.

In fact, William Kempner, M.D., put rice in the news as never before. It was Dr. Kempner's idea to treat patients suffering from high blood pressure with a diet of rice and fruit—and in many subjects blood pressure (and weight, too) fell dramatically. Dr. Kempner believed that the low sodium content of the rice and fruit accounted for the positive effect on blood pressure. His colleagues were slow to accept his idea, but further research proved him right. Today, his work has attained classic status—and the rice diet is still in use.

Of course, this hardly means that if you have high blood pressure, rice should be the mainstay of your diet. But including more rice in your diet is obviously a step in the right direction. Brown rice is especially good because it provides all the fiber and nutrients that nature put in the grain. With these whole grain nutrients, plus 5 grams of protein per cup, rice is clearly a lot more than "just starch."

At the Market: Choose brown rice according to the intended use. The most popular kind is "long grain," which is about five times as long as it is wide. When cooked, the grains become separate and light, not gluey, making it well suited to pilafs, paellas, stuffings, rice salads, fried rice, and casseroles.

"Medium grain" is plumper and stickier than long grain but nevertheless can be used interchangeably in most recipes. Some medium grains will require slightly less cooking water than long grains, so always check package instructions.

Almost round when cooked, "short grain" is very sticky and heavy. The Chinese like it in soups and gruels and the Japanese use it for sushi. Short grain is also used in many southeast Asian cuisines to make dumpling doughs and pasta. An especially interesting variety of brown rice is called wehani. It has huge amber grains and smells like popcorn when it's cooking.

Regardless of type, determine freshness by smelling the rice. Pass up any rice with even a trace of mustiness or rancidity. Even packaged rice can

Thai Fried Rice with Vegetable Ribbons

1 carrot, cut into
   julienne strips
1 leek, cut into
   julienne strips
½ cup snow peas, cut
   into julienne strips
2 teaspoons peanut oil
2 cloves garlic, minced
2 cups cooked rice
   juice and pulp of
   1 lime
1 teaspoon honey
¼ teaspoon hot pepper
   sauce, or to taste
1 tablespoon peanut
   butter
2 tablespoons minced
   fresh basil or mint
   (optional)

Set a strainer in the sink and place carrot, leek, and pea strips in it. Pour boiling water over vegetables for about 12 seconds. Set vegetables aside.

In a large nonstick skillet, heat oil over medium heat. Add vegetables, garlic, and rice and sauté until heated through and fragrant, about 4 minutes. (Don't crowd the pan; cook in two batches, if necessary.)

In a small bowl, whisk together lime juice and pulp, honey, hot pepper sauce, peanut butter, and basil or mint, if used. Add to rice mixture and toss well to combine. Serve hot as a side dish. It also makes an enjoyable main dish when accompanied by a clear soup and some wontons or egg rolls.

Makes 4 servings

sometimes be smelled through the box. If you get the rice home and discover it's not fresh, return it.

Kitchen Tips: Store brown rice in tightly covered glass jars in the refrigerator, where it will last for up to six months.

Variables–the type of heating element you're using, the material of your saucepan, humidity, temperature, grain size, and age of rice–will affect its cooking time. In general, though, the best way to cook brown rice (except for risotto and sushi) is to bring about 2 cups of water to a boil. Add about 1 cup of rice and let it boil, uncovered, for 5 minutes. Then reduce the heat to a very gentle simmer and cover, leaving a little "smile" open on the side of the pan. The rice is done when all the water is absorbed, in about 20 minutes.

To reheat refrigerated rice, scoop it into a tight mesh strainer and steam it over boiling water until heated through.

Accent on Enjoyment: Brown rice is not only healthful but also delicious and fun to eat. Here are three easy ideas to try.

- Sauté shelled shrimp in olive oil with garlic, shallots, and minced fresh mint and basil. Sprinkle with lime juice, then toss with cooked rice and serve warm in lettuce leaves.
- Place a mound of cooked rice before pouring hot soups into bowls. Gumbos and tomato soups are particularly nice when done this way.
- Toss cooked rice with diced cooked chicken, peanuts, chopped sweet pepper, ginger, garlic, and hot pepper sauce to taste. Serve at room temperature or chilled as a main dish salad.

SHELLFISH

Haute and Healthy

Clams: 86 calories per 4 ounces (shelled)

Crab: 105 calories per 4 ounces (cooked)

Lobster: 108 calories per 4 ounces (cooked)

Mussels: 107 calories per 4 ounces (canned)

Oysters: 103 calories per 4 ounces (shelled)

Scallops: 127 calories per 4 ounces (cooked)

Many nutritionists still promote the Basic Four approach to nutrition. But as far as we're concerned, the Basic Four needs a major overhaul. We've met many people who can tell us everything there is to know about food groups, yet know very little about which dairy and meat products, for instance, are high in fat and sodium.

The "meat group" of the Basic Four is a case in point. Such nutritionally diverse things as shellfish and hot dogs come under this group. What the Basic Four doesn't tell you is that shellfish have the edge over meats on the very points that concern us most.

For starters, shellfish tend to be far lower in calories; a 4-ounce serving of shucked clams, for instance, weighs in with fewer than 100 calories. The same amount of the leanest red meat contains far more. Naturally, the extra calories in meat come mostly from fat; while a serving a clams has only 2 grams of fat, a serving of beef typically has from 7 to 20 grams–sometimes even more.

Unlike the flesh of land animals, shellfish are also a modest yet significant source of calcium–something that most of us can use more of. And while many meats are similar in zinc content to shellfish, not one comes close to oysters.

So, as you can see, what the Basic Four doesn't tell you can hurt you. Use it, if you like, as an introduction to nutrition. But be sure to investigate which foods within each group are the most nutritious and wholesome. You may be in for some surprises.

Clams

At the Market: For hard-shell clams, select only those that are tightly closed. Soft-shell clams, however, may be slightly opened because of their necks. The flesh of good clams is plump, clean smelling, and cream colored, regardless of whether the clams are in the shell or shucked. It's best to buy these highly perishable shellfish the same day you plan to eat them.

Kitchen Tips: Refrigerate clams immediately, and try to use them the same day. If the clams appear sandy, soak them in cold water for a short time, then scrub and cook. Discard any clams that float.

Incidentally, if you like to shuck your own clams but find them difficult to open, soak them in ice water for about 5 minutes, then shuck.

Accent on Enjoyment: Clams offer countless eating adventures. For instance:

• Soft-shell clams are good steamed or baked.
• Littleneck clams can be used for clambakes or microwaved, covered loosely, on full power until open. Cherrystone clams can be microwaved the same way.
• Olive oil and garlic are classic seasonings for shucked clams.
• Clams are also excellent shucked, tossed with hot pasta and topped with freshly grated Parmesan cheese.

Crab

At the Market: When buying whole crabs, choose live ones only. (Dead crabs deteriorate very rapidly.) "Slabs" or "whales" are the largest crabs, followed by jumbo or prime. Medium crabs are smaller still. Soft-shell crabs actually are a type of blue crab; they have temporarily shed their shells so that a larger one can form.

From the standpoint of flavor, blue crabs, Dungeness, and Alaskan King crabs are the most popular. Male crabs are favored over females. Packaged crabmeat takes some of the work out of selecting crabs. When buying it, check the date on the label to ensure freshness.

Sodium under the Shell

A word to sodium watchers about shellfish is in order. The amount of sodium that occurs naturally in shellfish falls far below the amount found in processed meats and fish. Nevertheless, the sodium content of some shellfish is higher than that of many fresh animal foods.

Here's the full story, from the U.S. Department of Agriculture. Values are for a 3-ounce serving.

Shellfish	Sodium (mg)
Hard-shell clams, raw	174
Soft-shell clams, raw	30
Crab, canned, drained	425
Crab, steamed	314
Lobster, boiled	212
Mussels, raw	243
Oysters, fried	174
Oysters, frozen	323
Oysters, raw	113
Scallops, raw	217
Scallops, steamed	225
Shrimp, canned	1,955
Shrimp, fried	159
Shrimp, raw	137

Kitchen Tips: To keep crabs alive, you can store them for a short period of time on ice or in the refrigerator. Discard any that die. To cook, drop the live crabs into a pot of boiling water; add aromatics such as bay leaf, allspice, or lemon if desired. Boil until the shells turn bright red, about 10 minutes. Remove the lungs and intestinal tissue before eating.

As for packaged crabmeat, it may have some bits of shell that must be removed before eating. For easy removal, spread the crab out on a baking sheet and place it under a broiler briefly. The bits of shell will turn white and you can easily pick them out.

Accent on Enjoyment: Crab is naturally delicious, and even more so with mustard sauce, horseradish sauce, lemon, mild cheeses, and dill. Also consider adding crab to stir-fries, quiches, and omelet fillings. And for an ultra-elegant dish when cost is immaterial, sauté crabmeat with tender asparagus spears. Toss in minced shallot and celery and serve warm.

Lobster

At the Market: North American lobster should always be bought fresh. As you approach the lobster tank, keep an eye out for the liveliest ones, as these tend to be freshest.

Once in tanks, lobsters don't feed, and as a result they lose flesh rapidly. Accordingly, those that have been around for a few days have less meat.

Next, consider geography. Maine lobster is the best—tender and full-flavored, with snow-white flesh. Florida lobster and lobsters from around Honduras are good but tend to be a bit tough and stringy. Their flesh is tinged with yellow, because of the iodine in their waters, and this affects the taste, too. Lobsters from Tasmania, if you can find them, will take your breath away. They're crisp in taste and texture, gently briny, and pure white. One tail can weigh 3 pounds, and every ounce is a tender morsel.

Most North American lobster available for sale weighs between 1 and 3 pounds. But the 1½- to 2-pound lobsters have the most consistently sweet and tender flesh. The color of the shell, which can be white to blue to green-black, is not an indication of what's inside.

Kitchen Tips: Don't store fresh lobster. When you get them home, plunge them headfirst into a huge kettle of boiling water. Cover and continue to boil for 9 to 15 minutes, depending on the size. A 1½-pounder, for example, will take about 12 minutes. Lobster shells turn red when cooked.

When the lobster is cool enough to handle, use lobster crackers or nut crackers and picks to remove the flesh. Lobster liver, called tomalley (it's the green part; you can't miss it) is a wonderfully aromatic treat that tastes something like sea urchin. And the discovery of lobster roe, also called coral because of its color, will please a lobster gourmet for sure.

Cholesterol Chaos

Twenty-five years ago, when concern about cholesterol was just beginning, the U.S. Department of Agriculture (USDA) published tables showing shellfish to be very high in cholesterol. It was an alarm heard round the world, and as a result shellfish became a no-no for cholesterol watchers who had been advised to limit their cholesterol intake.

But it was a false alarm in a sense. A decade later, it became clear that the method used to calculate the cholesterol content of shellfish was flawed. So the USDA scientists went back to the laboratory and tried again. Their new results–which have been confirmed recently–showed that most shellfish contain cholesterol in amounts similar to common meats such as beef and poultry. Besides, shellfish contain almost no saturated fat, which we now know influences our blood cholesterol levels even more strongly than the cholesterol in our diet.

Unfortunately, to this day, some people remain unaware of all this and still consider shellfish unfriendly to the heart. Here are some new numbers to set the record straight, along with the original, but incorrect estimates.

	Cholesterol (mg)	
Food	Revised	Original
Clam meat	114 per cup	not available
Crabmeat	125 per cup	314 per cup
Lobster meat	123 per cup	290 per cup
Mussels	56 per 4 oz.	171 per 4 oz.
Oyster meat	114 per cup	456 per cup
Scallops	60 per 4 oz.	not available
Shrimp, canned*	164 per cup	138 per cup

*The cholesterol content of shrimp varies considerably from one type to another. The amount in a shrimp cocktail or dish containing small amounts of shrimp (less than ½ cup), however, should not be excessive.

Accent on Enjoyment: Lobster needs few embellishments, particularly when eaten outside with fresh sea air tickling your face. But if you're in the mood for variation, consider:

- Trying Dijon mustard instead of butter for dipping.
- Using lobster meat in seafood salads, crepes, or omelets.
- Seasoning with herbs or tart flavors, such as tarragon, basil, thyme, or citrus.

Mussels

At the Market: Blue mussels, the kind North Americans are used to eating, are frequently farm-raised and are more consistent in quality than wild mussels. Their shells are gently ridged and blue-black, with occasional splashes of white; they have less of a beard than wild mussels. They're also usually evenly sized, making them easier to cook.

If you can't find farm-raised mussels, wild ones are in season from June to December. Choose smallish, younger mussels that are evenly sized and tight lipped, with shells that are intact, not broken.

Kitchen Tips: It's hard for us to imagine mussels sitting in the refrigerator for long. And that's a good thing, because mussels don't keep well and are best cooked at once.

First, scrub them under cool water with a stiff brush. Then pull off the beards. Then steam or simmer the mussels until open, about 4 minutes, discarding any that refuse to open on their own.

Accent on Enjoyment: Mussels are great with onions, garlic, leeks, shallots, and most other aromatic seasonings. These quick and healthful ideas will get you started.

- Steam mussels, then sprinkle with fresh crushed herbs, such as basil.
- Chop steamed mussels and add to chowders or sauces for pasta.
- Marinate steamed and shelled mussels in garlic, olive oil, and lemon juice. Serve chilled on endive leaves.

Oysters

At the Market: Oysters are best to eat when they're not spawning, and should be purchased from September through April. Long Island Blue Point, Chincoteague, and Cape Cod Wellfleet are familiar East Coast varieties; many unusual and tasty ones are being spawned on the West Coast.

Oyster shells should be tightly closed or willing to close when gently coaxed. If not, don't buy them. Shucked oysters should be plump and cream colored in a clear liquor.

Kitchen Tips: If kept iced, oysters can be stored overnight in the coldest part of the refrigerator, but for maximum flavor and freshness, use them at once. Shucked oysters should be stored in their liquor.

Accent on Enjoyment: Serve oysters raw on the half-shell with lemon, or bake, grill, or sauté them. Some other ideas:

- Substitute oysters for clams in soups, sauces, and stews.
- Sprinkle oysters on the half-shell with a bit of lime juice, broil until opaque, and serve hot with tomato sauce.
- Season oysters generously with garlic, parsley, coriander, mustards, and leeks. Add a bit of a creamy cheese if you like.

Scallops

At the Market: Bay scallops are the tiny ones that come about 35 to a pound. They have the finest flavor and texture. Sea scallops are larger–about 12 to a pound–and also are good, but to ensure even cooking, take care to purchase ones that are similar in size. Both bay and sea scallops should smell sweet and be creamy ivory to pink in color and relatively free of liquid.

Occasionally, sea scallops still in their curly shells are available. Buy only those whose shells are tightly closed and have a sweet aroma.

Kitchen Tips: Enclose fresh scallops in heavy, tightly closed plastic bags and store them in the coldest part of the refrigerator; they will last for about three days. Scallops can also be wrapped in freezer wrap and frozen for about six months.

Bay scallops can take as little as 1½ to 2 minutes to cook through when sautéed. For tender results, sea scallops can be sliced horizontally into coins and sautéed in the same amount of time. Scallops in their shells can be baked open in a 400°F oven. Both the scallop and its lovely coral roe are eaten–unless the latter is prohibited on your diet.

Accent on Enjoyment: To keep scallops tender, sauté or steam them and don't expose them to long or high heat. For instance:

- Sauté scallops in a bit of sweet butter along with chopped scallions, minced shallots, julienne strips of carrot, and a pinch of grated orange peel. Serve hot.
- Steam scallops, then toss with chunks of avocado, chopped pink grapefruit, and minced sweet onion. Serve in lettuce leaves as a main dish salad.
- Sauté scallops in olive oil with chopped ripe tomato and minced garlic. Toss with freshly grated Parmesan cheese and serve hot.

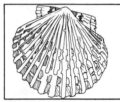

Mediterranean Scallop Sauté

1 tablespoon olive oil
2 cloves garlic, minced
¼ cup chopped onions
2 tomatoes, peeled, seeded, and chopped
juice and pulp of 1 lemon
splash of hot pepper sauce, or to taste
1 pound sea scallops
1 teaspoon dried basil
1 teaspoon dried oregano
crumbled feta cheese

In a large skillet, heat oil over medium heat. Add garlic and onion and sauté over medium heat until soft, about 4 minutes. Add tomatoes, lemon juice and pulp, and hot pepper sauce and continue to sauté until cooked down slightly, about 1½ minutes.

Stir in scallops, basil, and oregano and sauté until cooked through, about 4 minutes. Serve hot over pasta or rice, sprinkled with feta.

Makes 4 servings

Clams with Aromatic Rice and Peas

1½ cups water
1 cup rice, preferably
   aromatic or
   basmati (not quick
   cooking)
¼ cup freshly grated
   Parmesan cheese
1 tablespoon minced
   fresh basil
1 tablespoon minced
   fresh thyme
1 tablespoon minced
   fresh lovage or
   celery leaves
1 cup shelled peas or
   sugar snap peas
20 to 24 littleneck clams

In a large skillet or paella pan, bring water to a boil. Add rice and cook, uncovered, for about 7 minutes. Add cheese, basil, thyme, lovage or celery leaves, peas, and clams. Loosely cover the skillet with foil and cook until all clams have opened and rice has absorbed all the liquid, about 7 minutes. Serve immediately.

Makes 4 servings

Soft-Shell Sauté

¼ cup cornmeal
8 fresh soft-shell crabs
1½ teaspoons olive oil
1½ teaspoons sweet
   butter
¼ cup apple juice
¼ cup white grape juice
2 tablespoons raspberry
   vinegar
pinch of dry mustard
pinch of dried thyme

Spread cornmeal out on a sheet of waxed paper and lightly dredge crabs in it.

In a large nonstick skillet, heat ¾ tablespoon of oil and ¾ tablespoon of butter. When butter is melted, add 4 crabs and sauté until they turn reddish in color, about 3 minutes on each side. Repeat with remaining oil, butter, and crabs. Set cooked crabs aside and keep warm.

In a small saucepan, combine juices, vinegar, mustard, and thyme and boil until fragrant and reduced by half. Pour over crabs and serve.

Makes 4 servings

SKIN PROBLEMS

What Nutrition Can and Cannot Do

Nutrition and healthy skin have been linked in people's minds since the first vitamin was discovered almost 80 years ago. Vitamin pioneers showed that too little vitamin A brought on a long list of symptoms. Among them were lumps of hard skin resembling the texture of fingernails, which would develop where soft skin was the norm.

As more vitamins were discovered, however, it became clear that deficiencies of vitamin A weren't alone in their effects on the skin. Two other well-known deficiency syndromes–scurvy and pellagra–also made their presence known in the form of skin troubles. Vitamin C and niacin–the vitamins needed to correct these deficiencies–proved capable of correcting the ill effects on the skin.

Americans, however, usually get enough of these nutrients to avoid the skin troubles that accompany deficiency. Nevertheless, that's no reason to close the book on nutrition as it affects the skin. Rather, it's time to turn to a new chapter–one that focuses on nutritional approaches to skin problems other than those caused by low intakes of vitamins or minerals.

Soothing the Scales of Psoriasis

Fish oils have won our hearts, but it's possible that their benefits extend beyond the health of our circulatory system. One of the most fascinating possibilities now being investigated is for the treatment of psoriasis. This skin disease has long been frustrating for its victims and doctors alike.

At the Royal Hallamshire Hospital in Sheffield, England, S. B. Bittiner and associates treated psoriasis patients with ten MaxEPA fish oil capsules a day or with a placebo capsule filled with olive oil. No one knew who had which treatment. After eight weeks, the fish oil group had significantly less itching and also less of the scaling, reddened skin that is the hallmark of psoriasis. The research team also noted a reduction in the size of the scaly areas.

Science, of course, demands that results like these be confirmed. So far, we've found two other studies like this one, both reporting some benefit from fish oil treatment. We know that a total of three studies doesn't prove anything, yet we're impressed that none of the studies so far has been completely negative.

There's another very important side to this fish oil story. Some psoriasis patients are treated with prescription drugs called etretinate or isotretinoin. These drugs can adversely affect the blood fat profile; increases in triglyceride and cholesterol levels and decreases in the level of "good" (HDL) cholesterol can occur. But researchers such as Roslyn Alfin-Slater, Ph.D., of the University of California have reported that by using fish oil, psoriasis patients who take these drugs can minimize this effect. We'll bet that doctors would see that alone as a reason to consider fish oil.

The Agony of Acne

We all know that old notions die hard, and beliefs that diet causes acne simply prove the point. We've had our own experience with this belief. Some years ago, it occurred to us that teens might adopt heart-healthy eating habits more readily if doing so would also help rid them of acne. So we went to the library looking for documentation that high-fat foods such as chocolate and french fries contribute to acne. To make a long story short, we didn't find it.

We did learn, however, that dermatologists were experimenting with another nutritional approach to acne—supplementation with very high doses of zinc. But the side effects made the treatment impractical; the large doses used caused digestive complaints such as nausea, diarrhea, and vomiting. As for the effect on acne, the results were far from spectacular, although a minority of patients experienced some improvement.

The most impressive results against acne have come from treatment with prescription drugs such as Retin-A and Accutane. Because both are chemical cousins of vitamin A, you could say that their success demonstrates that nutrition affects acne after all. However, these drugs differ from the vitamin A in food—enough so that the link is at most a distant one.

Some Bits and Pieces

There are skin conditions besides psoriasis that are related to nutrition in some way. Although these conditions are not nearly as well known, if you have any of them, you should be aware of their nutritional components.

Dermatitis herpetiformis. Many of the patients who suffer from this little-known condition improve on a gluten-free diet. (See the entry on celiac disease, beginning on page 110, for details).

Angular stomatitis. This condition, marked by cracks around the corners of the mouth, sometimes responds to supplementation with large doses of riboflavin, a B vitamin.

Xanthomas. These yellowish nodules on the skin go hand in hand with extremely high levels of triglycerides in the blood. Dietary approaches vary from one patient to the next, depending on the particular blood fat disorder; some patients will need a very low fat diet not unlike those used for gallbladder disease; others will need a triglyceride-lowering diet. (See the entry on triglycerides, beginning on page 395, for more about diet and trigylcerides.)

Skin wounds are another condition that can be influenced by nutrition. You'll find more about how nutrition affects them in the entry on wound healing, beginning on page 416.

SOYBEANS

Soy to the World

234 calories per cup (cooked)

Once sold only in health food stores, soybeans are now on the shelves at the local supermarket. We suspect that in coming years, more and more soybean products will join the plain bean. The reasons are many: Soybeans are inexpensive, popular, and very nutritious. Consider just a few nutritional facts.

- Soybeans are amazingly high not only in protein but also in key minerals. Calcium, potassium, and iron are all present, the latter two in large amounts.
- The fat in soybeans is mostly unsaturated, making them great for cholesterol-lowering diets. Coupled with their low sodium content and the calcium and potassium mentioned above, the balance of fats in soybeans makes them perfect when blood pressure is a concern.
- In large doses, the fiber in soybeans has shown a cholesterol-lowering effect. Research done by Grace Lo and associates at Washington University found that cholesterol levels fell by an average of 13 milligrams when patients with high cholesterol levels were fed cookies containing 25 grams of soy fiber.
- Contrary to the long-held belief that vitamin B_{12} is present only in animal foods, preliminary research has suggested that fermented soyfoods such as miso and tempeh may also contain it. Delores D. Truesdell and associates at Florida State University have detected the presence of B_{12} in some samples of miso and tempeh. They believe that more samples will need testing, to ensure that this was not a chance occurrence.

It's little wonder that so many new foods made with soybeans are appearing every year. Of course, many people prefer to buy uncooked soybeans and prepare them at home. Certainly, that's the best way to ensure that lots of fat and salt won't be added.

At the Market: Choose small round beans that are smooth and unbroken. They range in color from pale buff to black, and buying in see-through packages or in bulk makes it easier to check for even shading.

Kitchen Tips: Keep soybeans in tightly covered jars in the refrigerator. They will last for about six months.

Soybeans should always be cooked! To get started, soak 1 cup of beans in hot water to cover overnight. Drain and add to a large saucepan with about 5 cups of water. Bring to a boil, then cover loosely and simmer until tender, about 3 hours. One cup of raw soybeans yields just under 3 cups cooked.

Accent on Enjoyment: Soybeans are a meaty addition to casseroles, green salads, and pâtés. You can also:

- Sauté onions, garlic, and bell peppers in olive oil, then toss in cooked soybeans and rice. Flavor with hot pepper sauce, cumin, and coriander and serve hot as an entrée.
- Add cooked soybeans to stews, gumbos, and vegetable soups.
- Substitute soybeans for the navy beans in your favorite Boston Baked Bean recipe.

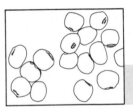

Chicken with Beans and Vegetables

1 tablespoon vegetable oil
1 tablespoon butter
1 chicken (broiler-fryer, about 3 pounds), cut into serving pieces
2 cups chopped leeks or onions
¼ cup chopped fresh parsley
1 large clove garlic, minced
1 cup sliced carrots
1½ cups water or chicken stock
4½ teaspoons soy sauce
3 cups cooked soybeans, drained

In a large heavy skillet or Dutch oven with a tight-fitting lid, heat oil and butter over medium heat. Add chicken pieces and brown evenly on all sides. Add leeks or onions, parsley, garlic, carrots, water or stock, and soy sauce. Cover and cook for about 1 hour, or until chicken is tender. Add soybeans and continue to cook until beans are heated through.

To serve, spoon beans and vegetables onto a heated serving platter and arrange chicken on top.

Makes 4 to 6 servings

SQUASH, WINTER

Color It Carotene

82 to 114 calories per cup (cooked)

The squashes of winter–butternut, hubbard, and acorn–are among the group of all-around protector foods that stand out as sources of a trio of anticancer nutrients: vitamin C, fiber, and carotene. The latter occurs in all three, but only hubbard and butternut have amounts that give you more than a day's recommended allowance in a single serving.

With very low levels of fat and sodium, squash are also ideal for heart-healthy diets. Hubbard squash even contains some protein that deserves mention. It's not the only one that has an unexpected nutritional asset; a cup of acorn squash, for instance, has almost 100 milligrams of calcium.

All squash are not created equal, however, when it comes to nutrition. Summer squash–the pale green-fleshed zucchini and yellow crookneck–don't even come close to their winter brethren as a source of carotene. They are, of course, low in sodium and fat, making them worthwhile for controlling blood pressure and weight. But for nutritional density, look to winter squash.

At the Market: Different kinds of winter squash vary dramatically in appearance yet belong to the same family. Acorn is roundish, lobed, and deep green with orange splotches, or bright orange all around. Butternut is shaped like a long bell and is toasty tan in color, and some varieties have green pinstripes that run down their sides. Hubbard is bright orange and lumpy and can be huge, medium, or small.

Regardless of type, squash should have a hard rind and feel heavy for its size. Picking ones that still have stems will help you avoid ones that are rotted inside. All squash should be free of gashes, mold, or soft spots.

Kitchen Tips: Store squash in a cool, dry place with good circulation. If conditions are good, it may keep all winter. About 55 degrees is ideal, but colder temperatures are not advised.

Cooking times will vary, depending on how small you cut the pieces and the density of the squash. Thin slices generally take about 10 minutes to simmer; ½ pound (about half an acorn squash) takes about 6 minutes when wrapped in waxed paper and microwaved on full power. In a conventional oven set at 400° F, halved squash will bake in about 35 minutes.

Accent on Enjoyment: As you might have guessed, these squashes differ in taste and texture just as they do in looks. Acorn is best when halved and baked. Because of its drier texture, butternut is great simmered and pureed. Hubbard, because it's a bit watery itself, tastes best when chunked and added to soups and stews. So stock your pantry with all three kinds and try these ideas:

- Bake halved acorn squash, then fill with cooked rice, chopped spinach, and freshly grated Parmesan cheese. Serve hot as a vegetarian entrée.
- Use pureed butternut squash in recipes for spice cookies, quick breads, or muffins.
- Add chunks of peeled hubbard squash to mushroom barley soup and simmer until tender. Hubbard is also great in Caribbean-type stews with pork, onions, and black beans.

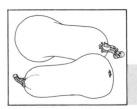

Spicy Squash Puree

1½ pounds butternut
   squash
¼ teaspoon ground
   mace
¼ teaspoon ground
   allspice
   seeds of 2 cardamom
   pods, ground
1 tablespoon maple
   syrup
2 teaspoons sweet
   butter or margarine

Using a large chef's knife, cut squash in half, then scrape out and discard the seeds (or save for roasting). Slice squash into manageable chunks (about 1½ to 2 inches) and boil in enough water to cover until tender, about 20 minutes.

When squash is cool enough to handle, remove the skin and spoon flesh into a food processor or blender. Add mace, allspice, ground cardamom seeds, maple syrup, and butter and process until smooth. Serve hot as an accompaniment to roast turkey or chicken.

Makes 4 servings

STROKE

The Nutrition Connection Grows Stronger

A stroke can be devastating. It can also be avoided.

A stroke is caused by a decrease in the blood supply to part of the brain. When blood and oxygen cannot get to the brain, cells die, leaving the victim faced with possible permanent paralysis and loss of speech or memory.

One of the leading causes of this debilitating condition is high blood pressure, the silent killer we discuss thoroughly beginning on page 247. If you have high blood pressure, you also face a high risk of having a stroke. Lower your blood pressure and you lower your risk.

How Good Nutrition Can Help

Of course, high blood pressure isn't the only cause of stroke. And, although stroke is usually thought of as a disease of old age, some kinds can strike the young and old equally. A history of rheumatic heart disease, a weakened blood vessel known as an aneurysm, the heart condition endocarditis, or abnormal heart rhythms make for higher risk regardless of age.

The typical stroke, though, comes from the same process that causes most heart attacks–a blood clot that cuts off the blood flow. So it's no surprise to find that study after study links common heart attack risk factors to stroke. The list bears repeating:

- High blood pressure.
- High blood cholesterol.
- Overweight.
- Smoking.
- Diabetes.

For heart attacks, experts don't quibble over whether high blood pressure or high cholesterol is worse; both are considered very guilty parties. But in the case of stroke, high blood pressure is by far the most powerful of the risk factors.

384

The well-known Honolulu Heart Study, for instance, is but one of many that has documented the influence of blood pressure. According to researchers Yo Takeya, M.D., and Jordan S. Popper, M.D., who looked at stroke risk factors among residents of both Japan and Hawaii, high blood pressure was clearly the number one risk factor—even more important than age, which came in second.

Obviously, then, nutritional approaches that help control blood pressure are the best ones for combatting stroke. A complete explanation of the dietary requirements and a seven-day meal plan can be found, beginning on page 247.

The Signs and Symptoms

A disorder affecting the brain has noticeable symptoms. Because a stroke can come on suddenly and because quick medical attention is imperative to the progress of recovery, we feel you should become familar with the common signs. They include:

- Impaired (or fluctuating) state of consciousness.
- Headache or stiff neck.
- Dizziness, seizures, or convulsions.
- Nausea and vomiting.
- Tingling sensations or visual disturbances.
- Inability to speak or move the limbs.

What happens after a stroke depends on many factors. Some victims recover, others are disabled, and some do not survive. It's this risk of long-term disability or death that makes preventive efforts so important.

SWEET POTATO

If You Must Puff, Eat This Stuff!

103 calories per ½ cup (mashed)

Sweet potatoes have plenty of nutritional oomph. But focusing on anything but their vitamin A value is like finding buried teasure and counting the coins rather than the $100 bills.

Sweet potatoes are so rich in vitamin A that even a few bites a day can put you on the nutritional safe side. In fact, sweet potatoes have so much vitamin A that 1 cup of mashed sweets delivers more than 43,000 international units! That's eight times the recommended allowance.

The vitamin A in sweet potatoes comes in the form of carotene, and its potential to reduce the risk of lung cancer actually has some researchers worried. While acknowledging that the carotene/cancer link offers so much hope for preventing the disease, they worry that many smokers will simply increase their carotene intake instead of quitting cigarettes. Charles Hennenkens, M.D., a Harvard researcher involved with this project, points out that "even if beta-carotene were effective in reducing deaths from lung cancer by as much as 50 percent, lifelong smokers would still have a risk 10 to 15 times greater than nonsmokers, rather than 20 to 30 times greater than they do now."

As we see it, there's more good in this than bad. Anything that can reduce a risk factor even a little is something to be grateful for. Especially when it tastes so good!

At the Market: Choose sweet potatoes that are firm and nicely shaped and have lively color. The color, by the way, can be tan, toast, brownish red, or burgundy red.

Kitchen Tips: Store sweets unwrapped in a cool, dry place. They will last for up to two months.

Southern-type sweets will have light to bold orange flesh and are best simmered, steamed, or microwaved. In other words, moist cooking enhances their texture. Northern-type sweets can have bold orange to ivory flesh and are best baked.

Chunked and steamed, sweets will take up to 15 minutes to cook. One sweet, punctured and wrapped in waxed paper, will take 4 to 5 minutes to

I Yam What I Yam

Is it a yam or a sweet potato? Here's the lowdown on how to distinguish the two.

A yam is a huge tuber that grows in very hot areas such as Central America and parts of Africa. It does not grow in the continental United States, but it is occasionally imported and sold in big chunks in Latin markets and some supermarkets.

Sweet potatoes are any of the almost 50 varieties of tuber that find their way to our holiday tables each year. Like yams, most sweet potatoes have creamy orange flesh, but they're much smaller, moister, and easier to find than yams.

Many supermarkets refer to sweet potatoes as yams, and although it's technically a mistake, the two names have almost become interchangeable. Some people speculate that the name overlap started with slaves who came from Africa. They missed their native yams and adored the ones that grow in the southern United States. The name may have stuck because it's friendly and easy to say, and no one but the most uppity of culinary experts really minds.

Just one caution: If you're in Africa and someone offers you a yam, bring your wagon. You'll need one to haul it home!

microwave on full power. At 450° F, sweets will take about 55 minutes to bake in a conventional oven.

Accent on Enjoyment: Those who pass up sweet potatoes have probably only had them covered with marshmallow goo. Little wonder they aren't aware that sweets are a delicious and fragrant addition to many meals. For example:

- Toss cooked, chunked sweets with pecans, raisins, and a dot of sweet butter. Serve with roasted chicken.
- Add cooked, diced sweet potato to curried chicken. Serve warm.
- Grate or slice sweet potatoes and use to add color and sweetness to vegetable soups and stews.

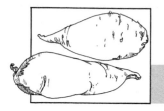

Sweet Potato Soup with Celery

1 tablespoon peanut oil
½ cup chopped onions
1 cup sliced celery
1 pound sweet potatoes,
    peeled and chopped
2 cups chicken stock
1 bay leaf
½ teaspoon dried basil
    toasted croutons for
    garnish

In a large stockpot, heat oil over medium heat. Add onion and sauté until just golden, about 3 minutes.

Add celery, sweet potatoes, stock, bay leaf, and basil and bring to a boil. Reduce heat and simmer, loosely covered, until vegetables are very tender, about 25 minutes. Remove bay leaf, then puree in batches in a food processor or blender. Serve hot, garnished with croutons.

Makes 4 servings

TANGERINES

Oriental Oranges

37 calories per tangerine

Some people think tangerines are a newfangled version of the sweet orange we know so well. Actually, tangerines belong to the mandarin orange family that has flourished in the Orient for centuries. Produce experts often refer to tangerines simply as "mandarins," and in the United States, tangerines are the most common of this family of more than a dozen members.

Count on the tangerine when you crave a change of pace from oranges but still want the nutrition they provide. Like oranges, tangerines are notable for their vitamin C: Just two fruits provide the Recommended Dietary Allowance (RDA). The tangerine, however, bests the orange for vitamin A; the same two-fruit serving will give you almost a third of the RDA for this nutrient.

We think that tangerines are great for weight watchers. Owing to their small size, a typical fruit contains fewer than 40 calories. It makes for a filling snack without guilt!

At the Market: Most tangerines are orange to red in color, but some may have greenish patches, and that's okay. Color does not indicate sweetness or juiciness. The best sign is a sweet scent–often impossible to detect if the fruit is cold. A tangerine that is heavy for its size, however, is probably juicy. Skins should be loose but not shriveled.

Kitchen Tips: Store tangerines in the crisper drawer of the refrigerator. They will last for about two weeks. You can turn them into tangerine juice using the same method you use for making orange juice. In fact, tangerine juice can replace orange juice in most beverages and other recipes.

Accent on Enjoyment: Chilled tangerine sections are a refreshingly sweet way to end a meal. They're also great in fruit salads, green salads, and spinach salads. And for more adventurous pursuits:

• Add seeded tangerine sections to poultry stuffing. This is especially nice with roasted turkey.

- Add tangerine juice to the water when simmering chunks of winter squash.
- Substitute tangerine juice for the lemon juice in a vinaigrette. Then toss with tangerine sections, blanched mushroom caps, and thin slices of red onion.
- Use scooped-out tangerine halves as cups for tangerine mousse or vanilla yogurt.

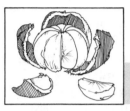

Tangerine and Chicken Salad

½ pound cooked chicken cutlets
4 tangerines, seeded and sectioned
3 tablespoons chopped pecans
2 tablespoons raisins
3 scallions, chopped
1 tablespoon olive oil
2 tablespoons orange juice
½ teaspoon minced fresh rosemary

Shred chicken into bite-size pieces, then place them in a medium bowl along with tangerines, pecans, raisins, and scallions.

In a small bowl, whisk together oil, juice, and rosemary. Pour over salad and toss well until all pieces are lightly coated. Serve at room temperature as a main dish salad.

Makes 4 servings

TOFU

East Meets West

About 86 calories per 2½-inch square piece

When discussing the virtues of tofu–also known as soybean curd–the biggest problem is deciding where to start. The best place to do so probably depends on your nutritional priorities.

Protein? Tofu has plenty–9 grams per piece. Calories? Tofu wins again, with fewer than 100 in a typical serving. Minerals? Tofu has impressive amounts of calcium and iron–with almost no sodium. So as you see, it's as well rounded a food as any.

We're most impressed, though, with the role tofu can play in controlling cholesterol. Research by Michael Liebman, Ph.D., and Carolyn Dunn, of the University of North Carolina at Greensboro, serves as a perfect example. Dr. Liebman and Dunn recruited volunteers who followed two special diets. On one diet, the subjects ate their normal fare with the addition of about 2 ounces of cheese a day. In the other phase, they replaced the cheese with tofu–enough to supply the same calorie count as the cheese.

The result? After switching from cheese to tofu, their average blood cholesterol levels dropped 16 points. The explanation is obvious, of course: Tofu contains very little cholesterol-raising saturated fat, while cheese contains quite a bit.

At the Market: Supermarket tofu is usually sold in 10- or 12-ounce packages in the produce section. The firm type is best for stir-frying; the soft type is good for pureeing and mashing. Oriental markets often sell tofu from large open containers, yet it's usually fresh because the turnover is high. Tofu in aseptic packages is also available at oriental markets and some health food stores. It's usually the soft type and is shelf-stable.

Recently, tofu has appeared in spicy and herbed flavors, which are interesting when chopped and added to salads. These flavored tofus, like their unflavored cousins, come in blocks.

Kitchen Tips: Packaged tofu should be kept refrigerated until the expiration date. If the package is open, continue to keep the tofu in water, which should be changed daily. Ditto for bulk-bought tofu, which will last for about a week.

To prepare tofu, drain it first. If using it uncooked, as in salad dressings or dips, it should be blanched. To do this, set the block of tofu in a strainer and pour boiling water over it for about 20 seconds. When stir-frying or sautéing, shake the pan instead of stirring to keep the tofu from crumbling during cooking.

Accent on Enjoyment: Tofu has a gentle nutty flavor that harmonizes with many foods. Here are some tofu tips to get you started.

* Slice blocks of tofu in half horizontally. Then marinate in stock, soy sauce, ginger, garlic, and minced scallions. Simmer both the marinade and tofu in a nonstick skillet until heated through. Serve hot.
* Cut tofu into julienne strips and add to clear or vegetable soups about 5 minutes before serving.
* For a creamy texture without the cream, add a bit of blanched tofu to a vinaigrette and process in a blender until creamy.

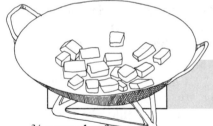

Braised Tofu with Shiitake Mushrooms

¾ pound tofu
1 clove garlic, minced
½ teaspoon minced gingerroot
1 tablespoon soy sauce
1 tablespoon rice vinegar
1 cup sliced fresh shiitake or button mushrooms
1½ cups beef stock
1 teaspoon toasted sesame oil
2 scallions, coarsely chopped

Cut tofu into chunks and place in a flat dish with sides. In a small bowl, combine garlic, ginger, soy sauce, and vinegar. Pour marinade over tofu and toss to coat. Marinate for an hour.

Spoon tofu and marinade into large skillet and add mushrooms and stock. (Handle tofu carefully so it doesn't crumble.) Bring to a boil, then reduce heat to low. Simmer, uncovered, until tofu is cooked through and stock is reduced by half, about 10 minutes.

Add sesame oil and serve hot, sprinkled with scallions. This makes a nice main dish when served over rice with a side dish of clear soup and a marinated vegetable salad.

Makes 4 servings

TOMATOES

Vine-Ripe and Very Right

23 calories per 2½-inch tomato

Here's an amazing story for you.

Graham A. Colditz, M.D., and his associates at Harvard Medical School interviewed more than a thousand people about their diets, then tracked their health for five years. Are you ready for what they found? The chances of dying of cancer was lowest among those who ate tomatoes or strawberries every week.

Is this another nonsense correlation–a scientific fluke? We suppose that it's possible. But the nutrient profile of the tomato–rich in vitamins A and C, and containing some fiber, too–fits right in with the cancer-prevention recommendations that the National Cancer Institute and other groups have issued based on our current knowledge of how diet affects the disease.

So we suspect that there's nothing odd about the results of this study. But we've been tomato fans all our lives–and we've been sold on their heart-healthy benefits for a long time. Like some of our other garden favorites, tomatoes are low in fat and sodium–and rich in potassium.

At the Market: Good tomatoes are smooth, well formed, and fragrant. Big round ones are ideal as salad tomatoes, plum types are good for sauces, and tiny cherry-types are bought for salads and snacks. All three kinds range in color from robust red to pink to yellow.

Fresh tomatoes are at their worst in midwinter. Their poor color, texture, and flavor can ruin a recipe in no time. Use canned tomatoes, instead, but be sure to check the label for purity.

Kitchen Tips: For the finest flavor, keep fresh tomatoes at room temperature. They actually ripen at temperatures between 50° and 85°F, but keep them out of the sun or they'll lose flavor. Tomatoes will also ripen in a fruit ripener or when tucked in a brown paper bag with a piece of ripe fruit.

To freeze fresh tomatoes, blanch them in boiling water for about 2 minutes, then plunge them quickly into ice water and drain. Remove skins, or chop if you like, and freeze in recipe-size portions for up to a year.

To peel tomatoes, blanch them in boiling water for about 30 seconds, then plunge quickly into ice water and drain. When cool enough to handle,

393

remove the peels with a paring knife. To prevent bitterness, you should remove skins from tomatoes that will be cooked for a long time.

Accent on Enjoyment: Want to add color, flavor, and bloom to soups, sauces, salads, and sautés? Add tomatoes! For instance:

- Create a salad of chopped red and yellow tomatoes. Toss with minced scallions, fresh snipped dill, and lemon vinaigrette.
- Layer thick slices of tomato in a baking dish. Sprinkle on some basil, oregano, and olive oil, then bake in a medium oven until soft and fragrant, about 20 minutes. Serve hot as a side dish.
- Combine chopped tomato, minced sweet onion, and minced sweet pepper with a splash each of olive oil and robust vinegar. Let stand for about 30 minutes, then serve as a sauce with tortillas, omelets, or pasta.

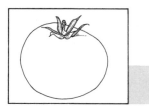

Garlic-Scented Sautéed Tomatoes

2 teaspoons olive oil
2 cloves garlic, minced
½ teaspoon dried basil
1 pound firm tomatoes, cored and cut into eighths
minced fresh chives
freshly grated Asiago or Romano cheese

In a large nonstick skillet, heat oil over medium heat. Add garlic, basil, and tomatoes, and sauté over medium heat until just wilted, about 2½ minutes. Add chives and Asiago and serve hot as an accompaniment to entrées such as grilled chicken.

Makes 4 servings

TRIGLYCERIDES

Cholesterol's First Cousin

Triglycerides aren't exactly a household word like their well-known cousin, cholesterol, but they're still getting some serious attention.

Like cholesterol, triglycerides are fatlike substances found in the blood. And as with cholesterol, an elevated triglyceride level in the bloodstream is believed to put you at risk for heart disease.

Not all doctors, of course, are sold on the notion that high triglyceride levels contribute directly to heart disease. But impressed with the possibility, most favor the better-safe-than-sorry approach and take action whenever the triglyceride level is high. Perhaps the best reason for doing so is that high triglycerides are often accompanied by low levels of HDL cholesterol, the type that is good for the heart. For that reason alone, it is a good idea to have your triglycerides checked.

Truth in Testing

Before you have your triglycerides tested, allow us to say just one word about doing it right. That word is fast. In order to put faith in your results, you really do need to fast before the test. Eight hours is usually recommended.

Unfortunately, not everyone takes this advice to heart. So we'd like to explain a little more. Because triglycerides are are a kind of fat, the amount present in the blood is affected by how much fat you have eaten recently. At the Sports Science Center, University of Capetown Medical School, Jonathan C. Cohen and his co-workers have shown that after a meal containing fat is eaten, the blood triglyceride level goes up–and stays up–for several hours.

What's more, the blood triglyceride level rises in proportion to the amount of fat eaten. So if you eat a hearty, high-fat breakfast right before your test, it may give a false impression of your true triglyceride level. Research by Bjarne K. Jacobsen and others at the University of Tromso in Norway shows that the triglyceride level in people who have just eaten is more than 20 percent higher than among those who have fasted 8 hours before the test.

That extra 20 percent could be enough for some people with normal trigylcerides to be labeled abnormal. Surely fasting for 8 hours on those rare days when you have your triglycerides tested is not too much to ask to ensure that the results represent the real you.

Fish First!

Jacobsen's study of heart health not only linked recent food intake to higher triglyceride levels but also revealed that levels of this blood fat went down in proportion to the amount of fish consumed. Sure enough, the fish factor has shown up in research throughout the world.

The team of David Robinson and Jose Day of BUPA Medical Research, London, for instance, studied East African tribesmen living in two separate locations. They compared how the men scored on a wide variety of health factors. All things considered, the most striking difference was in triglyceride levels. The average level was 31 percent lower among the tribesmen who ate lots of fish–an extraordinary difference, to be sure.

The effect of fish on triglycerides is now a hot issue in research circles. Accordingly, a recent issue of *Nutrition Reviews* included an overview of laboratory research on this topic which concluded that the omega-3 fatty acids in fish have a strong triglyceride-lowering effect in test animals. Add the results of studies with humans and we think you have a strong case for making fish part of a triglyceride-lowering diet.

More Food Factors

Like the blood cholesterol level, triglycerides are sensitive to not just one nutrient, but many. Unfortunately, some of these sensitivities can differ from one person to the next. Some people who have high triglycerides are sensitive to alcohol, others to sugars, and still others benefit most from losing extra pounds. In short, there is no one diet for high triglycerides; rather, the ideal approach is a personalized one based on what works best for you.

It isn't known, by the way, if fish works equally well for everyone with high triglycerides. We recommend it nonetheless–and with reason. Those on triglyceride-lowering diets are also advised to cut back on saturated fat and cholesterol in hopes of keeping the blood cholesterol level under control. As you know, fish fills the bill beautifully on this count, too.

Down-with-Triglycerides Dining

As we've already explained, the best triglyceride-lowering diet is tailored to personal needs. Nevertheless, we offer here a week's worth of sample menus that illustrate the basic principles—that is, low fat, low calories, and a generous amount of fish.

Day 1

Breakfast
  ½ cup cooked cream of wheat cereal
  1 slice Italian bread
  1 teaspoon margarine
  ½ white grapefruit
  ½ cup orange juice
    coffee

Lunch
  3 ounces chicken breast (without skin)
  2 slices whole wheat bread
  ½ cup butterhead lettuce
  6 cucumber slices
  ½ cup brown rice
  ½ cup fresh raspberries
  1 cup skim milk

Snack
  1 ounce cheddar cheese

Dinner
  3 ounces salmon fillet
  ½ cup broccoli
  1 small baked potato
  1 slice Italian bread
  1 tablespoon margarine
  ½ cup unsweetened applesauce
  1 cup skim milk
  ½ cup honeydew melon chunks
  ½ cup cantaloupe chunks

(continued)

Down-with-Triglycerides Dining–Continued

Day 2

Breakfast
½ cup cooked corn grits
1 slice raisin bread
1 cup skim milk
½ cup orange juice
   coffee

Lunch
3 ounces water-packed tuna
½ tablespoon reduced-calorie mayonnaise
2 slices Italian bread
1 small apple

Snack
1 cup nonfat yogurt
4 graham crackers

Dinner
2½ ounces sirloin steak (trimmed of fat)
½ cup brown rice
½ cup brussels sprouts
½ cup carrots
1 tablespoon margarine
1 cup skim milk
½ cup fresh peach slices

Day 3

Breakfast
1 ounce 100% natural cereal, plain
⅓ cup skim milk
½ cup fresh blueberries
1 piece whole wheat bread
1 teaspoon margarine

Lunch
Spinach salad (¾ cup fresh spinach, ½ cup celery, 4 radishes, ¼ cup
   onions, 6 cucumber slices, 1 tablespoon Italian dressing)

2 pieces raisin bread
1 fresh pear
1 cup skim milk

Snack
½ cup grapes

Dinner
3 ounces white meat turkey
¾ cup cooked okra
½ baked potato
2 pieces whole wheat bread
½ tablespoon margarine
½ cup canned pineapple juice
1 cup skim milk

Day 4

Breakfast
¾ cup unsweetened cereal
2 pieces Italian bread
1 tablespoon jam or preserves
1 cup grapefruit juice
   coffee

Lunch
3 ounces water-packed tuna
½ tablespoon reduced-calorie mayonnaise
2 pieces whole wheat bread
1 cup skim milk
½ cup lima beans
1 cup fresh raspberries

Snack
1½ cups air-popped popcorn

(continued)

Down-with-Triglycerides Dining–Continued

Dinner
  3 ounces oysters
  ½ cup eggplant
  ½ cup brown rice
  ½ cup asparagus
  ½ cup unsweetened applesauce
  1 piece Italian bread
  1 tablespoon margarine
  ½ cup cubed fresh apricot
  1 cup skim milk

Day 5

Breakfast
  ¾ cup spoon-size shredded wheat cereal
  1 papaya
  2 pieces raisin bread
  ½ tablespoon margarine
    coffee

Lunch
  3 ounces chicken breast (without skin)
  ½ tablespoon reduced-calorie mayonnaise
  ½ cup noodles
  2 pieces Italian bread
  ½ cup butterhead lettuce
  1 cup fresh strawberries

Dinner
  3 ounces swordfish or salmon steak
  1 small baked potato
  ½ cup cooked spinach
  ½ cup green beans
  1 piece whole wheat bread
  1 tablespoon margarine
  1 cup skim milk
  ½ cup watermelon chunks

Day 6

Breakfast
   1 cup oatmeal
   ⅓ cup skim milk
   1 piece Italian bread
   1 tablespoon jam or preserves
   1 cup grapefruit juice
      coffee

Lunch
Spinach salad (¾ cup fresh spinach, ¼ cup canned water chestnuts,
   6 cucumber slices, 4 radishes, ¼ cup onions, 1 tablespoon Italian
   dressing)
   2 slices French bread
   1 cup skim milk
   ½ cup juice-packed peaches

Snack
   1 apple
   1 ounce Swiss cheese

Dinner
   3 ounces baked flounder
   ¾ cup lettuce and tomato salad
   ½ baked sweet potato
   ½ cup brussels sprouts
   ½ cup Great Northern beans
   ½ tablespoon margarine
   1 cup melon fruit salad
   ¾ cup skim milk

(continued)

Down-with-Triglycerides Dining–Continued

Day 7

Breakfast
   1 cup cooked cream of wheat cereal
   1 banana
   ½ cup apple juice

Lunch
   3 ounces turkey breast (without skin)
   ½ tablespoon reduced-calorie mayonnaise
   ¾ cup butterhead lettuce
   2 pieces whole wheat bread
   ½ cup pinto beans
   1 small apple
   1 cup skim milk

Snack
   2 graham crackers

Dinner
   3 ounces veal cutlet
   ¾ cup broccoli
   ½ cup mashed potatoes
   ½ cup baked winter squash
   1½ tablespoons margarine
   1 piece rye bread
   ½ cup fresh strawberries with ¼ cup fruit ice

TURKEY

Here's to Pilgrim's Progress

193 calories per 4 ounces (without skin)

The basic foods of Thanksgiving–turkey, sweet potatoes, green beans, and pumpkin–deserve an image of healthfulness. Yet because of how we prepare and overeat them on the holiday, they've become a symbol of gluttony instead. That's a shame. Prepared with an emphasis on health, this is the kind of meal that can do us a world of good.

Nutritionally, turkey is similar to chicken–a lower-fat alternative to fatty meats that contains less saturated fat, too. As with chicken, the light meat has fewer calories and less fat than the dark, but feel free to enjoy both unless you must cut your fat intake dramatically.

Forego the skin if you can, for that's where most of the fat lurks. You'll get more nutrition from the meat, where the nutrients that turkey excels in–like zinc and niacin–are found.

Most people know that a roast turkey is a better choice than a fatty roast of red meat. But many are unaware of the versatility of ground turkey, which can often be found in the freezer section of the supermarket. It makes a delicious alternative to ground beef in everything from spaghetti sauce to meat loaf. You can even make it yourself to control leanness.

Four ounces of ground turkey meat contains about 145 calories and only about 5 grams of fat–about as much as in a teaspoon of butter or margarine. Compare that to the 313 calories and 23 grams (more than 4 teaspoons of fat) in an equal amount of ground beef. Don't worry about losing out on protein; both choices contain about the same amount. Even traditional ground meat lovers have been known to be pleased with the taste, too.

At the Market: Fresh whole turkey should have creamy white, smooth skin with no purple patches. It should be plump, firm, and clean smelling. When buying a frozen turkey, check the wrapper to make there are no tears in it.

To decide how much to buy, figure on about a pound per person. In other words, a 12-pound turkey will feed 12 people.

You can also buy turkey parts, such as drumsticks, thighs, and cutlets. Purchase the same amount as you would if using chicken.

Kitchen Tips: Fresh whole turkey can be refrigerated and stored for up to two days. If frozen, defrost it in the refrigerator overnight–longer if the bird weighs more than 12 pounds.

403

If you must stuff a turkey, pack it loosely so it will cook through. We prefer to cook stuffing separately, as stuffing made in a turkey tends to get full of fat, soggy, and gray. In addition, there is the problem of salmonella contamination from mishandling and improper storage. And speaking of salmonella, be sure not to leave cooked turkey out for longer than 30 minutes. It's best to refrigerate it as soon as possible.

Whole turkey needs 20 minutes of cooking time per pound. For example, a 12-pound turkey will take about 4 hours to roast. To be sure it's done, check the internal temperature with an oven thermometer. It should read 185°F.

Accent on Enjoyment: Turkey goes with a wide range of flavors, from basil and rosemary to orange and berry. Here are some ideas to help you prepare a perfect bird:

- Instead of basting turkey with fatty liquids, try fruit juice or stock instead.
- For aroma and flavor with no calories, stuff a whole turkey with whole lemons and onions.
- Put cooked cold turkey to good use by shredding and adding to salads, sandwiches, or antipasto trays.

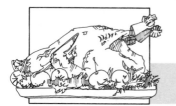

Turkey Breast with Chutney Glaze

1 turkey breast (about
    6 pounds)
⅓ cup prepared chutney
2 teaspoons Dijon
    mustard
juice and pulp of
    1 orange
juice and pulp of
    1 lime

Preheat the oven to 450°F.

Place turkey breast on a raised rack in a roasting pan. To prevent smoking when hot fat hits the roasting pan, pour in about an inch of water.

In a small bowl, combine chutney, mustard, orange juice and pulp, and lime juice and pulp. Rub over turkey, then place the roasting pan in the oven and immediately lower the temperature to 325°F. Roast, basting occasionally, until internal temperature registers 185°F on a meat thermometer, about 2½ hours. Let stand for about 20 minutes before carving.

Makes 12 servings

TURNIPS

The Root to Health

28 calories per cup (cooked)

If cabbage and other green vegetables are wasted on your family, consider the lowly turnip. Hardly anyone would expect that the turnip–with its texture just right for the meat-and-potatoes crowd–is related to the cabbage. But it is–and that means that turnips come with the seal of approval from countless expert panels on cancer prevention.

The turnip's membership in the cabbage family clan is its most impressive asset. But it also provides some vitamin C and a starchy taste reminiscent of potatoes–but with fewer calories.

If you're counting every milligram of sodium, though, stick with the potato; turnips apparently have more naturally occurring sodium than most vegetables–about 78 milligrams per cup.

At the Market: The ideal turnip measures no wider than 2 inches in diameter and is round, firm, and creamy white to violet. The very freshest ones are sold with their greens attached. Avoid those that are wrinkled or spongy.

Kitchen Tips: Separate the turnips from the greens and store in tightly closed plastic bags in the refrigerator. They'll last for about a week. If turnips are young and tender, there's no need to peel them before cooking.

To microwave turnips, cut 1 pound into ½-inch chunks. Place in a 9-inch glass pie plate and sprinkle on 2 tablespoons of stock. Cover with vented plastic wrap and microwave on full power until tender, about 4 minutes. Let stand for 4 minutes before serving.

Accent on Enjoyment: Turnips fit into all kinds of culinary undertakings. They're good braised, steamed, stewed, scalloped, or sautéed. Here are some of our turnip favorites.

- Steam turnips until tender, then puree. Stir in a bit of parsley and dill and serve hot as an accompaniment to roasted meats.
- Dice and add to vegetable soups.
- Arrange whole turnips around a roast instead of the usual carrots and potatoes. Toss in a bay leaf or two and roast as usual.

405

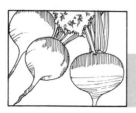

Gratin of Turnip with Dill and Shallots

1 pound turnips, peeled
    and sliced
1 cup milk
1 egg
1 teaspoon dillweed
1 shallot, minced
¼ cup freshly grated
    Parmesan cheese

Preheat the oven to 350°F. Lightly oil a 9-inch pie plate.

Arrange turnips in the pie plate.

In a medium bowl, whisk together milk, egg, dill, and shallot, and pour over turnips. Sprinkle with Parmesan and bake uncovered until golden on top, about 50 minutes. Serve hot as an accompaniment to roast pork or other meats.

Makes 4 servings

ULCERS

Calming the Chaos

It's funny how we connect certain disorders with personality.

Migraine sufferers, for instance, are thought of as detail oriented and high-strung. Likewise, the ulcer sufferer has an image as a stressed-out bundle of nerves.

But despite the stereotype, the evidence that stress causes stomach ulcers is not nearly as strong as the case against other factors such as smoking or chronic use of aspirin.

The Signs of Trouble

So you think you have an ulcer? Certainly, if you have pain in the stomach, you could be right. But there are lots of other factors that might be responsible for such pain. To get a better idea of whether your symptoms suggest ulcer or something else, ask yourself these questions.

- Does the pain have a gnawing or burning quality?
- Does the pain occur a few hours after eating, or at night?
- Does the pain subside if you eat or take antacids?
- Have you had nausea, vomiting, or weight loss?
- Do any close relatives have ulcers?
- Are you a smoker?
- Have you used a lot of aspirin or steroid drugs?

The more you answer in the affirmative, the more likely that your suspicion of an ulcer may be right. Realize, though, that diagnosing and managing an ulcer is a job for your doctor. You should make an appointment for an evaluation of your pain as soon as you can.

Food Facts and Fallacies

If your doctor confirms that you have an ulcer, you'll want to be up on the latest nutritional findings. Dietary advice for ulcer patients has changed dramatically since the days of bland milk-rich diets, so old advice is likely to be bad advice.

407

Contrary to old ideas about what the ulcer patient should eat, nutrition-ists now recommend that you eat normally but avoid any foods that trigger symptoms. The list of forbidden foods should include those that in your experience simply don't agree with you. If your doctor gives you more specific advice–for instance, to eat smaller, more frequent meals–take it to heart. Here is an update on current thinking about how specific foods affect ulcers.

Milk. The milk-rich diet is ancient history! We have learned that contrary to our old beliefs, drinking loads of milk does not benefit the ulcer patient, and may actually hurt. Nirmal Kumar, M.D., gastroenterologist at G. B. Pant Hospi-tal in New Delhi, India, has reported that a high-milk diet actually makes matters worse, inhibiting the healing of ulcers in a group of patients.

Coffee. Both decaffeinated and regular coffee have been found to stimu-late the production of stomach acid. But whether avoiding coffee will reduce acid secretion enough to speed the healing of an ulcer is debatable.

Spices. Black pepper and chili powder appear to stimulate the stomach to secrete acid, and some ulcer patients may find that avoiding them is useful. Nevertheless, avoiding all seasonings is generally unnecessary; whether they provoke symptoms should be evaluated on a case-by-case basis.

Alcohol. Beer and wine strongly stimulate acid secretion. Most doctors will advise you to avoid alcohol.

Vegetable oil. Preliminary findings suggest that the linoleic acid in polyun-saturated vegetable oil may help protect against ulcer formation. Research by Daniel Hollander, M.D., professor of medicine at the University of California, shows that linoleic acid helps guard against the ill effects of ulcer-inducing substances such as aspirin. Because only tiny amounts of linoleic acid are needed for this effect, however, he sees no reason to pour on more oil than we already use.

Many people are under the impression that coffee and spicy foods cause ulcers, but this just isn't so. While avoiding these items may help once an ulcer exists, decades of suspicion about their role in causing ulcers has given way mostly to skepticism.

The Salt Link

There's another food substance that has been linked to ulcers and one that we find particularly intriguing: salt.

Amnon Sonnenberg, M.D., of Harvard Medical School, reports that the worldwide death rate from stomach ulcer is closely tied to deaths from stroke. Salt, of course, is widely accepted as a contributor to strokes because of its ill effects on blood pressure.

Dr. Sonnenberg writes: "Gastric ulcer used to be a rare disease in Europe before the onset of the 19th century. The incidence of gastric ulcer rose steadily during the 19th century and reached a peak in the generation born at the turn of the 20th century. During the past decades the frequency of gastric ulcer has again declined. This rise and fall of gastric ulcer is paralleled by a rise and fall in the dietary salt consumption." We think his theory deserves serious consideration.

Should You Use Supplements?

Having focused on the food aspect of ulcer management for so many years, nutritionists have often overlooked the issue of supplementation for ulcer patients. As a result, there isn't much on which to base recommendations. We're struck, however, by the work of E. Harju of the University of Oulu, Finland.

Dr. Harju studied 14 patients whose stomach ulcers brought them into the hospital's surgery department. One striking finding was a very high incidence of iron depletion. Dr. Harju attributed the problem to reduced food intake, because ulcer patients often avoid eating to prevent their unpleasant symptoms.

Here's an excerpt from this important report: "The present results show that the patients with gastric ulcer are in danger of malnutrition due to their low intake of food, energy, and nutrients. One may ameliorate the situation by increasing the quality of their diet, which may, due to their problems related to eating, be difficult. Thus the use of vitamins and mineral supplements is recommended for the patients with gastric ulcer to achieve a rapid and sure way to an increased level of nutrient intake."

We agree that starting a sensible supplementation program is very wise for ulcer patients who aren't already using a multivitamin and multimineral supplement. As a precaution, we suggest taking them with food because stomach irritation occurs more readily when drugs or supplements–especially minerals–are taken on an empty stomach. Nevertheless, digestive upset generally occurs only with high doses–not the amounts you find in typical multiples. We have read one report of zinc reactivating a patient's ulcer when taken in a very high dose, so we'd like to stress that our recommendation here–supplementation to meet normal needs–is not a suggestion that you use very large doses without a physician's advice.

To us, the rule for using supplements should be the same as for food. If a product triggers symptoms, don't use it.

VEAL, LEAN

Good Health, Gourmet-Style

244 calories per 4 ounces (cooked)

Just like some other forms of life you can think of, cattle put on fat with age. That's why veal, which is from the calf, is the leanest form of beef you can buy–and also one of the most expensive. But nutritionally, you get your money's worth.

Lean veal is loaded with protein, niacin, and iron–nutrients that you'll find in other foods but often at the price of excessive calories and fat. Although veal breast tends to be fatty, other cuts are usually lean. So you can count on them for plenty of these nutrients without gobs of fat. Do trim away any obvious chunks of fat of course, before eating.

At the Market: The most tender veal is milk-fed and will be creamy ivory to buff with barely a blush. Grass-fed veal, which is older and a bit tougher, will be baby pink to rose. Both types should feel moist and springy.

Kitchen Tips: Wrap veal in waxed paper and store in the coldest part of the refrigerator; it will last for up to five days. It can also be wrapped in freezer paper and stored frozen for about three months.

Because veal is naturally lean, keep it tender by using cooking methods that are quick or moist. For instance, scallops can be sautéed; most large pieces of veal can be pot roasted or cooked in oven cooking bags. Veal leg, which has a bit more fat, can be roasted; it will take about 25 minutes per pound. For the most tender results with this very lean meat, always slice it against the grain.

Accent on Enjoyment: Veal is delicate and best made with clear, uncomplicated seasonings. Lemon, mustards, tomatoes, or sweet peppers are classic with veal. Here are some nonclassic yet delicious alternatives.

• Lightly flour veal scallops, then sauté quickly in olive oil. Just before the veal is cooked through, toss in chopped artichoke hearts, minced shallots, and capers. Serve hot.

410

- Rub lean veal chops with a bit of olive oil, then grill. Before serving, and while the chops are still very hot, dot with pesto.
- Have the butcher make a pocket in a breast of veal. Stuff it with cooked rice, shredded unsweetened coconut, and raisins. Roast until cooked through, then serve hot or chilled with chutney on the side.

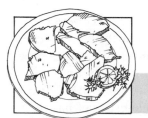

Veal Piccata

1 pound veal scallops
2 tablespoons flour
1½ teaspoons olive oil
1 teaspoon sweet
    butter or margarine
juice and pulp of
    1 lemon
1 tablespoon freshly
    grated Parmesan
    cheese
1 tablespoon freshly
    grated Romano
    cheese
1 tablespoon minced
    fresh parsley

Dredge veal in flour.

In a well-seasoned cast-iron skillet, heat oil and butter over medium heat. (If you don't have a cast-iron skillet, use a nonstick one.)

Add veal to the pan and sauté over medium-high heat until cooked through, about 1 minute on each side. (Do not overcook. If necessary, cook in two batches.)

Add lemon juice and pulp, then remove to heated plates and sprinkle with cheeses and parsley. Serve immediately.

Makes 4 servings

VENISON

Fair Game? No, Better Than That!

143 calories per 4 ounces (uncooked)

The nutritional tables on venison are not complete; the keepers of this information at the U.S. Department of Agriculture haven't analyzed it for every nutrient. But we've seen enough to say that even if the unknown values prove to be insignificant, venison still has what it takes to qualify as a winner.

Its best attribute, of course, is a fat content to make beef cattle blush. A 4-ounce piece has only 4 grams of fat—and even the leanest beef has more. Yet, venison compares favorably with beef for the "Big Three" B vitamins—riboflavin, thiamine, and niacin. It has plenty of protein, too, and some iron to boot.

At the Market: Venison varies in flavor depending on its species and the food eaten by the animal. Wild whitetail deer, for instance, often eat leaves and weeds and can taste unpleasant. Sex can make a difference, too. The male fallow deer, which is either rutting or starving itself most of the year, will not make tasty meat. But, deer that have fed on corn from fields, or have been ranch-raised eating grass, will result in a more tender, pale, and delicate meat.

Luckily, when sold in stores, venison is usually labeled as to variety. Look for axis deer, blackbuck antelope, sika deer, or nilgai antelope and you'll be most likely to get tasty, tender meat. Choose pieces that are a lively brown in color and free of any dark patches. If you have a choice, the buck (except fallow deer) is tastier than the doe.

Kitchen Tips: When a hunter presents you with a chunk of venison, first remove any visible fat with a sharp knife. To store both hunted and purchased venison, wrap in waxed paper and store in the coldest part of the refrigerator for up to five days. Venison can also be wrapped in freezer paper and frozen for up to nine months.

The saddle or loin sections are best roasted. Bucks will take about 25 minutes per pound; does will take about 20 minutes per pound. Other cuts can be gently braised or stewed, and if you have a tender steak, grill it.

If you know you've got a very gamey piece of meat, marinate it in milk for a couple of days, changing the milk each day. Then cook as usual.

Accent on Enjoyment: Bold, sharp flavors harmonize well with venison. Try mustard, rosemary, tarragon, sage, citrus, vinegars, garlic, leeks, plums, or cranberries. If your venison is tender, try it in beef recipes such as curries or stews. You can also:

- Grind venison and use it with beef or by itself in pâtés, meat loaves, or meatballs.
- Brown venison bones in the oven until rich in color. Then toss into a stockpot with onions, carrots, celery, bay leaf, and water to cover. Simmer for a couple of hours, then strain and chill. Scrape off the fat and use the stock in soups or stews.
- Substitute tender venison steak for beef in steak au poivre.

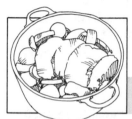

Egyptian Venison Stew

1 pound boneless
  venison, cut in
  chunks
2 tablespoons flour
1 tablespoon olive oil
1 teaspoon ground
  cinnamon
1 teaspoon saffron
  threads, crushed
¾ teaspoon coriander
  seeds, ground
2 cloves garlic, minced
2½ cups beef stock
½ teaspoon hot pepper
  sauce, or to taste
1½ cups chopped onion

Dredge venison in flour.

In a large stockpot, heat oil over medium heat. Add venison and sauté until just brown, about 7 minutes. Then add cinnamon, saffron, coriander, garlic, and stock. Bring to a boil, then reduce to a gentle simmer. Cover and continue to simmer, stirring occasionally, over medium heat for about 45 minutes.

Add hot pepper sauce and onions, cover and continue to gently simmer for an additional 45 minutes. Serve hot with couscous or other tiny pasta.

Makes 4 servings

WHEAT GERM

The Gold of the Grain

25 calories per tablespoon

Wheat germ is standard fare for almost anyone who's been "into" nutrition for long. The germ, of course, is the part of the grain that contains the richest concentration of vitamins and minerals.

Wheat germ is a source of B vitamins, vitamin E, and protein. Although often eaten only by the tablespoon, a substantial serving will make a noteworthy dent in your protein needs. One-quarter cup of wheat germ, for instance, boasts 8 grams of protein—something that few plant foods do.

Most wheat germ users start out looking for its nutrients. In no time at all, though, they find that it's a nice way to add the crunch of nuts to their diet with much less fat. Of course, wheat germ also has almost no sodium to speak of.

At the Market: Buy wheat germ in small quantities, as it is prone to rancidity. If possible, smell it before buying. It should smell toasty and nutty, not moldy. Raw and toasted types are basically interchangeable in recipes, although for sprinkling, toasted is crunchier.

Kitchen Tips: Store wheat germ in tightly closed containers in the freezer. It will last for up to six months and can be used directly from the freezer, without defrosting.

Accent on Enjoyment: Wheat germ adds a wonderfully nutty crunch to many foods. For example:

- Combine yogurt, chopped hazelnuts, chopped apples, and wheat germ, and enjoy for breakfast.
- Spread whole grain toast with a mild, creamy cheese and chopped olives. Sprinkle with wheat germ and serve as a sandwich with soup or salad.
- Use wheat germ instead of flour for dredging fish and chicken before sautéing.

You can toast your own wheat germ, by the way. Simply sprinkle raw germ out on a baking sheet with sides and toast in a preheated 325° F oven for about 15 minutes, stirring occasionally. Then store and use as you would pretoasted wheat germ.

414

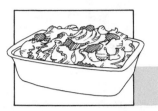

Toasty Apple-Rice Pudding

¼ to ⅓ cup maple syrup
2 tablespoons butter
¼ teaspoon ground
    cinnamon
⅛ teaspoon ground
    nutmeg
2 apples, cored and
    chopped
2 cups cooked rice
2 cups milk
⅔ cup raisins
⅓ cup toasted wheat
    germ

In a medium saucepan, heat syrup, butter, cinnamon, nutmeg, and apples until hot and bubbly. Add rice, milk, and raisins. Heat until mixture begins to bubble but has not reached a full boil. Reduce heat and simmer, stirring occasionally, until pudding thickens, about 15 minutes. Sprinkle with wheat germ and serve.

Makes 4 to 6 servings

WOUND HEALING

The Nutritional Recovery Discovery

"The surgery was a success."

Undoubtedly those are the best words you'll ever hear from your surgeon. But consider this thought: No matter how extraordinary the surgery may have been, you're really only halfway home. Recovery is the key to getting back on your feet. And a sound recovery, many scientists are discovering, depends a lot on sound nutrition.

Robert L. Ruberg, M.D., of Ohio State University, is one surgeon who recognizes just how much nutrition influences the healing process. "It is well recognized," says Dr. Ruberg, "that malnutrition slows the healing process, causing the wound to inadequately or incompletely heal."

The question that follows is obvious. Where do we draw the line between adequate and inadequate nutrition for the patient with an unhealed wound? Dr. Ruberg starts with the basics: a balanced diet that provides ample amounts of protein, carbohydrate, fat, vitamins, and minerals.

But that's just the beginning. Some nutrients are more directly involved in wound healing than others. Dr. Ruberg cites several B vitamins–B_6, riboflavin, and thiamine–as direct contributors to the wound-healing process, and names vitamin K as one that plays a background role.

Because it is essential to the blood-clotting process, he says, vitamin K helps prevent abnormal bleeding that could lead to an abnormal swelling or mass of clotted blood called a hematoma. This is potentially dangerous because it could inhibit the healing process by causing the wound to become infected or burst open.

As valuable as these nutrients are, however, they don't play quite the lead role that two other nutrients do. Those two–legendary for their effects on wound healing–are vitamin C and zinc.

The Vitamin C Victory

The essential role that vitamin C plays in healing has been recognized for many years. Without enough vitamin C, the whole wound-healing process may go awry. With too little on hand, the amino acids needed for rebuilding the tissue are produced in the "wrong order." As a result, the body tries to make healing happen without the right material to do so.

416

What's more, old wounds have been known to "fall apart" even when C deficiency develops long after healing has occurred. But don't despair! Diagnosing the problem and treating it with vitamin C can quickly bring things under control and allow for normal healing.

Surgical cuts are not the only kind of wounds that require vitamin C for healing. As the authoritative British textbook *Human Nutrition and Dietetics* explains, "Injuries of any sort, especially burns and including surgical operations, increase utilization of ascorbic acid [vitamin C]. Such a patient needs a good supply of the vitamin. Visitors to the hospital who bring fresh fruit and fruit juices contribute to meeting his need."

If some vitamin C is good for wound healing, does this mean that more is better? Not necessarily. In fact, the authors say evidence of such a benefit is lacking. But before major surgery, they say, "it is advisable to give a dose of up to 250 milligrams of ascorbic acid for a few days and to continue this until the patient is eating well."

Think Zinc

Serious deficiencies of vitamin C are uncommon in Westernized countries. In fact, common food and supplement habits in the United States probably ensure that many Americans have enough vitamin C to tide them over while a wound heals. By contrast, deficiencies of zinc–the mineral best known for its wound-healing role–don't seem to be nearly so rare. In the United States, for instance, mild zinc deficiency has been documented even in children from affluent families.

It's certain that zinc plays a role in the healing process. Studies show clearly that wounds heal more slowly if zinc deficiency is present and that correcting the deficiency makes a difference.

Dr. M. W. Greaves and Dr. A. W. Skillen of Britain's University at Newcastle upon Tyne illustrated this effect among 18 patients whose leg ulcers simply did not respond to the standard medical treatments. Sure enough, those slow-to-heal patients proved to have lower blood zinc levels than a group of speedier recoverers. After four months or more of zinc therapy, however, some healing occurred in all 18 patients, and in 13 of them, the leg ulcers healed completely.

As for surgical incisions, there is one notable report that zinc helps. Walter J. Porries, M.D., chief of surgery for the hospital at the Wright-Patterson Air Force Base in Ohio, and several co-workers prescribed supplemental zinc to airmen recovering from removal of pilonidal sinuses. The incisions healed more quickly in those who received zinc than in those who did not. Other studies, however, have failed to show a benefit of zinc on the healing of surgical wounds.

Making sense of the conflicting findings has been a challenge. The best explanation we've heard is that additional zinc makes a difference for patients who are low on the mineral, but not for those who already have plenty on hand.

A Bad Time to Diet

Doctors have long recognized that the risk of surgery is greater for obese patients than for those of normal weight. It's not unusual, in fact, for doctors to demand that obese patients lose some weight before going through with surgery. One study, however, raises questions about sharply restricting food intake during the week or so immediately before surgery.

J. A. Windsor of the University of Auckland School of Medicine in New Zealand interviewed patients about their food intake during the week before surgery. Their food intake was classifed as inadequate if they had eaten no more than half as much food as usual during the week prior to surgery. Not surprisingly, Dr. Windsor found that the wounds of these patients healed more slowly than those of patients who did not sharply restrict eating before their operations.

Based on these findings, Dr. Windsor urges that patients eat normally prior to surgery. We have no argument with that.

YOGURT, LOW-FAT

Catch Some Culture!

144 calories per cup (plain)

Yogurt is not only a handy breakfast or snack but also one of the most versatile foods to use in cooking.

Nutritionally, low-fat yogurt is a winner. Lots of protein, but not too much fat; lots of calcium, and some zinc and riboflavin. It's the calcium, of course, that earns yogurt the most praise.

Many adults lose their taste or tolerance for milk with age, but yogurt continues to agree with them on both counts. That makes it an ideal calcium source for the over-21 set. (Of course, it's great for kids and teenagers, too.)

Nutritionists have long known that yogurt contains as much calcium as milk. Recently, though, Theresa M. Smith, M.D., of the Veterans Administration Medical Center in Minneapolis, looked at how well lactose-intolerant people absorb this calcium. Her study found that the calcium in yogurt was absorbed as well as the calcium in milk.

A frequent question about yogurt relates to claims that it's associated with long life. When asked to comment, we're always at a loss for words. No one seems to have seriously studied the notion using the kind of scientific methods considered valid these days. But just for the record, we want to mention one report that linked eating yogurt–along with whole grain bread, porridge, vegetables, fish, and fruit–to longer life. It comes from Erasmus University in the Netherlands, where Maarten Nube and associates surveyed 3,000 government workers. They found that men who ate more of these wholesome foods had better survival rates.

At the Market: Yogurt now comes in more varieties than ever before. The most nutritious are those made from skim or low-fat milk; we don't recommend whole-milk yogurts because of their fat content. To control calories and sugar, buy plain low-fat yogurt and add fruit yourself.

Kitchen Tips: Yogurt must be refrigerated. The date stamped on the container will tell you how long it should keep.

In salad dressings, dips, and potato toppings, plain yogurt often replaces fattier sour cream beautifully. If put into hot liquids or heated with any

419

intensity at all, however, yogurt will curdle. Avoid using it to enrich sauces and whisk it into soups only after they're cool.

Accent on Enjoyment: No kitchen should be without a container of plain yogurt. It's a perfect way to add flavor to chicken or sweet, juicy fruits without adding a lot of fat. Some suggestions:

- Marinate lamb in yogurt, garlic, and lemon juice. Then grill and serve hot or cold.
- Combine yogurt with a bit of orange juice concentrate and use as a dessert sauce for poached fruit, fruit compotes, or cakes.
- Combine yogurt with a bit of Dijon mustard and use as a sauce for broccoli or green beans.
- Combine yogurt, fresh snipped dill, and minced shallots and use as a sauce for cold poached fish.
- Combine yogurt with chopped cucumber and minced fresh mint and serve as an accompaniment to spicy curries.
- Substitute thin yogurt for buttermilk in baking.

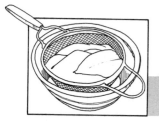

Yogurt Cheese

4 cups plain low-fat yogurt

Line a strainer with good-quality paper towels and set it in the sink. Add the yogurt and drain overnight. If you must refrigerate, set the strainer in a bowl and let it drain in the refrigerator. What's left in the strainer is yogurt cheese.

Makes about 1½ cups

Flavorful Ideas for Yogurt Cheese

Yogurt cheese can be used as you would cream cheese, but it has significantly less fat, calories, and cholesterol. Here are some suggestions for flavoring it.

- Stir in minced garlic, minced fresh parsley, and a splash of lemon juice. Serve as a dip for raw vegetables or pita chips.
- Stir in minced fresh spinach, fresh snipped dill, minced fresh parsley, and toasted pine nuts. Spread on toasted bagels for brunch, lunch, or snacks.
- Stir in orange juice, minced shallots, tarragon, and a pinch of grated orange peel. Serve as a sauce for poached fish.
- Stir in chopped dried apricots, raisins, and pecans. Serve with warm muffins or toast for breakfast.

APPENDIX

The Finest Food Sources of Vitamins and Minerals

More than 70 foods have merited our attention as the healing foods—the best of the best, the superfoods, so to speak, when it comes to eating for the health of it.

They've earned this special distinction for several reasons; foremost, they are especially high on one or more nutrients—bone-strengthening calcium or cancer-fighting carotene, for example. But they fit other criteria, too: They're low in fat, cholesterol, and sodium, and many of them are also particularly low in calories and high in fiber. These foods were selected because you can eat them any time and, in most cases, in any sensible amount, without fear of a less-than-healthy backlash.

Due to lack of space, however, it was impossible to list all of the best food sources of the major vitamins and minerals each and every time a nutritional health benefit of a specific nutrient was called out in this book. So, for easy reference, we've devised lists of the major foods containing the major vitamins and minerals. Unless otherwise noted, foods listed as "good" provide 20 to 45 percent of the U.S. Recommended Dietary Allowance (USRDA); "better" foods provide 50 to 75 percent, and "best" foods provide 80 percent or more.

We have, however, been somewhat selective in our choices. We've called out only the foods we consider the *best* for your health—those that fall under the umbrella of the healing foods that you've just read about. There are some high-nutrient foods—liver and nuts are perfect examples—that didn't make our lists because of their negative factors. Those foods (like liver and nuts) may be high in fat and cholesterol, or high in sodium or calories. After all, why bother eating foods that balance the good with the bad when there are so many just-plain-good-for-you foods to choose from?

For easy reference, we've also summarized the important role each of the major nutrients plays in your health and some of the healing promise that many of them hold for your future health.

Here's to good health *and* good eating!

Vitamin A: First and Foremost

If you value healthy eyes, healthy skin, and good resistance to infection, thank all forms of vitamin A for making them possible.

These Foods Rate an A

Good

1 cup brussels sprouts

⅔ cup Buc Wheats

1 cup Cheerios

1 cup yellow corn

⅔ cup Cracklin' Oat Bran

⅔ cup 40% Bran

⅔ cup Fruit & Fibre

⅓ cup granola

⅓ cup Grape-Nuts

⅔ cup Grape-Nuts flakes

1 cup peas

1 packet Quaker
  Instant Oatmeal

1 cup romaine lettuce

⅔ cup Special K

⅔ cup Team

1 tomato

½ cup tomato sauce

¾ cup vegetable juice
  cocktail

⅔ cup Wheaties

Better

1 cup apricot nectar

3 fresh apricots

1 cup crabmeat

1 cup minestrone
  or vegetable soup

1 nectarine

1 cup papaya

⅔ cup Total or
  Corn Total

1/16 watermelon

Best

1 cup canned apricots

1 cup beet greens

1 cup bok choy

1 cup broccoli

½ cantaloupe

1 large carrot

1 cup kale

⅔ cup Most

1 cup dried peaches

¾ cup Product 19

1 cup spinach

1 sweet potato

½ cup canned pumpkin

1 cup turnip greens

1 cup winter squash

1 cup mixed vegetables

NOTE: The USRDA for vitamin A is 5,000 international units.

All forms? you may ask. That's right. Vitamin A has the unique distinction of being two nutrients in one. Animal foods contain retinol, or preformed vitamin A. Plant foods contain the nutrient in its precursor form, which is converted to vitamin A in the body. These precursors are known as carotenoids, and the best known of the bunch is beta-carotene, or carotene, for short.

Among cancer researchers, carotene has gained the most fans. Although some studies link all forms of vitamin A to prevention of some common forms of cancer, carotene-rich foods have the longest list of credits. Why? Possibly because of the antioxidant properties that carotene has and retinol lacks. Researchers have identified antioxidants as capable of inhibiting the development of cancer.

We're fans of carotene for another reason: High intakes of it are safer than high intakes of supplemental preformed vitamin A or even foods that are high in preformed A. Taken in very large amounts, performed A can lead to toxic symptoms—a syndrome that begins with peeling skin, headaches, and digestive complaints.

Although excess carotene is deposited in the organs and skin, giving it a yellow-orange appearance, it has never led to vitamin A toxicity. The discolored skin will clear within a few weeks or months, by the way, if your intake is cut back.

Multivitamins or fortified foods that provide vitamin A almost always contain the preformed kinds, not carotene. Although potentially toxic if greatly overdone, they should cause no trouble when used as intended. One precaution, though: Recent reports link moderately high intakes of preformed vitamin A (in the range of 25,000 international units or more) to birth defects. With this in mind, we recommend that pregnant women (and women who are likely to become so) should take doses in the five-figure range only if prescribed by a doctor for a specific purpose.

B Complex: Getting Down to Basics

This group of nutrients boasts some of the most familiar as well as some of the least familiar vitamins. We like to call them the B Majors and the B Minors. Please understand, however, that we use these terms only to reflect how well the vitamin is known—not how important it is. The B Minors are every bit as important to health as the B Majors. They simply haven't become household words quite yet.

The B Majors

The Majors include thiamine, riboflavin, and niacin, also known as B_1, B_2, and B_3 respectively. The trio functions at a very basic level, helping the body to metabolize protein, carbohydrates, and fats. Severe thiamine deficiency, known as beri-beri, still occurs in some parts of the world, and niacin deficiency, or pellagra, was once a problem in the United States. Both conditions are so rare here that physicians rarely order lab tests to check for deficiencies.

The B Minors

As for the B Minors, the list is fairly long, so we're just going to mention a few that are getting more and more attention from nutritional scientists. The first is folate, also called folic acid, a nutrient that's so important, we'd all be lost without it. It is essential for making blood, for normal growth, for healthy pregnancies, and for protein metabolism.

At one time nutritionists were smug about the adequacy of folate nutrition in the United States, but they now believe that elderly Americans, in particular, are prone to borderline inadequacies. Moreover, the problem may be worsened by reliance on processed or overcooked foods. Folate is a temperamental nutrient that is easily lost in cooking and storage.

Another notable member of the B Minor group is vitamin B_6. It's in the news regularly–and getting both good and bad press. The good news is that some women report that the vitamin helps relieve their premenstrual symptoms. The bad news concerns reports of nervous system damage from very high doses of supplemental B_6–hundreds to thousands of milligrams daily. So taking B_6 also requires a dose of caution, and you should contact your doctor if you experience tingling and numbness, two noted side effects.

Our vote for "most fascinating" piece of B_6 research goes to a report linking low levels of B_6 to depression and obsessive-compulsive behavior. It may sound a little far out, but we wouldn't dismiss the notion entirely. Vitamin B_6 is needed for the body to make serotonin, an important brain chemical. In fact, serotonin is the focus of intense research right now among scientists seeking biological explanations for depression and obsessive-compulsive disorder.

What about B_{12}? It's important to be sure, with a varied list of roles that includes helping in the metabolism of fats and carbohydrates and in the production of cells, blood, and nerve fiber coverings.

Vitamin B$_{12}$ deficiency is rare among westerners who eat ample amounts of animal products that supply so much of this vitamin. Overdoing alcohol, though, may boost the need for this vitamin, and in some other cases, deficiency develops because of an underlying disease that prevents absorption of the

Thiamine

Good

⅔ cup Bran Chex

2 slices bread

⅔ cup Buc Wheats

1 cup Cheerios

⅔ cup Corn Bran

1 piece corn bread

1 cup Corn Chex

1 cup cowpeas

1 cup crabmeat

1 packet instant cream of wheat

1 cup egg noodles

1 English muffin

⅔ cup 40% Bran

⅔ cup Fruit & Fibre

⅓ cup Grape-Nuts

⅔ cup Grape-Nuts flakes

1 Italian sandwich roll

Good

⅔ cup Life

1 cup lima or Great Northern beans

⅓ cup 100% bran

⅔ cup Product 19

1 packet Quaker Instant Oatmeal

1 cup soybeans

⅔ cup Special K

1 cup split peas

¼ cup sunflower seeds

⅔ cup Wheat Chex

⅔ cup Wheaties

4 oz. veal

Better

4 oz. pork chop or roast

⅔ cup Total or Corn Total

vitamin from food. In such cases, B_{12} injections are sometimes in order.

The following tables list the "best of the B's." For easy reference, there is a list for each B vitamin individually.

Best

⅔ cup Most

⅔ cup Product 19

NOTE: The USRDA for thiamine is 1.5 milligrams.

Riboflavin

Good	Good	Better
1 cup asparagus	⅔ cup Life	⅔ cup Total or Corn Total
1 cup broccoli	4 oz. mackerel	
⅔ cup Buc Wheats	⅓ cup 100% bran cereal	
⅔ cup Corn Bran	4 oz. pork loin or roast	
1 cup Cheerios	4 oz. poultry	
1 cup collard greens	½ cup pudding or custard	
1 cup cottage cheese	4 oz. baked shad	
1 packet instant cream of wheat	⅔ cup Special K	
1 English muffin	1 cup spinach	
⅔ cup 40% Bran	⅔ cup Team	
⅔ cup Fruit & Fibre	1 cup turnip greens	
⅓ cup granola	⅔ cup Wheaties	
⅓ cup Grape-Nuts	1 cup winter squash	
⅔ cup Grape-Nuts flakes	4 oz. veal	
1 Italian sandwich roll	1 cup low-fat yogurt	
4 oz. lamb		

Best

⅔ cup Most

⅔ cup Product 19

Niacin

Good

4 oz. ground beef or ground round

1 cup most children's cereals

⅔ cup most commercial cereals

4 oz. cod

1 cup crabmeat

1 lamb chop

4 oz. leg of lamb

1 packet Quaker Instant Oatmeal

4 oz. pork roast

4 oz. pork roast

1 Italian sandwich roll

4 oz. red salmon

1 tin sardines

4 oz. turkey

Better

1 cup Kaboom cereal

4 oz. chicken breast

4 oz. broiled chicken

4 oz. mackerel

4 oz. pink salmon

4 oz. turkey breast

4 oz. veal scallopini

Best

⅔ cup Most

⅔ cup Product 19

4 oz. water-packed tuna

4 oz. veal rump roast

NOTE: The USRDA for niacin is 20 milligrams.

Folate

Good

⅓ cup All-Bran

1 cup asparagus

1 banana

1 cup pearled barley

1 cup broccoli

1 cup brussels sprouts

1 cup carrots

1 egg white

1 cup grapefruit

1 cup green beans

1 cup kale

1 cup lima beans

1 orange

1 cup peas

1 potato

1 tomato

Better

1 cup beets

1 cup broccoli

1 cup cabbage

1 cup cauliflower

1 cup cowpeas

1 cup pinto beans

1 cup romaine
  lettuce

Best

1 tablespoon
  brewer's yeast

1 cup chick-peas

1 cup orange juice

½ cup soybeans

1 cup spinach

NOTE: The USRDA for folate is 400 micrograms. Foods listed as "good" provide 10 to 20 percent of the USRDA; "better" foods provide 25 to 35 percent; and "best" foods provide 40 percent or more.

Vitamin B₆

Good

½ cup All-Bran

1 cup pearled
  barley

4 oz. beef

1 tablespoon brewer's yeast

1 cup broccoli

1 cup brussels sprouts

1 cup carrots

1 cup cauliflower

1 cup corn

1 cup crabmeat

1 cup Great Northern beans

3 oz. hamburger

4 oz. lamb

1 cup lentils

1 cup lima beans

1 cup peas

1 baked potato

4 oz. dark meat poultry

1 cup brown rice

4 oz. salmon

1 cup soybeans

1 cup spinach

1 cup tomatoes

4 oz. tuna

Better

4 oz. light meat
  poultry

⅓ cup sunflower
  seeds

Best

1 cup kidney
  beans

NOTE: The USRDA for vitamin B₆ is 2 milligrams. Foods listed as "good" provide 10 to 20 percent of the USRDA; "better" foods provide 25 to 35 percent; and "best" foods provide 40 percent or more.

Vitamin B$_{12}$

Good	Better	Best
4 oz. chicken	4 oz. haddock fillet	4 oz. beef
1 cup cottage cheese	1 cup ice milk	4 oz. halibut
4 oz. lobster	1 cup milk	3 oz. hamburger
4 oz. tuna		4 oz. lamb
1 oz. part-skim mozzarella cheese		4 oz. salmon
4 oz. pork roast		4 oz. veal
4 oz. turkey		

NOTE: The USRDA for vitamin B$_{12}$ is 6 micrograms. Foods listed as "good" provide 10 to 20 percent of the USRDA; "better" foods provide 25 to 35 percent; and "best" foods provide 40 percent of more.

Vitamin C: The Controversy Continues

If you take vitamins, you almost certainly take vitamin C. We doubt that there are any health-conscious individuals who haven't been curious about what this now-famous vitamin might do for them.

Some of C's benefits go without question. If you praise the way that it aids iron absorption, metabolism of folate and proteins, or healing open wounds, no one will argue with you. Should you also know of its role in the formation of collagen—the stuff that "holds" cells together—or in the manufacture of the brain chemicals norepinephrine and serotonin, again you're still on non-controversial ground.

Bring up the issue of vitamin C and the common cold, however, and you've reopened the door on the great debate. A majority of nutritionists, we'd guess, would deny its value for preventing colds. We're impressed, though, with evidence that taking vitamin C when a cold appears helps you feel better sooner. And whether it actually prevents colds has become something of a moot point for us now that a strong case has been made for preventing cancer with vitamin C.

Although some still protest that C is unproven for preventing cancer, we're quite taken with the notion because evidence comes from so many directions. In the laboratory, vitamin C reduces formation of cancer-causing agents such as the notorious nitrosamines. Out in the real world, researchers have found that populations at high risk of digestive tract cancers have low

(continued on page 436)

Here's Where C Is Better Than Average

Good	Good	Better
3 fresh or 1 cup canned apricots	1 cup pineapple	1 cup apricot nectar
1 artichoke	1 potato	1 cup asparagus
1 banana	1 cup hash brown potatoes	1 cup raw green cabbage
1 cup beet greens	1 cup romaine lettuce	½ grapefruit
1 cup beets	⅔ cup Special K	⅒ honeydew melon
1 cup blackberries	⅔ cup Team	1 plantain
1 cup blueberries	⅔ cup Wheaties	1 cup mashed sweet potato
1 cup bok choy	5 oz. raspberries	1 cup canned tomatoes
⅔ cup Bran Chex or Wheat Chex	1 cup Rice Chex	1 cup tomato juice
⅔ cup Buc Wheats	1 cup rhubarb	⅔ cup Total or Corn Total
1 cup carrots	1 cup raw spinach	1 cup turnips
1 cup sour cherries	1 cup squash	
1 cup or one ear of corn	1 sweet potato	
1 cup Corn Chex	1 tangerine	
½ cup mixed fruit	1 tomato	
1 cup green beans	1 cup stewed tomatoes	
1 cup Kix	¾ cup vegetable juice cocktail	
⅓ cup 100% bran cereal	1 cup mixed vegetables	
1 nectarine	1 cup wax beans	
1 cup parsnips		
½ cup dried peaches		
1 cup peas		

Best

1 cup broccoli

1 cup brussels sprouts

1 cup cooked cabbage

½ cantaloupe

1 cup cauliflower

1 cup collard greens

½ grapefruit

1 cup grapefruit juice

1 cup mango chunks

⅔ cup Most

1 cup mustard greens

1 orange

1 cup orange juice

1 cup papaya chunks

1 cup pineapple juice

⅔ cup Product 19

1 cup cooked spinach

5 oz. strawberries

1 cup turnip greens

NOTE: The USRDA for vitamin C is 60 milligrams.

levels of vitamin C. There's more evidence—much more than can fit here—and certainly enough to support the recommendation of expert committees who tell us to get ample amounts of vitamin C in our diet. The table that follows shows how easy that can be.

Vitamin D: Unsung Hero of Healthy Bones

The word has been out for a while that osteoporosis can be prevented with calcium—a mineral you'll read more about in a few pages. Oddly enough, though, all the attention to calcium hasn't been matched by equal time for its essential co-worker, vitamin D.

Without vitamin D, calcium would be unable to do its job effectively, because the body can't metabolize calcium without vitamin D. No amount of calcium is likely to be enough without it!

But vitamin D is more than an essential vitamin. It is a hormone, too. And like other hormones, vitamin D is powerful. That's the reason for warnings about its toxicity; of all the vitamins, it's the easiest to overdo. Such overdoses, however, are uncommon and require intakes far above what you'd get from using vitamin D-rich foods and/or normal amounts of a supplement.

Vitamin D's friendship with calcium is also likely to help reduce cancer risk. New research links both calcium and vitamin D to lower rates of colon cancer. Calcium is probably doing the work inside the digestive tract—binding to harmful substances. But because vitamin D helps calcium absorption in the first place, it, too, appears to play a vital role.

You'll notice that the following list of foods rich in vitamin D is on the short side. And there's good reason for that: Our primary source of vitamin D is the sun. A little sunlight each day goes a long way toward supplying your daily allotment of D.

Searching for Vitamin D

Good	Better	Best
1 oz. dry cereals	4 oz. mackerel	4 oz. salmon
1 oz. super-fortified cereals	4 oz. sardines	
1 cup milk	4 oz. tuna	

NOTE: The USRDA for vitamin D is 400 international units. Foods listed as "good" provide 35 to 100 I.U., "better" foods provide 101-500 I.U., and "best" foods provide 501 to 994 I.U.

Vitamin E: Moving into the Major Leagues

Nutritionists used to joke that vitamin E was a "vitamin in search of a disease." But not anymore. Breast lumps are no laughing matter. Nor is preventing cancer. And vitamin E is part of the picture for both of these.

Of course, nutritionists have long acknowledged that vitamin E is essential for metabolism of polyunsaturated fats. It's just that beyond that, they saw little to be impressed about. And they couldn't find a vitamin E deficiency disease anything like scurvy or beri-beri. So they considered vitamin E rather ho-hum stuff.

That was until cancer research became focused on antioxidants such as carotene and vitamin C. It only followed that if these two antioxidants have value in cancer prevention, vitamin E probably does, too, for it also has antioxidant effects. Right now, serious cancer research with vitamin E is finally under way, as is follow-up work on vitamin E's value in treating benign (but not painless) breast lumps.

Sorry, but we can't offer a table of foods rich in vitamin E. Foods that contain polyunsaturated fat have a little bit, but that's about the extent of it. Only supplements can supply large doses of this vitamin.

Potassium: A Major Mineral in Its Own Right

Potassium is to sodium what Burns was to Allen or Laurel was to Hardy. It takes both of them to stage a winning act.

For a long time, it was believed that sodium acting alone had an effect on blood pressure. But that's not the case any longer. Researchers now believe that it is a balance between sodium and potassium that keeps blood pressure in check.

But potassium isn't solely dependent on sodium for work. It goes out on its own in helping other nutrients keep muscles and nerves functioning, in synthesizing protein, and in storing carbohydrates.

Getting more potassium in your diet is easy and delicious—just take a look at the list that follows. And food is not only the best-tasting source of potassium but also the safest way to get more.

Iron: A Strange Problem

If there's a lesson to be learned from the iron story, it's that talking about nutritional problems isn't enough to solve them. Preventing and treating iron deficiency has been a top priority of nutritionists for decades. Yet in the United States, inadequate iron continues to be a major problem, mostly among young children and women of childbearing age.

(continued on page 440)

Primary Sources of Potassium

Good

1 cup dried apples

1 cup apricot nectar

3 apricots

1 medium banana

4 oz. beef

1 cup sliced beets

1 cup bok choy

⅓ cup Bran Buds

1 cup broccoli

1 cup brussels sprouts

1 cup cauliflower

4 oz. broiled chicken

1 cup yellow corn

1 cup fruit cocktail

4 oz. goose

1 cup grapefruit juice

4 oz. lamb

1 cup milk

1 nectarine

1 cup peach slices

1 cup pineapple juice

Good

1 pomegranate

4 oz. pork

1 cup hash brown
potatoes

5 prunes

4 oz. canned salmon

1 sweet potato

1 tomato

4 oz. water-packed tuna

1 cup turnips

1 cup mixed vegetables

¹⁄₁₆ watermelon

1 cup low-fat fruit yogurt

Better

½ cup dried apricots

1 cup beet greens

½ cantaloupe

4 oz. cod

1 cup collard greens

1 cup cowpeas

10 dates

4 oz. flounder

1 cup kidney beans

1 cup lentils

1 cup orange juice

1 cup parsnips

1 cup split peas

1 potato

1 cup mashed potatoes

1 cup prune juice

½ cup pumpkin seeds

1 cup rhubarb

4 oz. fresh salmon

4 oz. scallops

½ cup soybeans

Better	**Best**
1 cup spinach	1 cup Great Northern beans
½ cup sunflower seeds	1 cup lima beans
1 cup canned tomatoes	1 cup navy beans
1 cup tomato juice	1 cup dried peaches
½ cup tomato puree	1 plantain
1 cup plain, low-fat yogurt	1 cup winter squash

NOTE: There is no RDA for potassium, but the Safe and Adequate Range, set by the Committee on Dietary Allowances, is 1,875 to 5,625 milligrams for adults. Foods listed as "good" provide 350 to 500 milligrams; "better" foods provide 500 to 750 milligrams; and "best" foods provide 750 to 1,350 milligrams.

Loading Up on Iron

Good	Good	Better
½ cup dried apricots	1 cup kidney beans	⅔ cup instant cream of wheat
4 oz. beef round	1 cup lentils	1 cup Kix
4 oz. ground beef	⅔ cup Life	⅔ cup Total or Corn Total
⅓ cup Bran Buds	1 cup lima beans	
⅔ cup Buc Wheats	½ cup dried peaches	
1 cup Cheerios	4 oz. pork roast	
1 cup shucked clams	½ cup pumpkin seeds	
4 oz. Cornish hen	1 packet Quaker Instant Oatmeal	
1 cup cowpeas	4 oz. scallops	
⅔ cup quick cream of wheat	4 oz. sirloin steak	
⅔ cup Crispy Wheats 'n Raisins	1 cup soybeans	
1 cup farina	⅔ cup Special K	
⅔ cup 40% Bran	½ cup sunflower seeds	
⅔ cup Fruit & Fibre	1 veal chop	
⅔ cup Grape-Nuts flakes	4 oz. veal cutlet	
1 cup Great Northern beans	⅔ cup Wheat Chex	
⅔ cup Honey Bran	⅔ cup Wheaties	

Like all of us, they need iron to build healthy red blood cells. It's also part of some enzymes. The body stores some iron, but for many, especially menstruating women, stores are too low for comfort. Needless to say, bolstering iron stores before they dwindle completely is preferable to waiting until a full-blown case of anemia sets in.

Best

²/₃ cup Most

²/₃ cup Product 19

NOTE: The USRDA for iron is 18 milligrams.

For those in the high-risk groups, a daily supplement that provides the RDA for iron is a good preventive measure. (Be sure to keep these supplements out of children's reach, though, as iron poisonings are most common among curious children who get their hands on the supplement bottle and swallow a handful of pills.) In addition, here is a list of iron-rich foods to enjoy.

Zeroing In on Zinc

Good	Good	Better
1 cup cooked beans	1 cup brown rice	4 oz. lamb
2 slices rye bread	4 oz. salmon	4 oz. lean pork
2 slices whole wheat bread	7 oz. spaghetti and meatballs	4 oz. dark turkey meat
½ chicken breast	1 cup spinach	
4 oz. chicken meat	1 oz. shredded wheat	
4 to 5 hard-shell clams	4 oz. white turkey meat	
8 oz. surf clams	1 tablespoon toasted wheat germ	
1 cup cottage cheese		
1 oz. 40% Bran cereal	4 oz. whitefish fillet	
1 cup lentils	1 cup plain low-fat yogurt	
1 cup lima beans		
1 cup lobster meat		
1 cup milk		
1 cup oatmeal		
1 oz. puffed oat cereal		
1 cup peas		
1 medium baked potato		

Zinc: The Healing Mineral

Zinc serves some basic purposes for all of us. It's part of certain enzymes, some of which metabolize protein, carbohydrate, and alcohol. It helps in making protein and building bones, affects the senses of smell and taste, and aids in healing wounds.

Although severe zinc deficiency is rare in the United States, nutritionists suspect that the mild form may be more common than realized, especially in children. Symptoms of mild deficiency are poor appetite, suboptimal growth, and reduced sense of taste and smell. Scaly skin, delayed wound healing,

Best

4 oz. lean beef

1 cup crabmeat

1 cup cowpeas

4 oz. oysters

NOTE: The USRDA for zinc is 18 milligrams. Foods listed as "good" provide 10 to 20 percent of the USRDA; "better" foods provide 25 to 35 percent; and "best" foods provide 40 percent or more.

fatigue, hair loss, diarrhea, and reduced resistance to infection are also symptoms and can affect all ages.

Some of us have special needs for zinc. Supplemental zinc is used to treat acrodermatitis enteropathica, a rare gastrointestinal and skin disease of childhood. A number of chronic health problems may interfere with zinc nutrition; these include alcoholism, chronic infections or inflammatory diseases, diabetes, kidney disease, pancreatic disease, psoriasis, and certain kinds of anemia. Large amounts of zinc may be lost due to surgery, burns, or multiple injuries–making supplementation with therapeutic doses a necessity.

For those of you with more routine need for zinc, though, the following foods are your best bets.

Calcium: The Mineral King Conquers New Ground

When it comes to taking a role in nutrition, calcium always plays a lead. It's been linked to heart health, cancer prevention and, of course, better bones.

Here we present a list of calcium-rich foods for those who want more of it as well as for those plagued by kidney stones who may be need to avoid it. Remember that as beneficial as calcium-rich foods generally are, they will reduce absorption of the antibiotic tetracycline. Try to allow at least an hour–and preferably two–between taking these medications and eating any of these foods.

Magnesium: Growing in Importance

We suspect that magnesium is another mineral that offers more benefits to health than realized by nutritionists, who've long considered magnesium as essential to the nervous system. It's also a part of some key enzyme systems.

It's possible, though, that magnesium has an important role in preventing heart disease. Low levels of the mineral have been linked to higher risk of heart attack. What's more, magnesium is found in bone, raising concern that a healthy intake of the mineral may help in the war against osteoporosis, too.

On both of the latter counts, we'd have to say it's too soon to tell. But we're not waiting to enjoy our favorite magnesium-rich foods from the list that follows.

Selenium: A Soiled Reputation

Selenium is nutrition's ugly duckling. For decades, nutritionists damned it with faint praise–conceding that the body does require some of the mineral while stressing that, taken in large amounts, it's toxic. It earned its bad name in earlier times when agriculture experts determined that selenium-rich pastures (the result of selenium-rich soil) were responsible for the deaths of thousands of livestock in the Midwest.

Some scientists have been so suspicious of selenium ever since that they have had trouble seeing that selenium isn't all bad. It's essential to the health of

Getting Rich in Calcium

Good	Better	Best
8 oz. baked beans	1 cup bok choy	1 cup Calcimilk
1 cup beet greens	1 cup collard greens	1 oz. Dairy Crisp cereal
1 cup broccoli	1 cup mackerel	1 tin sardines with bones
1 bean burrito	1 cup milk	1 cup low-fat protein-fortified yogurt
1 cup creamed cottage cheese	1 milk shake	
1 cup ice milk	⅔ cup canned pink salmon with bones	
1 cup kale	1 cup plain yogurt	
1 cup mustard greens		
1 cup okra		
½ cup oysters		
4 oz. scallops		
1 cup soybeans		
4 oz. tofu		
1 cup turnip greens		
1 cup vegetables in cheese sauce		
1 cup frozen yogurt		

NOTE: The USRDA for calcium is 1,000 milligrams. Foods listed as "good" provide 10 to 20 percent of the USRDA; "better" foods provide 25 to 35 percent; and "best" foods provide 40 percent or more.

the heart muscle; without it, a kind of congestive heart failure known as Keshan's disease occurs. The name comes from the Chinese province of Keshan, where the disease once was epidemic among children and women of childbearing age.

Selenium also helps maintain the health of hair, nails, muscles, and red blood cells. And it is part of an enzyme, glutathione peroxidase, now believed to help detoxify harmful chemicals and reduce risk of cancer.

A few decades ago, public health experts documented that people living in areas of the country having selenium-rich soil had certain symptoms suggestive of excessive selenium intake. Among the most common were bad teeth, brittle fingernails, skin discoloration, dizziness, fatigue, garlic odor of the breath, gastrointestinal complaints, brittle or lost hair, irritability, jaundice, and skin inflammation. There have been no similar reports lately–probably because Americans tend not to depend on locally grown foods anymore.

Magnesium: Getting the Max

Good	Good	Better
1 medium banana	4 oz. flounder	1 cup cowpeas
1 cup frozen green beans	½ grapefruit	1 cup kidney beans
1 cup blackberries	1 cup grapefruit juice	1 cup lima beans
⅓ cup bran	½ cup dry lentils	1 cup pork and beans
1 slice pumpernickel bread	1 cup milk	
1 cup broccoli	⅔ cup oatmeal	
1 cup brussels sprouts	1 cup orange juice	
1 cup carrots	1 cup oysters	
1 cup cauliflower	1 cup peas	
1 cup chopped celery	1 baked potato	
1 cup canned cherries	4 oz. salmon	
4 oz. chicken	1 cup spinach	
1 cup corn	1 cup tomatoes	
½ cup dates	4 oz. turkey	
	½ cup Wheatena	

The selenium content of food varies so much depending on where it is grown that a list of food sources would not be something in which to put much stock. Suffice it to say, however, that nutritionists credit beef, garlic, asparagus, and mushrooms as the best sources of this mineral, and seafood, too, is generally good.

Best

½ cup dry soybeans

NOTE: The USRDA for magnesium is 400 milligrams. Foods listed as "good" provide 10 to 20 percent of the USRDA; "better" foods provide 25 to 35 percent; and "best" foods provide 40 percent or more.

INDEX

Page references in *italic* indicate tables.